LF

EXERCISE
TESTING&TRAINING

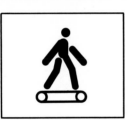 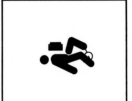

VICTOR F. FROELICHER, MD
Associate Professor of Medicine
University of California, San Diego, School of Medicine
University Hospital
Director
Cardiac Rehabilitation and Exercise Testing
San Diego, California

Year Book Medical Publishers, Inc.
Chicago

IV

Library of Congress Cataloging in Publication Data

Froelicher, Victor F.
    Exercise testing & training.

    Bibliography: p.
    1. Exercise tests.   2. Heart function tests.   3. Heart
—Diseases—Diagnosis.   4. Radioisotope scanning.
I. Title.   II. Title: Exercise testing and training.
RC683.5.E94F76   1984   616.1′2   84-2364
ISBN 0-8151-3332-4

Printed in the United States of America

ISBN 0-8151-3332-4

To my teachers and my students and
especially to those who have been both;
to my daughter Beth, and to Erika

Preface

THE ORGANIZATION of the book is straightforward and complete. References are listed at the end of the book by each chapter and section heading. Almost one half of the book addresses standard clinical exercise testing—all of which is contained in chapter I. Chapter II presents the key concepts of radionuclide exercise testing beginning with basic radiation physics. Chapter III is entitled "Responses to Chronic Exercise" and consists of a review of animal, hemodynamic, echocardiographic, and exercise electrocardiographic studies. Chapter IV is a review of the data available on the prevention and management of coronary heart disease using exercise. Chapter V presents the pilot studies and design of the University of California, San Diego (UCSD), randomized trial using radionuclide exercise tests to evaluate the effects of one year of exercise on myocardial perfusion and function. The appendix contains forms that my group at UCSD have designed and have found to be helpful for exercise testing and cardiac rehabilitation.

Why another book on exercise? As I look back on the last ten years of my career, the unifying feature has been the subject of exercise. This experience began in research and in writing in 1971 when my mentor, Joe Reeves, suggested that we write a book together. At the time, I was a Cardiology Fellow at the University of Alabama, in Birmingham. I promptly wrote three chapters, all aided by Joe, and another on epidemiology that Al Oberman guided. Joe left the University of Alabama and went into private practice, and so our book never was completed. However, the three "chapters" were subsequently published in two different journals and one book. Also at this time, Joe and Tom Sheffield helped me start my research on the clinical utilization of treadmill testing. Next followed four good years of research at the United States Air Force School of Aerospace Medicine spent evaluating apparently healthy pilots. I had the good fortune to find good colleagues there, including Frank Yanowitz and A.J. Thompson, and I was able to take advantage of the work started by Larry Lamb, Keith Cohn, Paul McHenry, and Hank Brammell. Then there was one year with no time for research as Assistant Chief of Cardiology at USAF Wilford Hall Medical Center. During that time, I wrote a monograph in the series "Current Problems in Cardiology" on treadmill testing with my colleagues there, which formed the skeleton for my subsequent reviews of treadmill testing, including chapter I of this book. For the past five years, I have been at UCSD where my efforts have been supported and directed by Dr. John Ross, Jr. Both Joe and John have been giants in my life. At UCSD, I have concentrated on cardiac rehabilitation, computerized exercise electrocardiography, and radionuclide exercise testing. Dr. William Ashburn has graciously taught me all that I know about nuclear medicine. He is a skilled and patient teacher from whom I continue to learn.

Considering this fortunate and broad experience, it seemed like a good time to bring all of my previous works up-to-date and to tie them together. Also, in my fortieth year, it was an appropriate time to fulfill one of my lifelong dreams, that is, to write a creative work—this preface. In addition to this personal indulgence, I feel my experiences have been unique—providing the basis for an exceptional book. It is designed as a basic textbook for anybody performing exercise testing; in addition, it is a specialized text for devotees of the clinical uses of exercise and those interested in how exercise impacts on the health care system.

This book contains much of my work but also includes my analysis of others' works. Personal biases will stand out, for instance, the presentation on using the work load achieved rather than total treadmill time as the best means of estimating aerobic capacity. I feel that the use of total time and nomograms has impeded physicians in understanding exercise testing and exercise physiology. My bias tends toward the work Alex Battler and I did regarding R waves, which disproved Ellestad's work. But I want to make clear that I appreciate the incredible impact that many admirable researchers have had on my work. Exercise testing would not be as widely used in the United States today if it were not for the "giants whose shoulders I sit on," and any differences or disagreements I have are in a very friendly, admiring fashion. Certainly, I owe much to Bob Bruce. He is a friend who first helped me long ago with the epidemiologic terms used in the original paper I published on screening asymptomatic men with maximal treadmill testing. Another point to remember is that because much of the methodology of exercise testing has not been validated, my biases are presented often without scientific support. When this is so, I try to make it clear that this is the case.

It is appropriate to acknowledge other co-workers. Roger Wolthuis, PhD, and I worked together for three years at the School of Aerospace Medicine and published papers on treadmill testing. Roger is a careful and perceptive researcher, who now is pursuing a productive career in the medical instrumentation industry. Jim Whinnery and I had much fun studying the response of bundle branch block to exercise. His training as an MD and PhD and his excellent research background are apparent when one realizes the care he took to cut out examples of many of the patients with bundle branch block to include as "data" in our papers. I told him they would not be published because they took up too much space, but Jim proved me wrong. Mikky Bhargava, PhD, is the most talented engineer-computer scientist I have ever worked with. He quickly picked up the concepts of computerized exercise electrocardiography and personally has made new contributions. He has the potential of influencing positively this field even more. Dave Mortara, PhD, is a gifted engineer working in industry, but still highly research oriented. Mikky and I would never have accomplished the computer work that we have at UCSD without Dave's interest. Actually, I think that history will show that electrocardiography has been advanced by Einthoven, Wilson, Pipberger, Bonner, and Mortara. He truly belongs in this elite group.

I have adapted several sections from writings I had done elsewhere in collaboration with colleagues. Eddie Atwood, MD, and I wrote the section on test agreement, and several figures are of his original design. Paul Gamble, II, MS, helped with the computerized electrocardiographic figures. Julio Tubau, MD, initially wrote the section on radionuclide techniques of measuring left ventricular volume and the associated figures were done by him. Kiyoshi Watanabe, MD, and I summarized the other computerized exercise electrocardiographic programs together and did our computerized pre/post exercise training study. Roy Ditchey, MD, completed the pre/post echocardiographic study and published the results. The cross-sectional area approach for estimating left ventricular mass was his idea.

Certainly, our rehabilitation group has been a big help in my professional progress and has helped make this book possible. Dave Jensen, MS, has been my right hand for nuclear medicine studies, and Dan McKirnan PhD, has been the same for the exercise program. Thanks must also go to MaryLou, Julie, Pam, Susan, Liz, and Mike. Also to my secretary, Lou

Smith, who has most directly made it possible for these past four years to be so productive. She patiently puts my garbled speech and scribbled writing into our word processor and then outputs a finished product. Finally, Julie Scharf has edited each work for grammatical and technical accuracy and moved things around on the word processor. Her unique combination of skills and knowledge has greatly facilitated the development of this book.

To quote Osler—"the teacher's life should have three periods: study until twenty-five, investigation until forty, profession until sixty at which age I would have him retired on a double allowance." I think that these ages should be moved up about ten years, which would give me ten more years of investigation. By then, I hope to be a "Master Teacher" and to rewrite this book. I do hope this is enjoyable reading and helpful to those interested in the clinical aspects of exercise.

VICTOR F. FROELICHER, JR., M.D.

VICTOR F. FROELICHER, MD, is currently Associate Professor of Medicine at the University of California, San Diego, and Director of Cardiac Rehabilitation and Exercise Testing. He is in the Cardiology Division directed by John Ross, Jr, MD.

He received his MD degree from the University of Pittsburgh in 1967. He had his internship and Internal Medicine Residency at Wilford Hall USAF Medical Center in San Antonio, Texas, and then was a Fellow in Cardiology and Instructor in Medicine for two years at the University of Alabama, in Birmingham, under Dr. T.J. Reeves. For four years, he was at the USAF School of Aerospace Medicine in San Antonio, Texas, and for one year was Assistant Chief of Cardiology at Wilford Hall USAF Medical Center.

He is a Fellow in the American College of Cardiology, the American College of Physicians, the American College of Sports Medicine, and the American Heart Association Councils on both Epidemiology and Clinical Cardiology. He is also a member of the AHA Subcommittee on Exercise and Cardiac Rehabilitation. Board certifications include Internal Medicine and Cardiology.

His main interests are in exercise testing, cardiac rehabilitation, exercise physiology, health care delivery systems, and computerized electrocardiography.

He is on the editorial boards of *Circulation, Cardiology,* the *Journal of the American College of Cardiology,* and the *American Heart Journal* and co-editor of the *Journal of Cardiac Rehabilitation.*

Contents

CHAPTER I. STANDARD EXERCISE TESTING

1   INTRODUCTION
1   Basic exercise physiology

4   METHODOLOGY
4   Safety precautions
7   Consent form
7   Legal implications of exercise testing
8   Recording instruments
10   Exercise test modalities
10   Supine versus erect exercise testing
12   Protocols
12   Submaximal versus maximal exercise testing
14   Skin preparation
14   Electrodes and cables
15   Lead systems
20   Blood pressure
20   Measurement or estimation of maximal oxygen uptake
22   Postexercise period
23   Indications for treadmill test termination
23   Computerized exercise electrocardiographic analysis

32   INTERPRETATION
38   Functional capacity
41   Heart rate and blood pressure response
45   The electrocardiographic response to exercise
50   Q-wave, R-wave, and S-wave amplitudes

52 ST slope, J-junction depression, and T-wave amplitude

56 Percent R-wave changes

57 Abnormal segment changes

57 ST-segment elevation

60 ST-segment normalization or absence of change

61 ST-segment depression

63 Exercise-induced ST-segment depression not due to coronary artery disease

66 Exercise-induced ventricular dysrhythmias

67 Subjective responses

68 Observer agreement in interpretation

74 Summary

74 APPLICATIONS

75 Diagnosis of chest pain and other cardiac findings

82 Determination of prognosis and severity

87 Evaluation of functional capacity

88 Evaluation of treatment

88 Evaluation of dysrhythmias

89 Evaluation for an individualized exercise program

89 Exercise testing soon after acute myocardial infarction

93 Screening apparently healthy individuals

94 Exercise testing as a screening tool

102 Maximal or near-maximal exercise testing with coronary angiography

103 New electrocardiographic criteria

104 Thallium-201 exercise testing

105 Radionuclide left ventricular angiography during exercise

107 Cardiokymography

108 Coronary artery calcification on fluoroscopic examination

109 Lipid screening

109 Gated chest x-rays

109 Computerized probability estimates

110 Systolic time intervals

110 Prognosis in asymptomatic coronary disease

111 Summary

114 CONCLUSION

117 REFERENCES

CHAPTER II. RADIONUCLIDE EXERCISE TESTING

137 INTRODUCTION

137 RADIATION PHYSICS

141 MYOCARDIAL IMAGING WITH POTASSIUM-LIKE RADIONUCLIDES (COLD-SPOT IMAGING)

145 Cold-spot exercise imaging with angiographic correlation

151 RADIONUCLIDE VENTRICULAR ANGIOGRAPHY DURING BICYCLE EXERCISE

156 Ejection fraction response to exercise in normal subjects and in patients with coronary heart disease

158 Detection of wall motion abnormalities

161 Right ventricular ejection fraction response to exercise

162 Ejection fraction response in valvular heart disease

162 DETERMINATION OF LEFT VENTRICULAR VOLUME

162 Ventricular volume using the first-pass method

163 Ventricular volume using the equilibrium gated technique

168 CONCLUSION

171 REFERENCES

CHAPTER III. THE CARDIOVASCULAR EFFECTS OF CHRONIC EXERCISE

179 INTRODUCTION

181 ANIMAL STUDIES OF THE EFFECTS OF CHRONIC EXERCISE

181 Myocardial hypertrophy

182 Myocardial microcirculatory changes

184 Coronary artery size changes

184 Coronary collateral circulation

187 Cardiac mechanical and metabolic performance

191 Skeletal muscle mitochondria and respiratory enzyme changes

191 Myocardial mitochondria and respiratory enzyme changes

193 Effects on atherosclerosis and risk factors

196 Changes in peripheral blood flow in response to acute exercise

196 Summary

197 HEMODYNAMIC STUDIES OF THE EFFECTS OF AN EXERCISE PROGRAM

200 Studies of normal subjects

202 Studies of coronary heart disease patients

207 Discussion

210 ECHOCARDIOGRAPHIC STUDIES OF THE EFFECTS OF AN EXERCISE
PROGRAM

210 Cross-sectional studies comparing echocardiographic measurements of
normals and of athletes

212 Echocardiography before and after an exercise program

217 Discussion

220 Summary

220 EXERCISE ELECTROCARDIOGRAPHIC STUDIES

227 CONCLUSION

228 REFERENCES

237 **CHAPTER IV. EXERCISE IN THE PREVENTION AND MANAGEMENT OF
CORONARY HEART DISEASE**

238 RETROSPECTIVE STUDIES OF PHYSICAL INACTIVITY AS A RISK FACTOR

243 PREVALENCE STUDIES OF PHYSICAL INACTIVITY AS A RISK FACTOR

245 PROSPECTIVE STUDIES OF PHYSICAL INACTIVITY AS A RISK FACTOR

252 POSTMORTEM STUDIES OF PHYSICAL INACTIVITY AS A RISK FACTOR

253 MARATHON HYPOTHESIS

254 CARDIAC REHABILITATION STUDIES

254 Early ambulation after acute myocardial infarction

258 Prognostic indicators

259 Intervention studies

260 Complications of an exercise program

261 Summary

262 CONCLUSION

263 REFERENCES

269 **CHAPTER V. THE USE OF EXERCISE RADIONUCLIDE TESTING TO EVALUATE
CARDIAC REHABILITATION**

270 INITIAL CORRELATIVE AND VALIDATION STUDIES

280 PREEXERCISE AND POSTEXERCISE TRAINING STUDIES

283 PERFEXT—A RANDOMIZED TRIAL OF THE EFFECTS OF EXERCISE ON HEART
PERFUSION AND PERFORMANCE

287 Exercise testing

287 Electrocardiographic and vectorcardiographic techniques

287 Radionuclide gated left ventricular imaging
287 Exercise training
288 CONCLUSION
289 **REFERENCES**

APPENDIX: EXERCISE TESTING AND CARDIAC REHABILITATION FORMS

291 TESTING FORMS AND ILLUSTRATIONS
292 Report of Treadmill Test
294 Treadmill Test Worksheet
295 Treadmill Form
297 Thallium-201 Imaging Data Sheet
298 Radionuclide Imaging Worksheet
299 Thallium Interpretation
300 Report of Supine Bike Radionuclide Exercise Test
300   Data Page
301   Interpretation Page
302 Exercise Heart Function Study
303 Exercise Heart Function Worksheet
304 Computer Output from the UCSD Exercise ECG/VCG Program
305 Exercise Test Responses
306 Women and Exercise Testing
307 Left Main Disease and Exercise Testing
308 Computerized Exercise ECG Angiographic Studies
309 Frank X Lead and Frank Frontal Plane
310 Frank Horizontal Plane and the Eigen Plane
311 Use of the Cubic Spline Technique to Smooth Baseline Wander
311 The Effect of the Improper Placement of the Fiducial on the Average Waveform
312 Effect of Averaging on Noise (RMS = Root Mean Square)
313 Comparison of the Use of the Median and the Mean when Averaging Signals Containing Baseline Discontinuity
314 ST-Segment Vectors and an Illustration of the Effect of Changing Discriminant Value on Sensitivity and Specificity
315 Computer ECG Criteria

APPENDIX: EXERCISE TESTING AND CARDIAC REHABILITATION FORMS

317 TRAINING FORMS
318 Cardiovascular Rehabilitation History Questionnaire
319 Cardiovascular History and Exercise Test Summary

320   History/Physical Form
321   Cardiovascular History and Exercise Test Responses
322   Cardiac Rehabilitation Exercise Training Report Worksheet
323   Work Load Record for Exercise Classes
324   Phase III Daily Exercise Training Form
325   UCSD Cardiac Rehabilitation Program Physical Activity Diary
326   UCSD Cardiac Rehabilitation Strength and Flexibility Assessment
327   PERFEXT Symptom Checklist
338   UCSD Cardiac Rehabilitation Exercise Training Form #1
330   Activity Preference Form
331   UCSD Cardiac Rehabilitation Physical Activity Guidelines
332   UCSD Cardiac Rehabilitation Program Warning Symptoms
333   University Hospital Informed Consent for Exercise Treatment
334   You are PERFEXT!
334   Supervised Exercise
335   Home Exercise
336   UCSD Certificate of Appreciation

337   **INDEX**

CHAPTER

I
Standard Exercise Testing

INTRODUCTION

Exercise, a human being's most common physiologic stress, can bring out cardiac abnormalities not present at rest. For this reason, exercise can be considered the most practical test of cardiac perfusion and function. This chapter will present the methodology, interpretation, and applications of standard exercise testing, as it is performed in most clinical exercise laboratories.

Basic Exercise Physiology. If the two basic principles of exercise physiology (Table I) are understood, much confusion can be avoided. The first is a physiologic principle: total body oxygen consumption and myocardial oxygen consumption are distinct in their determinants and in the way they are measured or estimated. Total body, or ventilatory, oxygen consumption ($\dot{V}O_2$) is the amount of oxygen that is extracted from inspired air as the body performs work. Accurate measurement of $\dot{V}O_2$ requires gas analysis equipment, but it can be estimated from the work load performed because there is relatively small variation in the oxygen cost of a given work load. Maximal $\dot{V}O_2$ is equal to maximal cardiac output times maximal arteriovenous oxygen ($AV\,O_2$) difference. The maximal $AV\,O_2$ difference during exercise has a physiologic limit that cannot be exceeded; hence, if a maximal effort is given, maximal oxygen consumption can be used to estimate maximal cardiac output noninvasively. Since cardiac output is equal to the product of stroke volume and heart rate, it is of course related to heart rate. Total body oxygen consumption is best estimated by the aerobic work load performed rather than by total exercise time because the latter is very much influenced by endurance and muscular strength.

TABLE I
TWO BASIC PRINCIPLES OF EXERCISE PHYSIOLOGY

Myocardial Oxygen Consumption	$\cong$ Heart rate $\times$ systolic blood pressure (determinants include wall tension $\cong$ left ventricular pressure $\times$ volume; contractility; and heart rate)
Ventilatory Oxygen Consumption ($\dot{V}O_2$)	$\cong$ External work performed, or cardiac output $\times$ AV O_2 difference*

*AV O_2 difference is approximately constant at maximal exercise; therefore, $\dot{V}O_2$ max is a noninvasive method for estimating cardiac output.

Accurate measurement of myocardial oxygen consumption requires the placement of catheters in a coronary artery and in the coronary venous sinus to measure oxygen content. Its determinants include intramyocardial wall tension (left ventricular pressure times end-diastolic volume), contractility, and heart rate. It has been shown that myocardial oxygen consumption is best estimated by the product of heart rate and systolic blood pressure (double product). Angina usually occurs at the same double product rather than at the same work load. When this is not the case, the influence of other factors should be suspected, such as a recent meal or abnormal ambient temperature or coronary artery spasm.

The second principle is one of pathophysiology: aerobic capacity, systolic blood pressure, and heart rate response to exercise are closely related to left ventricular function, whereas the electrocardiographic response and angina are closely related to ischemia and coronary artery occlusion. These two can interrelate (i.e., exercise-induced ischemia can cause cardiac dysfunction, which results in aerobic work impairment and reduced systolic blood pressure), but in general, the above is true.

The response to dynamic muscular exercise consists of a complex series of cardiovascular adjustments designed to: (1) see that active muscles receive a blood supply appropriate to their metabolic needs; (2) dissipate the heat generated by active muscles; and (3) maintain the blood supply to the brain and the heart. There is an immediate dilatation of the arteries and arterioles in active muscle because of the sudden increase in metabolites. This results in a decrease in systemic vascular resistance proportional to the muscle mass involved. To maintain arterial blood pressure, there is an increase in sympathetic activity. This causes constriction of the resistance vessels in the splanchnic bed and the kidneys. The resistance vessels also constrict in non-working muscles. The generalized vasoconstriction in inactive tissues as well as the increased venous return result in an increase of maintenance of the heart's filling volume and pressure. As cardiac output increases, there is an increase in systemic arterial pressure. The increase in pulmonary blood flow causes a moderate increase in mean pulmonary artery pressure. The relationship of pressure, flow, and resistance is defined in Ohm's law. This physical law states that resistance is equal to pressure divided by flow. Peripheral resistance increases in the tissues that do not function in the performance of the ongoing exercise and decreases in active muscle. The total result is a decrease in overall systemic resistance. This is explained by the fact that while pressure only increases mildly, flow can increase by as much as five times during dynamic exercise. Since the denominator (flow) increases much more than the numerator (pressure) in the formula for resistance, the result is a decrease in systemic resistance.

The regulation of circulation during exercise involves the following adaptations: (1) Local—the resistance vessels dilate in the active muscle owing to the products of muscle metabolism. These products disconnect the sympathetic nerves from the muscle vessels so there will not be constriction. (2) Mechanical—during upright exercise the muscle pump returns blood from the legs to the central circulation. (3) Nervous—the sympathetic outflow to the heart and systemic blood vessels is increased; the vagal outflow to the heart decreases. This causes tachycardia, increased contractility, and constriction of the resistance vessels in the kidneys and gut. The increased sympathetic outflow is due in part to a central command from the cerebral cortex and to activation of receptors in contracting skeletal muscles. The arterial and cardiopulmonary mechanoreceptors prevent marked fluctuations in arterial pressure from normal values. As exercise continues and body temperature rises, the temperature-sensitive cells in the hypothalmus are activated. They inhibit the sympathetic outflow to the skin vessels and stimulate the cholinergic fibers to the sweat glands. This results in dilatation of the skin vessels. (4) Humoral—if exercise is severe, the cholinergic fibers to the adrenal medulla are activated and epinephrine is released into the bloodstream. This further increases the heart rate and myocardial contractility and tightens the constriction of the veins and renal arterial system.

There is a highly predictable relationship between oxygen consumption and the cardiovascular and respiratory responses to exercise. To explain this relationship, six major hypotheses have been advanced. First, the arterial baroreflex is based on the idea that vasodilatation of active muscle would cause a fall in blood pressure, which in turn would trigger a baroreflex and raise heart rate and cardiac output. However, a fall in blood pressure cannot be the stimulus for the exercise response. Second, the central nervous system excitation hypothesis—that outflow of motor impulses could interact with the centers that regulate the cardiovascular responses to exercise. The major problem with this hypothesis is that there is no feedback mechanism to the central nervous system to maintain the delicate relationship between these responses and exercising muscle. The third and fourth hypotheses are based on chemoreflexes in the arterial or central venous systems. However, there are little data to support the idea that changes in PO_2, CO_2, or pH are the mediators. Fifth, the skeletal muscle mechanoreceptors hypothesis—these receptors cannot be involved in the exercise reflex since there is no cardiovascular or respiratory response to muscle vibration, which is a potent stimulus to mechanoreceptors, and selective blockade of large mechanoreceptor afferents does not block the exercise response.

The sixth and most logical hypothesis is based on muscle chemoreceptors. The most current evidence suggests that some sensor within skeletal muscle detects small changes in the local chemical environment and serves to monitor the adequacy of muscle perfusion.

METHODOLOGY

The multitude of approaches to the methodology of performing exercise testing have been a drawback to its proper growth. Most laboratories agree on the use of safety precautions, but otherwise there are nearly as many methods as there are investigators.

Safety Precautions. The safety precautions indicated by the American Heart Association are very explicit in regard to the requirements for exercise testing. Everything necessary for cardiopulmonary resuscitation must be available, and regular drills should be performed to make certain that both personnel and equipment are ready for a cardiac emergency. A survey of clinical exercise facilities has shown exercise testing to be a safe procedure with approximately one death and five nonfatal complications per 10,000 tests. However, the literature contains reports of acute infarctions and deaths occurring secondarily to this procedure. Bruce has reported the relatively frequent association of exercise-induced hypotension and ventricular fibrillation. Though the test is remarkably safe, the population referred for this procedure usually is at high risk for coronary events. Shepard has hypothesized the following risk levels for exercise: (1) 3 or 4 times normal in a cross-country foot race; (2) 6 to 12 times normal in a coronary prone population performing unaccustomed exercise; and (3) as high as 60 times normal when exercise is performed by coronary disease patients in a stressful environ-

TABLE II
ABSOLUTE AND RELATIVE CONTRAINDICATIONS TO EXERCISE TESTING

Absolute	Relative*
Acute myocardial infarction or any recent change in the resting electrocardiogram	Any less serious noncardiac disorder
Unstable angina	Ventricular conduction defects
Serious cardiac dysrhythmias	Significant arterial or pulmonary hypertension
Acute pericarditis or myocarditis	Tachydysrhythmias or bradydysrhythmias < serious
Endocarditis	Moderate valvular or myocardial heart diseases
Severe aortic stenosis	Drug effect or electrolyte abnormalities
Severe left ventricular dysfunction	Fixed-rate artificial pacemaker
Acute pulmonary embolus or pulmonary infarction	Left main obstruction or its equivalent
Any acute or serious noncardiac disorder	Psychiatric disease or inability to cooperate
Severe physical handicap	

*Under certain circumstances, relative contraindications can be superseded.

ment, such as a physician's office. The risk of exercise testing to coronary artery disease patients cannot be disregarded even with an excellent safety record.

Table II lists the absolute and relative contraindications to performing an exercise test. Good clinical judgment should be foremost in deciding the indications and contraindications for exercise testing. Whereas the absolute contraindications are straightforward, in selected cases with relative contraindications, testing can provide valuable information even if performed submaximally.

Preparations for exercise testing include the following: (1) the patient should be instructed not to eat two to three hours prior to the test and to come dressed for exercise; (2) a brief history and physical examination should be accomplished to rule out any contraindications to testing (particularly outflow tract obstruction); (3) specific questioning should determine if there are any drugs being taken or possible electrolyte abnormalities; (4) if the reason for the exercise test is not obvious, the patient should be questioned and the referring physician contacted; and (5) a 12-lead electrocardiogram should be obtained. The latter is an important rule, particularly in patients with known heart disease, since an abnormality may prohibit testing. On occasion, a patient referred for a treadmill test will instead be admitted to the coronary care unit. There should be a careful explanation of the testing procedure with its risks and possible complications. The patient should be instructed on how to perform the exercise test, and treadmill walking should be demonstrated.

The treadmill should have front and side rails for patients to steady themselves, and some patients may benefit from the helping hand of the person administering the test. Patients should not grasp the front or side rails as this decreases oxygen uptake and work and increases exercise time and muscle artifact. It is helpful if patients take their hands off the rails, close their fists, and extend one finger touching the rails to maintain balance while walking after they are accustomed to the treadmill. The addition of isometric work should be avoided, but when the patient first steps on the treadmill it is best to allow him or her to hold on as much as is necessary.

Most problems can be avoided by having an experienced physician or exercise physiologist standing next to the patient, measuring blood pressure, judging skin temperature, and assessing the patient during the test. The exercise technician should operate the recorder and treadmill, take the appropriate tracings, enter data on a form, and alert the physician to any abnormalities that may have been missed on the monitor scope. If the patient's appearance is worrisome, if blood pressure drops or plateaus, if there are alarming electrocardiographic abnormalities, if chest pain occurs and becomes worse than the patient's usual pain, or if a patient feels he or she is being harmed in any way, the test should be stopped, even at a submaximal heart rate. In most instances, a symptom-limited maximal test is preferred, but it is usually advisable to stop if 0.2 mV of ST-segment elevation occurs. In some patients estimated to be at high risk because of their clinical history, it may be appropriate to stop at a submaximal level since it is not unusual for severe ST-segment depression, dysrhythmias, or both to occur only after exercise. If the measurement of maximal functional capacity or other information is needed, it is better to repeat the test later, once the patient has demonstrated a safe performance of a submaximal work load.

Exercise testing should be an extension of the physical examination. A physician obtains the most information by being present to talk with, to observe, and to examine the patient in conjunction with the test. In this way, patient safety and an optimal yield of information are assured. In some instances, such as when asymptomatic men are being screened, research studies are being performed, or a repeat treadmill test is being done on a patient whose condition is stable, a physician need not be present but should be in close proximity and prepared to respond promptly.

Prior to an exercise test, it is advisable to obtain an abbreviated medical history and a 12-lead electrocardiogram and to perform a cardiovascular examination even if the patient was referred by a physician. In this manner, patients with recent onset of an infectious disease or with worsening ischemic heart disease can be identified. Patients with a history of increasing or unstable angina should undergo exercise testing in certain circumstances. A cardiac examination should indicate which patients have valvular or congenital heart disease, particularly those with severe aortic stenosis, who should not be exercised.

Consent Form. In any procedure with a risk of complications, it is advisable to make certain the patient understands the situation and acknowledges the risks. Some physicians feel that informing patients of the risks involved will often make them overly anxious or discourage them from having a test performed. Because of this and the fact that a signed consent form does not protect a physician from legal action, there has recently been less insistence on consent forms. If those performing the exercise test carefully explain in detail the possible risks and complications of the test to each patient, a consent form should be superfluous.

Legal Implications of Exercise Testing. The legal implications of performing exercise testing include several considerations. Establishment of physician-patient communication before and after performance of the exercise test should be the first consideration. A test should not be performed without first obtaining the patient's informed consent, preferably in writing. In the process of obtaining informed consent, the patient should be made aware of the potential risks and benefits of the procedure. A physician may be held responsible in the event of a major untoward effect, even if the test is carefully done, if consent is not first obtained. The argument can be made that the patient would not have undergone the procedure had he or she been made aware of the risks associated with the test. After the test, responsibility then rests with the physician for prompt interpretation and consideration of the implications of the test. Communication of these results to the patient is necessary—with advice concerning adjustments in life-style—without delay. It would be of major concern if an untoward event occurred during such a delay.

The second consideration should be adherence to proper standards of care during performance of the test. Every test should be preceded by a physical examination and an electrocardiographic evaluation by the physician supervising the test or by the referring physician. Exercise testing should be carried out only by persons thoroughly trained in its administration and in the prompt recognition of problems that may arise. The patient must be instructed to report symptoms (i.e., angina, light-headedness) that may necessitate termination of the test. A physician trained in exercise testing and resuscitation should be readily available during the test to make the judgment to stop the study. Resuscitative equipment should always be available.

Recording Instruments. Many technologic advances in electrocardiographic recorders have taken place during the past decade. The medical instrumentation industry has promptly complied with specifications set forth by various professional groups. Machines with a high-input impedance ensure that the voltage recorded graphically is equivalent to that on the surface of the body despite the high natural impedance of the skin. There remains some concern about mismatching lead impedances, which can result in distortion. Optically isolated buffer amplifiers have ensured patient safety, and machines with a frequency response from 0 to 100 Hz are commercially available. The 0 Hz lower end is possible because dc coupling is technically feasible.

Some electrocardiographic equipment has monitoring and diagnostic modes, particularly that equipment used in coronary care units. The diagnostic mode follows diagnostic instrument specifications with a frequency response from 0.05 Hz to 100 Hz, whereas the monitor mode has a frequency range of 4 Hz to 50 Hz. In the monitor mode, there is distortion of the electrocardiogram. The monitor mode is available to lessen the effects of electrical interference, motion, and respiration in the electrocardiogram and should not be used for exercise testing. The type of distortion is affected by the electrocardiographic waveform that is presented. If the electrocardiographic waveform is a tall R wave without an S wave, the ST-segment distortion can be different than if there is an R wave followed by a large S wave. In general, an inadequate low-frequency response can greatly decrease the Q- and R-wave amplitude and create S waves. The middle-range frequency response of recorders is important and is particularly affected by stylus overpressure. Alteration of the 25 Hz to 45 Hz frequency response is the most common cause of ST-segment distortion found in tracings with abnormal ST segments. A simple office test is available for checking the 0.05 to 45 Hz frequency response of a recorder. It consists of recording approximately five seconds of the decay curve of a 1 cm/mV calibration pulse at the standard paper speed of 25 mm/sec. The time between the initial upstroke of this calibration pulse and the point at which the initial signal has decayed to 3.7 mm should be at least 3.2 seconds to meet the 0.05 Hz low-frequency end point. In this same recording, the presence of a sharp, square-cornered leading edge at the peak of the pulse reflects the existence of a high-frequency response of at least 45 Hz, because roundness at that junction becomes visually apparent below this frequency. Not all ambulatory electrocardiographic monitoring recorders or telemetry equipment meets diagnostic frequency requirements, which impairs the diagnostic usefulnesss of such instruments for ischemia.

Analog and digital averaging techniques have made it possible to average electrocardiographic signals to remove noise. There is a need, however, for consumer protection in these areas since most manufacturers do not specify how the use of such procedures modifies an electrocardiogram. Signal averaging can distort the electrocardiographic signal. These techniques are attractive since they can produce a pretty tracing in spite of poor skin preparation. However, the common expression used by computer scientists, "garbage in, garbage out," applies here. The clean-looking electrocardiographic signal produced may not be a true representation of the actual waveform and in fact may be dangerously misleading. Also, the instruments that make computer ST-segment measurements cannot be totally reliable since they are based on imperfect algorithms. For instance, the algorithm that measures QRS end at 70 or 80 msec after the peak of the R wave can hardly be valid, particularly with a changing heart rate.

It is advantageous to have a recorder with a slow paper speed of 5 mm/sec. This speed makes it possible to record all of an exercise test and reduces the likelihood of missing any dysrhythmias. A faster paper speed of 50 mm/sec can be helpful for making accurate ST-segment slope measurements. There are many different types of electrocardiographic paper that can be used. The most experience has been with wax-treated paper, which is known to retain an electrocardiographic image for 20 years or longer. However, it is pressure sensitive and easily marred. The relatively new thermochemical-treated paper is sturdy and not easily marred. There are many different types of such paper, and the life expectancy of images recorded on it is not yet known. There has been at least one instance of this paper losing recorded electrocardiographic images that subsequently resulted in legal action by a hospital against a manufacturer. Ceramic-coated paper is very sturdy and comparable in price; it has a hard finish with a high contrast, which makes it durable and easy to interpret. Untreated paper is the cheapest, but the ink jet and carbon-transfer technique characteristically produce fuzzy images. The ink jet and carbon-transfer recorders are available with six channels and are expensive, but they do have an excellent upper-frequency response for phonocardiography. The ceramic paper also requires an ink-jet stylus rather than a heat stylus. Ink-jet recorders are said to require more maintenance, but recent models appear reliable. Copying can be a problem since blues and reds are poorly copied by some xerographic reproduction machines. Z-fold paper has the advantage over roll paper in that it is easily folded, and the study can be interpreted in a manner similar to paging through a book. Exercise electrocardiograms can be microfilmed on rolls, cartridges, or in fiche cards for storage. They also can be stored in digital or analog format on magnetic media.

Exercise Test Modalities. Three types of exercise can be used to stress the cardiovascular system: isometric, dynamic, and a combination of the two. Isometric exercise, defined as constant muscular contraction without movement (i.e., handgrip), imposes a disproportionate pressure load on the left ventricle relative to the body's ability to supply oxygen. Dynamic exercise, defined as rhythmic muscular activity resulting in movement, initiates a more appropriate increase in cardiac output and oxygen exchange. Since a delivered work load can be accurately calibrated and the physiologic response easily measured, dynamic exercise is preferred for clinical testing. Using progressive work loads of dynamic exercise, patients with coronary artery disease can be protected from rapidly increasing myocardial oxygen demand. Although bicycling is a dynamic exercise, most individuals are more likely to give adequate muscular effort on a treadmill because of their greater familiarity with walking and the specificity of training.

Numerous modalities have been used to provide the dynamic exercise for exercise testing, including steps, escalators, and ladder mills. Today, however, the bicycle ergometer and the treadmill are the most commonly used dynamic exercise devices. The bicycle ergometer is usually cheaper, takes up less space, and makes less noise. Upper body motion usually is reduced, but care must be taken so that isometric exercise is not performed by the arms. The work load administered by the simple bicycle ergometers is not well calibrated and it is very dependent on pedaling speed. It is too easy for a patient to slow pedaling speed during exercise testing and decrease the administered work load. More expensive bicycle ergometers keep the administered work load at a determined level over a wide range of pedaling speeds. This latter type of instrument is particularly needed for supine bicycle exercise testing.

Supine Versus Erect Exercise Testing. European cardiologists have favored supine bicycle testing, because of safety reasons or because of their experience with this technique in the cardiac catheterization laboratory. There is a marked difference between the body's response to acute exercise in the supine and erect positions. In normal persons, stroke volume and end-diastolic volume do not change much during supine bicycle exercise from volumes obtained at rest, whereas in the erect position these values increase during mild work and then plateau. In patients with abnormalities, left ventricular filling pressure is more likely to increase during exercise in the supine position than in the erect position. When angina patients perform identical submaximal bicycle work loads in supine and erect positions, heart rate is higher in the supine position. The maximal work load is lower in the supine position, and angina will develop at a lower double product. ST-segment depression is often greater in the supine position because of the greater left ventricular volume.

The linear relationship of cardiac output to oxygen uptake during supine bicycle exercise has been demonstrated and has been used to separate heart disease patients from normal persons. Exercise factor, or the increase of cardiac output for an increase in oxygen uptake, is based on studies of normal persons. For every 100 ml increase in oxygen consumption, cardiac output should increase by 500 ml. Left ventricular filling pressure does not increase in proportion to work in normal persons but very often increases in patients with abnormalities. Radionuclide imaging has shown that the ejection fraction decreases during supine exercise in patients with coronary artery disease rather than increases as it does in normal persons. Patients with coronary artery disease, however, can have discordance between their disease and ventricular function and can respond normally to exercise.

In most studies comparing erect bicycle exercise with treadmill exercise, maximal heart rate values have been similar, whereas maximal oxygen consumption values were greater during treadmill exercise. However, these studies were based mostly on the performance of athletes and the results would be more comparable if higher pedaling speeds had been used (60 to 90 rpm). Niederberger and associates concluded that bicycle exercise constitutes a greater stress on the cardiovascular system, in terms of the double product at any given oxygen uptake, than does treadmill exercise. The clinical importance of their findings in relation to patients with cardiovascular disease undergoing exercise testing is that slightly higher maximal oxygen uptakes are achieved with slightly less hemodynamic stress when treadmill exercise is used. Oldridge and co-workers found similar electrocardiographic changes with treadmill testing as compared with bicycle testing in patients with coronary artery disease. Rather than for any medical reason, however, the treadmill is the most commonly used dynamic testing modality in the United States because patients are more familiar with walking than they are with bicycling. They are more likely to give the muscular effort necessary to adequately increase myocardial oxygen demand by walking rather than by bicycling.

Protocols. Some standardization of exercise testing is necessary to compare tests among patients and between subsequent tests in the same patient. Unfortunately, there are many different treadmill protocols in use. The most commonly used protocols are progressive, i.e, they are uninterrupted and the work load is increased in stages. Of note are branching protocols that increase grade and speed depending on the patient's heart rate response. In this type of protocol, patients of different functional capacity perform for approximately the same time period so that differences in endurance are minimized. This type of protocol is usually too complicated for clinical use.

When compared with other protocols, the Air Force School of Aerospace Medicine (USAFSAM) or other modification of the Balke-Ware protocol using a constant speed has many advantages. The USAFSAM protocol consists of a constant brisk walking speed (3.3 mph) with 5% increases in grade every 3 minutes. The constant treadmill speed requires only an initial adaptation in stride, reduces technician adjustment, and produces less electrocardiographic and blood pressure artifact than do protocols using multiple or higher treadmill speeds or a combination of both. This protocol provides a larger number of appropriate work loads for patients and increases in even increments of work load. Speed can be started at 2.0 mph for patients who find 3.3 mph too brisk. It is advisable to individualize any exercise protocol for the type of patient being tested. Three-minute stages are certainly not needed to achieve steady state at a low work load. Performance can be estimated with the oxygen cost of maximal work load achieved rather than in total treadmill time. In this way, performance in different protocols can be compared. After evaluating a number of protocols, this estimation has been found to be as accurate as predicting maximal oxygen uptake from maximal treadmill time. For individuals with above-average exercise capacity, it is better to increase the speed rather than the grade after reaching an incline of 25%. Figure 1 compares the USAFSAM protocol with the Bruce protocol. In stage 4 of the Bruce protocol, an individual can walk or run. Since running is much less efficient, the oxygen cost is greater than if the individual walks.

Submaximal Versus Maximal Exercise Testing. The most commonly used submaximal treadmill test is the graded exercise test of Sheffield and Reeves. They utilize the Bruce protocol, but the test is terminated when the patient reaches 90% of predicted maximal heart rate for age and level of training. Predicted maximal heart rate was determined from a study of normal individuals; in the study athletically trained subjects had a slightly lower maximal heart rate than did the others. Unfortunately, as in other studies, there is a wide spread of maximal heart rate around the regression line, declining with age (SD ± 12 beats/minute). Thus, the target heart rate is

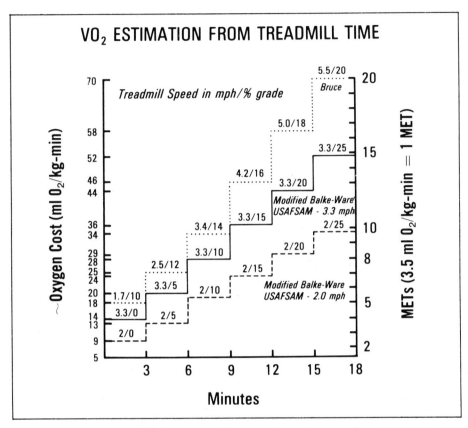

Figure 1. Three progressive continuous treadmill protocols are shown with the approximate oxygen cost to perform each stage. The Bruce protocol and modifications of the Balke-Ware protocol are the most commonly used treadmill protocols. Walking or running and holding on alter the oxygen cost of a work load. Uneven increases in oxygen cost and the motion artifact secondary to running are disadvantages of the Bruce protocol. Accelerated protocols using 5% or greater increments may require stages longer than two minutes to estimate aerobic capacity, particularly in cardiac patients.

maximal for some subjects, beyond the limits of others, and submaximal for others. This testing procedure has the advantage that patients can be tested in street shoes and clothes and are not usually uncomfortable during it since most patients are not stressed to a maximal effort. However, maximal sensitivity is not obtained and thus functional capacity cannot be accurately estimated or measured.

A test is considered maximal when the patient appears to give a true maximal effort or when other clinical end points are reached. A true maximal exercise test is achieved when measured oxygen uptake reaches a value that will not increase despite an increase in work load. When using submaximal tests, there exists a paradox that the most vulnerable patients are stressed to a relatively greater extent, whereas the less impaired are limited by submaximal target heart rates.

Skin Preparation. Proper skin preparation is essential for the performance of an exercise test. During exercise, because noise increases with the square of resistance it is extremely important to lower the resistance at the skin-electrode interface and thereby improve the signal-to-noise ratio. It is often difficult to make technicians consistently prepare the skin properly because doing so may cause the patient discomfort and minor skin irritation. The performance of an exercise test with an electrocardiographic signal that cannot be continuously monitored and accurately interpreted because of artifact is worthless and can even be dangerous.

The areas for electrode application are marked with a felt-tip pen, the mark serving as a guide for removal of enough of the superficial layer of skin. The electrodes are placed using anatomic landmarks that are found with the patient supine. Some individuals with loose skin can have a considerable shift of electrode positions when they assume an upright position. The marked areas are then cleansed with an alcohol-saturated gauze pad. The next step is to further remove the superficial layer of skin either with a hand-held drill or by light abrasion with fine-grain emery paper. Skin resistance should be reduced to 5,000 ohms or less, which can be verified prior to the exercise test with an inexpensive ac impedance meter driven at 10 Hz. Each electrode is tested against a common electrode with the ohmmeter, and when 5,000 ohms or less is not achieved, the electrode must be removed and skin preparation repeated. This maneuver saves time by obviating the need to interrupt a test due to noisy tracings.

Electrodes and Cables. The only suitable electrodes are constructed with a metal interface that is sunken to create a column that can be filled with either an electrolyte solution or a saturated sponge. These fluid column electrodes markedly decrease motion artifact as compared with those with direct metal-to-skin contact. There are many disposable electrodes that perform excellently. Silver plate or silver–silver chloride crystal pellets are the best electrode materials. Platinum is too expensive and the frequently used German silver is actually an alloy. If electrodes of different types of metals are used together, an offset voltage can be generated that makes it impossible to record an electrocardiogram. The disposable electrodes have the advantages of quick application and no need for cleansing for reuse. They are more expensive to use than nondisposable electrodes, however, and they require a wire connection on the electrode that may induce motion artifact. The better nondisposable electrodes can be used for over a hundred tests. Breakdown usually occurs in the wire connection as it goes through the electrode housing. This problem can be reduced if the electrodes are not removed by pulling the connecting wire. A recent development is an electrode that has an abrasive center that is spun by an applicator after the electrode is attached to the skin (Quickprep, Quinton Instrument Co.). This approach does not require skin preparation. A clever feature of the applicator is a built-in impedance meter that stops it from spinning when the necessary impedance is achieved.

A problem in gathering exercise data has been obtaining a suitable connecting cable between the electrodes and the recorder. The earliest versions of these cables were subject to wire-continuity problems, frequent failures, and motion artifact; they were improperly shielded and utilized inadequate connectors. Shielding of the electrode wires and cables is especially important in metropolitan areas or near high-voltage x-ray equipment. Several commercial companies have concentrated on solving these problems, and now there are exercise cables available that are constructed to avoid these problems. Buffer amplifiers carried by the patient are no longer advantageous.

Lead Systems. Electrodes have been placed in a variety of ways and in many different lead systems. This situation has complicated making comparisons of the ST-segment response to exercise. The four major exercise electrocardiographic lead systems are the bipolar, the Mason-Likar 12-lead, a simulation of Wilson's central terminal, and the three-dimensional (orthogonal or nonorthogonal systems).

Bipolar lead systems have been used because of the relatively short time required for placement, the relative freedom from motion artifact, and the ease with which noise problems can be located. Figure 2 illustrates the electrode placements for most of the bipolar lead systems. The usual positive reference is an electrode placed the same as the positive reference for V_5. The negative reference for V_5 is Wilson's central terminal, which consists of connecting the limb electrodes—right arm (RA), left arm (LA), and left leg (LL). The only other notable bipolar lead system is the roving bipolar lead, which was introduced by McHenry. In this system, beginning with a CC_5 placement, the electrodes are moved around to obtain the maximal R wave with a small S wave. McHenry feels that this type of left ventricular waveform is the most sensitive for ST-segment changes.

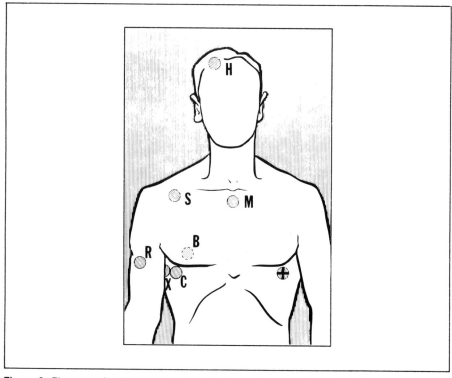

Figure 2. Placement for the negative electrode for most commonly used bipolar lead systems is shown. The letters on the torso represent the second prefix. The positive electrode is placed at the intersection of the level of the fifth intercostal space (determined at the midclavicular line) and the left anterior axillary line. Shown are CH_5, CS_5, CM_5, CR_5, CX_5, CC_5, and CB_5. (With permission of Chest.)

The problem with comparing the results of ST-segment analysis if different leads are used has been demonstrated by a computer analysis study. ST-segment depression and slope measurements were made on signals gathered simultaneously from CC_5, CM_5, and V_5. A common positive reference electrode was used. CM_5 consistently had a more negative J junction and a more positive slope than did V_5 and CC_5. V_5 and CC_5 were essentially identical, on the basis of standard analysis, but differed statistically when computer measurements were compared. This difference in the leads most likely explains why investigators using CM_5 have reported an inadequate ST slope to be as serious as horizontal depression.

Figure 3 illustrates the Mason-Likar torso-mounted limb lead system. The conventional ankle and wrist electrodes are replaced by electrodes

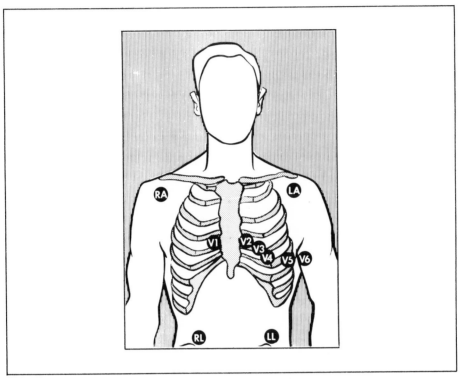

Figure 3. The Mason-Likar exercise electrocardiographic lead system is illustrated. The electrodes for the arms should be placed as far off the torso as possible so that the electrocardiogram most closely simulates the electrocardiogram obtained using standard wrist placement.

mounted on the torso at the base of the limbs. In this way, the artifact introduced by movement of the limbs is avoided. An electrocardiogram obtained in this manner shows a more rightward axis than that obtained with wrist and ankle electrodes. It offers the advantage of producing an electrocardiogram that supposedly does not differ essentially from the standard 12-lead electrocardiogram, especially if the limb electrodes are kept at the base of the limbs. Moving them onto the chest and abdomen further decreases motion artifact but distorts the electrocardiogram. The standard precordial leads use Wilson's central terminal as their negative reference, which is formed by connecting the right arm, left arm, and left leg. This triangular configuration around the heart results in a zero voltage reference through the cardiac cycle. The use of Wilson's central terminal for the precordial leads (V leads) requires the negative reference to be a combination of three additional electrodes rather than the single electrode used as the negative reference for bipolar leads. Simulation of Wilson's central terminal by other combinations of electrodes has not been validated, and therefore such alternate configurations should be avoided.

Few studies have correctly evaluated the relative yield or sensitivity and specificity of different electrocardiographic leads for exercise-induced ST-segment depression. Studies show that using other leads in addition to V_5 will increase the yield of abnormal responders by about 25%. The specificity of abnormal responses in these leads, however, is decreased.

Robinson and associates reported their results using 12-lead exercise tests in 39 patients with both abnormal exercise tests and abnormal coronary angiograms. Eighteen percent had an abnormal response in leads other than V_5. Patients with right coronary artery lesions usually showed ST-segment depression in inferior leads, and patients with left coronary system lesions usually showed ST-segment depression in leads I and aVL and in the chest leads. However, almost a third of the patients showed ST-segment depression in leads other than those anticipated from their angiographic anatomy. Tucker and colleagues reported their results using 12-lead exercise tests in 100 consecutive patients who were also studied with coronary angiography. Forty-eight had abnormal tests, with 30% of the abnormal responses occurring in leads other than V_5 (17% in aVF and 13% in other leads). Two false positives occurred in V_5 and two in aVF, whereas 16 positives occurred in leads other than V_5 or aVF. Of those abnormal in aVF alone, five had lesions in the right coronary or left circumflex artery and two had disease in the left anterior descending artery. It remains to be demonstrated what the specificity of leads other than V_5 eventually will be, but one has the impression that inferior leads have more false positives and may require different criteria. This apparent lack of specificity may be due to the effect of atrial repolarization in inferior leads, which causes depression of the ST segment. With adequate experience, atrial repolarization can be recognized in the PR segment and can be understood to cause ST-segment depression. Such findings also support the concept of an intercoronary artery steal during exercise, that is, ischemic areas obtain blood flow through collaterals. This phenomenon leads to a reduced ability of ST-segment depression in multilead exercise testing to predict the location and severity of coronary artery disease.

Chaitman and colleagues reported the role of multiple-lead electrocardiographic systems and clinical subsets in interpreting treadmill test results. Two hundred men with normal electrocardiograms at rest had a maximal treadmill test using 14 electrocardiographic leads and then underwent coronary angiography. This study included standard leads plus three bipolar leads. The prevalence of significant coronary stenosis was 86% in 87 men with typical angina, 65% in 64 men with probable angina, and 28% in 49 men with nonspecific chest pain. The predictive value of ST-segment deviation in any one of 14 leads was 45% in men with nonspecific chest pain versus 82% in men with probable angina and 100% in men with typical angina. The predictive value of a normal ST-segment response in 14 leads was 83% in men with nonspecific chest pain versus 70% in men with probable angina, and 55% in men with typical angina. The investigators found multiple-lead testing to be most valuable in the men with angina and least helpful in those with nonspecific chest pain. In the latter, recording a single lead such as CM_5 was adequate. In men with typical or probable angina, a normal response in 14 leads associated with treadmill work time longer than nine minutes reduced the chance of three-vessel disease to less than 10%. The likelihood of multivessel disease in a patient with an abnormal ST response and a treadmill time equal to or less than three minutes was approximately 90%. In patients with angina, the use of 14 leads increased sensitivity over that of V_5 alone from 52% and 65% to 75%. This value was increased even further to 86% by the additional consideration of bipolar leads.

There are a number of three-dimensional or vectorcardiographic lead systems that can be used during exercise. The corrected Frank lead system has the advantage that the electrical activity of the heart is orthogonally represented in the three derived signals. The relative ease of placement of only seven electrodes required for the Frank system has made it the most popular orthogonal lead system. Care should be taken so that the X and Z electrodes are placed as described by Frank in his original paper, at the fifth intercostal space level at the sternum. The vectorcardiographic approach makes it possible to evaluate the spatial changes of the ST-segment vector. The Frank X is a left precordial lead but is about 25% smaller in amplitude in V_5 because of the Frank network resistance, which is an attempt to electrically move the heart to the center of the chest. ST-segment criteria have not been adjusted for this fact, however.

The Dalhousie square is an eloquently simple way to assist with the proper and reproducible placement of the Frank electrodes and of the Wilson precordial electrodes. It is a simple right-angle device that is held to the chest. Proper placement is necessary for the application of electrocardiographic and vectorcardiographic interpretive criteria. Reproducible placement is essential to assess serial changes.

Since the question of how many leads need to be recorded during an exercise test has not been resolved, it seems advisable to record as many as economically and practically possible. In patients with a normal resting electrocardiogram, a V_5 or similar bipolar lead along the long axis of the heart may be adequate. In patients with electrocardiographic evidence of myocardial damage or with a history suggestive of coronary spasm, additional leads are needed. As a minimal approach, it is advisable to record three leads: a V_5 type lead, an anterior V_2 type lead, and an inferior lead such as aVF; or Frank X,Y, and Z leads may be used. This approach is also helpful for the detection and identification of dysrhythmias. It is advisable also to be able to record a second three-lead grouping consisting of V_4, V_5, and V_6. Sometimes abnormalites may be seen as borderline in V_5, whereas they will be clearly abnormal in V_4 or V_6.

Blood Pressure. Blood pressure should be taken at least at the midportion of each exercise stage and with the occurrence of chest pain. The following equipment is preferable to the commonly available automated blood pressure devices: (1) a mercury manometer or a damped anaeroid pressure gauge mounted on the treadmill, (2) either an anesthesiologist's stethoscope with long tubing or a crystal microphone attached over the brachial artery and amplified through stethophones, and (3) a pressure device that inflates and then deflates the cuff at the press of a button or a standard cuff inflator with a pushbutton bleed-off valve. The patient's arm should be held straight down and free of the treadmill rails when blood pressure is taken. The test should usually be stopped if the systolic blood pressure shows a sustained drop, especially if this drop is accompanied by chest pain. There has been a malpractice settlement over the failure to take blood pressure during the performance of an exercise test.

Measurement or Estimation of Maximal Oxygen Uptake. The guidelines to prepare for the measurement of maximal oxygen uptake are: (1) common dynamic exercise of a large portion of the muscle mass, (2) progressive increases in work load to fatigue, (3) precise gas measurement techniques, and (4) minimal testing time to lessen the effect of endurance. These guidelines have been followed using different treadmill protocols, and similar results were obtained.

To measure oxygen uptake, the concentration of oxygen in expired air and in inspired or room air must be determined by using gas analyzers. Flow can be measured using air bags or flow meters and then the amount of oxygen consumed by the body can be determined. Because the measurement of maximal oxygen uptake requires a nose clip, mouthpiece, breathing valves, weather balloons, and gas analysis equipment, it is not practical to perform in clinical practice. Only experienced patients do well with a mouthpiece in place, and it is not advisable to measure oxygen consumption during a first test. Automated systems have not been adequately validated and are very expensive; all are limited mainly by technical difficulties in measuring airflow during exercise.

Maximal oxygen uptake and treadmill work load are directly related. Linear regression equations for this relationship have correlation coefficients of + .8 to .9. There is, however, a wide scatter around the regression line that is due to wide variations in mechanical efficiency among individuals. Care should be taken so that patients do not support their weight or allow themselves to be dragged by the hand rails, since this reduces the amount of work performed. Bruce has suggested the following method of estimating functional aerobic impairment (FAI):

$$FAI = \frac{\text{Predicted} - \text{Observed maximal oxygen consumption}}{\text{Predicted} - \text{Maximal oxygen consumption}} \times 100$$

Normally FAI should be zero because observed maximal oxygen uptake should be the same as that predicted. Bruce constructed a nomogram to determine FAI. On one side is treadmill time in his protocol, and on the other is age. Between these two lines are sloped lines with percent increments of FAI for sedentary and active individuals. By lining up age (from which the maximal oxygen uptake can be predicted) with the treadmill time (from which observed maximal oxygen uptake can be estimated), an estimate of aerobic impairment can be read from the sloped lines. The nomogram is based on two relatively poor relationships, which thereby limit its ability to predict functional capacity. It is preferable to estimate an individual's maximal oxygen uptake from the work load reached while performing a treadmill test. This estimation facilitates comparison between different treadmill protocols and avoids the problem arising from the fact that the same performance time in different protocols does not mean that the same work load was performed. Serial treadmill testing is complicated by the occurrence of adaptation, which increases treadmill time without an increase in maximal oxygen uptake.

The use of total treadmill time as a measure of a patient's functional capacity and its subsequent introduction into medical practice have had advantages and disadvantages. The advantages are that an understanding of exercise physiology is not necessary for analyzing exercise test results and that, if the same protocol is used, test results can easily be compared. After some consideration, however, it is apparent that these advantages are far outweighed by many disadvantages.

A true test of aerobic capacity is best limited to a total exercise time of 9 or 10 minutes, as endurance really becomes the key factor thereafter. Endurance is much more difficult to assess and is much more impacted by peripheral factors than by central cardiac ones. Comparison of total treadmill time locks one into a fixed treadmill protocol, and for the best physiologic testing, one should adjust work loads to the individual patient, rather than the patient to the work loads. Some patients can reach higher functional capacities if the grade is mainly increased rather than the speed. At high levels of performance it is usually best to increase speed rather than grade, because of the mechanical difficulties of staying on a treadmill with a steep incline.

Cardiothoracic surgeons, in particular, will often ask "How long did the patient walk?" and not be concerned at all with what work load was reached. In performing serial treadmill tests, the improvement that a patient can achieve in total time because of learning makes it appear as if they have had functional improvement. Though it takes a greater understanding of exercise physiology and an active interaction with the patient, it would be much better to tailor each exercise test for the patient being tested. Rather than consider total time, which should be about ten minutes, functional capacity should be estimated from the highest treadmill speed and grade at which the patient equilibrates. Though the gross relationships between total treadmill time in a fixed protocol or the work load achieved and total body oxygen consumption are adequate for clinical purposes, it is to be hoped that in the near future a relatively inexpensive automated system for airflow and gas analysis will be developed that can accurately measure oxygen consumption. Such a system is very much needed for accurate estimation of maximum cardiac output (i.e., cardiac function) and for the evaluation of serial changes in functional capacity after interventions.

Postexercise Period. If maximal sensitivity is to be achieved with an exercise test, patients should be supine in the postexercise period. It is advisable to record about ten seconds of electrocardiographic data while the patient is standing motionless, but still experiencing near maximal heart rate, and then have him lie down. Some must be allowed to lie down immediately to avoid hypotension. Having the patient perform a cool-down walk after the test can delay or eliminate the appearance of ST-segment depression. This is not an important consideration when the test is not being performed for diagnostic purposes. According to the law of Laplace increased supine heart volume increases myocardial oxygen consumption. Investigators have reported that this relation enhances ST-segment abnormalities. Monitoring should continue for six to eight minutes after exercise or until changes stabilize. In the supine position four to five minutes into recovery, approximately 85% of patients with abnormal responses in a large series were abnormal at this time only or in addition to other times. An abnormal response occurring only in the recovery period is not unusual and may be due to reactive hyperemia. All such responses are not false positives, as has been suggested. Recent animal experiments confirm mechanical dysfunction and electrophysiologic abnormalities in the ischemic ventricle after exercise. A cool-down walk can be helpful when doing tests on patients with an established diagnosis undergoing testing for other than diagnostic reasons or when testing athletes.

Indications for Treadmill Test Termination. The following absolute and relative indications for termination of an exercise test have been derived from clinical experience. As before, absolute indications are clear-cut, whereas relative indications can sometimes be disregarded if good clinical judgment is used. Absolute indications include a drop in systolic blood pressure despite an increase in work load, anginal chest pain becoming worse than usual, central nervous system symptoms, signs of poor perfusion (such as pallor, cyanosis, and cold skin), serious dysrhythmias, technical problems with monitoring the patient, patient's request to stop, and marked electrocardiographic changes, e.g., more than 0.3 mV of horizontal or downsloping ST-segment depression, and 0.2 mV of ST-segment elevation. Relative indications for termination are other worrisome ST or QRS changes such as excessive junctional depression; increasing chest pain; fatigue, shortness of breath, wheezing, leg cramps, or intermittent claudication; worrisome appearance; hypertensive response (systolic pressure greater than 280 mm Hg, diastolic pressure greater than 115 mm Hg), and less serious dysrhythmias including supraventricular tachycardias. In some patients estimated to be precarious by their clinical history, it may be appropriate to stop at a submaximal level since the most severe ST-segment depression or dysrhythmias can occur only after exercise. If more information is required, the test can be repeated later.

Computerized Exercise Electrocardiographic Analysis. A digital computer was first used for electrocardiographic analysis by Taback and colleagues in 1959. They pointed out the advantages of digital versus analog data processing, including more precise and more accurate measurements, less distortion in recording, direct accessibility to digital computer analysis and storage techniques, rapid mathematical manipulation (i.e., averaging), avoidance of the drift inherent in analog components, digital algorithm control permitting changing analysis schema with ease (i.e., software rather than hardware changes), no degradation with repetitive playback, higher plotting resolution (i.e., not real time), and facile repetitive manipulation of data (i.e., plotting with different gains and filters).

The two critical problems posed by exercise electrocardiography are reduction of the amount of electrocardiographic data collected during exercise testing and elimination of the noise in the electrocardiogram secondary to exercise. The total period of an exercise test can exceed one-half hour, and many physicians want to analyze all 12 leads during and after testing. The three-lead vectorcardiographic approach would reduce the amount of data, but clinicians continue to favor the 12-lead electrocardiogram. The noise in the exercise electrocardiogram includes random and periodic noise of both high and low frequency that can be due to respiration, muscle artifact, electrical interference, wire continuity, and electrode-skin contact problems. In addition to reducing noise and facilitating data processing, computer techniques have the potential to make precise and accurate measurements, to separate and capture dysrhythmic beats, to perform spatial analysis, and to apply optimal diagnostic criteria for ischemia.

With the advent of large-scale integrated electronics, microcomputers have been developed so that now exercise electrocardiographic processing can be done without large, expensive digital computers. Without the assistance of microcomputers, conventional equipment can be used to digitize electrocardiographic signals and immediately apply digital techniques while the data are being gathered, that is, on-line. Earlier approaches to computer processing required that analog data be recorded, later digitized, and then analyzed (i.e., off-line).

In 1965, Blomqvist reported a computerized quantitative study of the Frank lead exercise electrocardiogram. He concluded that the electrocardiographic response during exercise contained more information than the electrocardiograms recorded after exercise and that the maximal information for the differentiation of patients with angina pectoris from normal males was located at ST 4, or the midpoint of ventricular repolarization.

In 1966, Bruce and colleagues reported using a computer of average transients to analyze exercise electrocardiographic data gathered from bipolar lead CB_5. They reported that in middle-aged apparently healthy men, the ST-segment depression with exercise was found in greater magnitude and prevalence than anticipated. In 1969, Hornstein and Bruce reported measuring the ST forces of the Frank leads and bipolar lead CB_5 using a computer of averaged transients and a large digital computer. They concluded that a single bipolar precordial lead appeared to be as reliable for purposes of classifying electrocardiographic response to maximal exercise as was the three-dimensional Frank lead system. In 1973, Neiderberger and Bruce reported on the spatial ST-T magnitudes at rest and immediately after maximal exercise.

They noted that in patients with ischemic heart disease the spatial magnitudes of late ST and T vectors at rest were smaller than those in a normal group. Somewhat contrary to the prior study, they reported that even if the electrocardiogram did not show an ischemic pattern, this spatial trend became more obvious with exercise.

McHenry and colleagues reported results with a computerized exercise electrocardiographic system developed at USAFSAM and later applied at the University of Indiana. ST-segment amplitude was measured over the 10 msec interval of the ST segment, starting at 60 msec after the peak of the R wave. The slope of the ST segment was measured from 70 msec to 110 msec beyond the R-wave peak. The PQ, or isoelectric, interval was found by scanning before the R wave for the 10 msec interval with the least slope (rate of change). If the ST-segment depression was 1.0 mm or greater and if the sum of ST-segment depression in millimeters and ST slope in millivolts per second equaled or was less than one during or immediately after exercise, the response was defined as abnormal. This measurement, called the ST index, was developed by comparing two groups of subjects, one with angina pectoris and the other consisting of age-matched clinically normal people. Used as a criterion for diagnosing coronary disease, they demonstrated a specificity of 83% and sensitivity of 95%.

Sheffield and co-workers reported an on-line approach in which V_4, V_5, V_6 and Frank X, Y, and Z leads were digitized at 500 samples per second. They computed the time-voltage integral of the ST segment beginning at QRS end and continuing until crossing the isoelectric line or until reaching 80 msec after QRS end. This integral expresses the area of ST-segment deviation from the baseline. An ST integral greater than minus 10 mV was found to be an abnormal exercise electrocardiographic response, and the normal range was from 0 to minus 7.5 mV. Results on 41 normal and 31 angina patients yielded a sensitivity of 81% and a specificity of 95%.

Wolf and colleagues reported their computer processing for rest and exercise electrocardiograms in 1972. The diagnostic criteria for exercise-induced ischemia were based on the vector analysis of the ST-T segment waveform according to the Dalhousie code. This code classified the ST segment into three categories by means of the orientation (W) and the magnitude (D) of the ST-slope vector; the difference vector between three eighths and one eighth of the ST-segment (ST 3–ST 1). The orientation of the slope vector was defined as the spatial angle W between the slope vector D and the reference angle (pointing in the direction of the left lower anterior octant). In 123 normal males, increases in ST-slope vector D was found to be in proportion to increases in heart rate during exercise. In 1973, they reported the normal values for Chebyshev waveform polynomials fitted to the ST segment during exercise.

Simoons and colleagues reported using a PDP-8E computer on-line to process the Frank orthogonal leads. The program, which Simoons wrote largely himself, consisted of four parts: (1) detection of the QRS complex, (2) selection of beats, (3) averaging of selected beats, and (4) waveform analysis. The interactive computer system also controlled the exercise test, which allowed the physician and technician to interact with the patient. In trying to decide the optimal criteria for the detection of ischemic heart disease, Simoons compared the computerized criteria of other investigators. These criteria included ST area, or integral; ST index; polar coordinates; time-normalized ST-T amplitudes; and Chebyshev polynomials. These criteria were applied to a population of 95 coronary artery disease patients and 129 healthy males. He obtained the best results with ST-segment amplitude at 60 msec after the end of the QRS complex. A range of amplitudes for exercise heart rates was established by considering the response of the normal group. This approach is a logical one since ST-segment depression increases in proportion to heart rate. He obtained a sensitivity of 81% and a specificity of 93% using this new criterion. In comparison, previous computer criteria were not superior to this ST-amplitude measurement adjusted for heart rate. He has also demonstrated that the ST shift during exercise in patients with coronary artery disease occurred in the direction of wall motion abnormalities.

In 1976, Werner and colleagues published a description of their rest and exercise computerized electrocardiographic system. Six Wilson precordial leads (V_{1-5} and V_7) and extremity leads I and II were recorded at rest. A computer algorithm reconstructed leads III, aVL, aVF, and aVR from I and II. Six chest-head leads were processed (CH_{1-5}, CH_7). The ST-T segment arbitrarily extended to 400 msec times the square root of 60, divided by the heart rate. The ST segment was reported by the amplitude and temporal position of the lowest point in the first two thirds of the ST-T segment, the amplitude at the J junction, the ST area, and early and late ST-segment slopes. ST area was calculated from 10 msec after the QRS end to crossing the isoelectric line or to the end of the ST segment. Early and late slopes of the ST segment were defined as the slope of the regression line between 20 to 120 msec and 120 to 180 msec after the end of QRS complex. The T wave was evaluated according to the Minnesota code. These investigators felt that their system reduced costs and performed high-quality exercise tests. It also enabled technicians to pay more attention to the patients since much of their job was automated. Werner and colleagues examined the reliability of their computer program by comparison of ST-segment and T-wave interpretation between their program and two observers. At rest, there was agreement in 75% of the computer-observer ST-code comparisons and in 71% of the interobserver ST codes. With exercise, the agreements decreased to 59%, whereas interobserver ST-code agreements decreased to 55%. They have not tested the utility of their approach for diagnosing coronary artery disease.

In 1977, Marquette Electronics introduced a commercial on-line exercise system using a LSI-11 computer (CASE). The computer performed test-control functions, signal conditioning, beat averaging, and on-line ST measurement. Instead of simple averages, a new technique of averaging was introduced in this system. Called incremental averaging by the developers, it is a method well suited to a continuous input with slow changes. In this method of averaging, each digital sample of a new, time-aligned cardiac cycle is compared with its corresponding member in the current average. Alignment is accomplished using frequency components of the QRS complex. Wherever the average is low (or high) it is incremented (or decremented) by a small, fixed amount (3.5 mV) independent of the size of the difference. ST-level and slope-measurements were displayed and recorded. These measurements were made from the average cycle, using the onset and offset of QRS determined during initialization. ST-slope measurements were made to correlate with visual impressions by dynamically adjusting the ST-slope interval with heart rate. This system is the only commercial system that actually determines QRS end rather than making ST measurements at a fixed point after the R-wave peak or S-wave nadir. The ST interval for slope measurement was one eighth of the average RR interval.

A recently introduced microprocessor-based commercial system is the Status 1000 made by Quinton Instrument. Analog electrocardiographic data are converted to digital data with a stated resolution of 0.1%. The computer programs used to analyze this digitized information are primarily coded in a structured higher-level language similar to PASCAL, which facilitates program modularity and ease of modifications. A few critical fast computations, such as real-time waveform averaging, are written in computer assembly language. These assembly language routines are written in modules and incorporated into the basic structure of the higher-level language. The strong point of this system is that the exercise-testing protocols and methodology can be easily programmed into the system by the operator.

The signal processing that is performed can be modified by replacing a microprocessor chip with a chip that has another new program in it, which could possibly avoid obsolesence. All parameters are available for display on the screen. In addition, time-histographs of all parameters are recorded on a summary report at the end of the test. The three leads from which this information is obtained are chosen by the physician prior to the test.

Sketch and colleagues conducted a study to evaluate the validity and usefulness of the Viagraph, a system made by International Medical Corp., for automated exercise electrocardiographic analysis. One hundred seven patients who were referred for evaluation for chest pain underwent a Bruce protocol exercise test and coronary angiography. Patients who had a previous myocardial infarction and those on digitalis were excluded. Twenty-nine patients were considered to have performed submaximal testing because of not reaching 85% of maximal heart rate predicted for age. V_5 was continuously sampled at 500 samples/sec, and 16 complexes were averaged sequentially. The system measured and stored the area of depression that was maximal during exercise and in recovery. This area measurement began at 60 msec after the peak of the R wave and extended for 80 msec. Postexercise areas were more specific, whereas areas measured during exercise were more sensitive. Also, as the criteria for ischemia were lessened, sensitivity increased while specificity decreased and these values varied over the range of ST-area criteria presented. It appeared that automated analysis of the ST area was valid and comparable to visual analysis. They concluded that it should not negate the need for visual confirmation or for the physician's consideration of hemodynamic responses. In the subgroup who performed maximal tests, a nomogram was constructed including duration of exercise and ST area used in predicting severity of disease.

Hollenberg and colleagues reported their use of CASE for developing a treadmill exercise score. Instead of using a single value, they integrated all ST-amplitude and slope changes that occurred during the test. Seventy patients who had coronary angiography and 46 healthy volunteers were included. By using the treadmill exercise score shown below, sensitivity and specificity were 85% and 98%, respectively.

$$\text{Treadmill exercise score} = \frac{\text{J-point amplitude and ST-slope curve areas}}{\text{Duration of exercise} \times \text{percent predicted max HR achieved}}$$

This score includes the following measures of severity: depth of J-point depression, slope, occurrence of depression in relation to heart rate, decreased heart rate response to exercise, and functional capacity. The areas under the curves were considered during hyperventilation and when ST-segment abnormalities were present at rest. In their hands, this technique was highly reproducible. They concluded that it greatly improved the diagnostic ability of exercise testing and provided the ability to quantify serially the extent of coronary disease.

Subramanian and colleagues used CASE to analyze the ST-segment response to exercise in angina patients treated with verapamil. They found a significant improvement in exercise-induced ST-segment depression while their subjects were on verapamil.

Computer approaches for exercise testing have grown more sophisticated over time, and recent reports have suggested that they can be clinically superior to standard techniques. There have only been limited attempts to validate systems or compare approaches. Though known to be more consistent, computers have not yet replaced the human observer. Many different computer criteria for ischemia including those listed in Table III and illustrated in Figure 4 have been recommended. Though they usually outperform standard criteria, few studies have compared computer criteria in the same data base and often they are not applied to the electrocardiographic waveform in the manner initially specified. In addition, the basic approaches to processing electrocardiographic signals have not been adequately compared and validated. The following is an explanation of the principles and approaches to computerized exercise electrocardiographic signal processing.

Figure 5 illustrates the principles of analog-to-digital conversion. An analog signal can be represented by a continuous signal that varies in amplitude with time. Converting into a digital signal requires sampling it periodically at fixed time intervals and converting the amplitudes at any point in time into binary numbers that have a time index or sequence. The digital signal is recorded as a binary number, because the basic computer unit is a switch that is either on or off.

The basic computer storage unit is the byte, or word, that has a certain number of bits for a given computer and reflects how large or small an integer can be represented on the computer. Analog-to-digital conversion resolution is determined in part by the word size. Storage-unit size effects the resolution by controlling the range of measurements that are possible, according to the formula 2^n minus 1 where n equals the number of bits in a word, or byte. An eight-bit digitizer divides the input range into 2^8 minus 1, or 255. In general, the more bits per word, the greater the resolution. Resolution is also dependent on the sampling rate. The greater the sampling rate, the greater the detail of the analog signal that is retained. The more points sampled, however, the more digital data that must be analyzed and stored. The usual sampling rates used for electrocardiography are 250/sec (4 msec

TABLE III
CRITERIA FOR ST-DEPRESSION ABNORMALITIES SEEN DURING OR AFTER
EXERCISE TESTING

Method	Criteria for Abnormal (Ischemia)
Classic ST-Segment Depression	With junctional depression of 0.1 mV (1 mm) or more: exercise-induced ST-segment depression must be flat or downsloping to be abnormal.
Upsloping ST 80	For upsloping ST segment with junctional depression of > 2 mm from the isoelectric baseline: abnormal if ST segment is depressed 2 mm or more at 0.08 sec (80 msec) after J point (QRS end); normal if less depressed at that point.
ST Midpoint (ST_4)	Blomqvist divided the ST segment from QRS end until the end of the T wave into 8 equal time periods. He found ST_4, or the midpoint, to provide the most discrimination between normal and abnormal. Simoons used a midpoint from QRS end until peak of the T wave, since peak is easier to identify than T end.
ST Index	If ST-segment depression is 1.0 mm or greater and the sum of ST-segment depression in mm plus ST slope in mv/sec equal to or greater than 1.0. (Mean ST depression measured at 60–70 msec after R-wave peak, slope in 40 msec window afterward.)
ST Integral	ST integral greater than -10 μv-sec (1 square mm on electrocardiographic paper at standard speed and calibration = 4 μv-sec). Sheffield originally described measuring the ST integral from the end of the QRS complex to the beginning of the T wave or where the ST segment crossed the isoelectric line. Commercial systems have implemented this by using the peak of the R wave and measuring the area from 60 to 140 msec after the R wave.
Spatial ST-T Magnitudes	Dower and Bruce analyzed magnitudes and slopes at time-normalized areas of $\sqrt{X^2 + Y^2 + Z^2}$.
ST 60	A range of amplitudes at 60 msec after QRS end for different exercise heart rates with abnormal being measurements outside of a normal band.

increments) or 500/sec (2 msec increments). In addition to sampling rate and word size, signal resolution is also determined by the analog input window. The analog window must be wide enough to accept the largest possible electrocardiographic signal amplitude, but a large window decreases the resolution possible for small electrocardiographic signals.

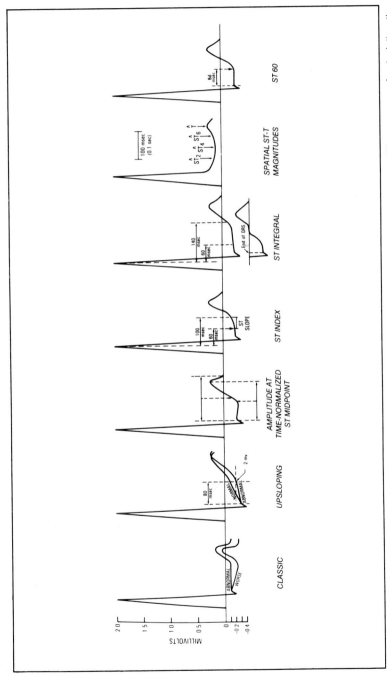

Figure 4. Here are the recommended computer criteria for categorizing ischemia. As shown, there are different ways of calculating the measurements. Blomqvist recommended using the end of the T wave for measuring the midpoint of the ST segment, but Simoons used the peak of the T wave. This change was made to have a more stable end point, since the end of the T wave is much more difficult to find than the peak of the T wave. ST integral, as defined by Sheffield, required that the end of the QRS complex, or J junction, be found and that the area measurement stop as soon as the ST segment crossed the isoelectric line or as the T wave began. The ST integral used by most commercial systems initiates the area at a fixed period after the R wave and then ends 80 msec thereafter.

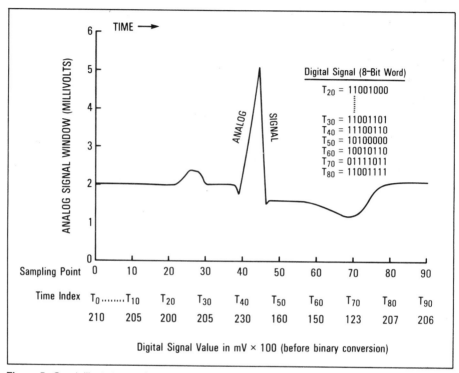

Figure 5. Graph illustrates analog-to-digital conversion of an electrocardiogram. An analog signal is characterized as a continuous signal of varying amplitude. Digital conversion involves sampling such a signal at predefined time intervals and converting the measurement at each sampling interval into a binary number that has a time index. (With permission of Progress in Cardiovascular Disease.)

Figure 6 illustrates the effects of analog-to-digital convertor resolution and input signal range, or window, on the details of the electrocardiogram. The top line is the actual electrocardiogram. The second line shows this electrocardiographic signal after being digitized and then being reconstructed as an analog signal. Five-bit resolution of the analog-digital convertor loses details but roughly follows the S, R, and T waves. The three-bit analog-digital convertor distorts the P, S, and T waves. When only half of the input range of the three-bit convertor is used, the P and T waves are completely lost and the S wave considerably distorted—roughly equivalent to a two-bit analog-digital convertor. The bottom line shows the effect of sampling rate on the resolution of the electrocardiogram. The original electrocardiographic signal shown on the top of the figures is digitized at different sampling rates and then reconstructed as an analog signal. Sampling at 100 samples/sec accurately represents the P-, R-, S-, and T-wave amplitudes but loses some

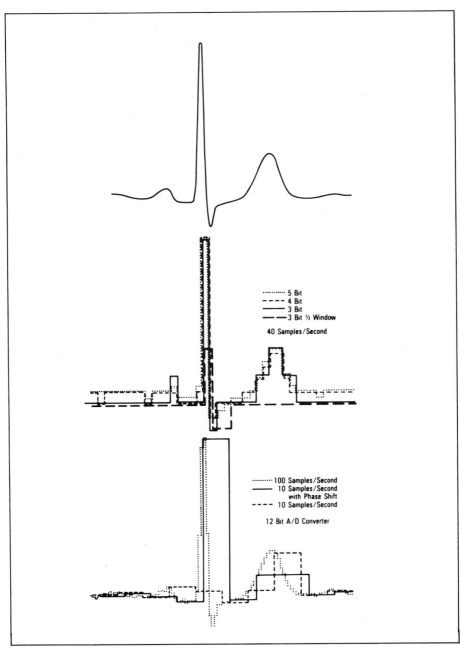

Figure 6. Examples of the effects of computer word size, input range, and sampling rate on electro-cardiographic signal resolution (see text for explanation).

detail. Sampling at 10 samples/sec loses either the P or R wave and distorts the T wave. A slight shift of the point in time when digitization begins (a phase shift) greatly effects resolution.

The American Heart Association and others have recommended that eight-bit resolution and 250 samples/sec are minimal digitizing specifications for computer processing of an electrocardiogram. High-frequency information can be lost, and so in the future, industry will probably deliver instruments with higher resolution. If future research indicates the value of higher-frequency components of the electrocardiogram, then more rigorous digitizing specifications will be necessary.

Mathematical constructs applied by computers to digital electrocardiographic data are used for three purposes: (1) to locate and characterize QRS complexes, (2) to obtain a reference, or fiducial point, in the QRS complex, and (3) to determine the beginning and the end of the P wave, QRS, and T wave. The crucial purpose of these constructs, however, is the definition of a reference point to align beats and thus permit averaging. Peak R wave was first used, but because of the rapid amplitude changes at peak, different peaks could be sampled during digitizing and result in misalignment of complexes. The point of most rapid change in electrocardiographic amplitude (dx/dt), which usually occurs in the downslope of the R wave or or in upslope of QS, can be consistently found and has been used. Particularly for one-lead analysis, the mathematical construct of maximal dx/dt can be a reliable and efficient fiducial point. More recently, investigators have used spatial constructs from three time-coherent leads to achieve alignment. Figure 7 illustrates the major spatial mathematical constructs.

Thresholds set in these mathematical constructs also permit the localization of a waveform's beginning and end. Intuitively the spatial recognition of the QRS, ST, and T waves that requires multiple leads would be more accurate than algorithms applied to only one lead. Electrical activity may appear to end in a single lead but continue in a perpendicular direction with activity seen in another lead.

There are many causes of noise in the exercise electrocardiogram that cannot be corrected, even by meticulous skin preparation. Noise is defined as an electrical signal foreign to the electrocardiogram or as anything that distorts the electrocardiographic waveform. With this definition of noise, the types of noise that can be present may be due to line frequency (60 Hz), muscle, respiration, contact, and continuity. Line-frequency noise is generated by the interference of the 60 Hz electrical energy with the electrocardio-

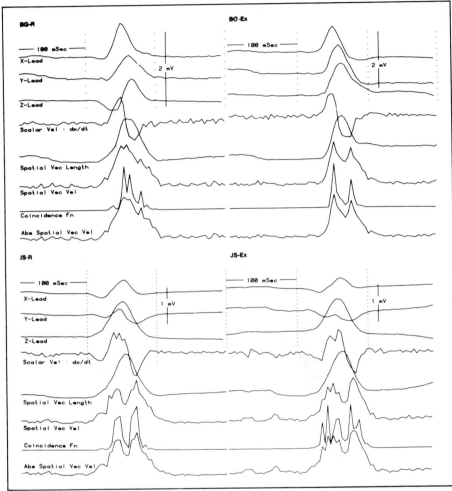

Figure 7. Illustrations of the mathematical constructs used for computer manipulations of electro-cardiographic signals are shown. The constructs are displayed in phase below the X, Y, Z signals from which they were derived using the equations below. Two patients are shown with signal from rest (left) and maximal exercise (Ex). Patient BG had an abnormal ST-segment response to exercise in the X lead, and patient JS had extensive anterior damage. Derivations:

Scalar first-derivative $= \frac{dx}{dt}$

Spatial vector length $= \sqrt{X^2 + Y^2 + Z^2}$

Spatial vector velocity $= \sqrt{\left(\frac{dx}{dt}\right)^2 + \left(\frac{dy}{dt}\right)^2 + \left(\frac{dz}{dt}\right)^2}$

Absolute spatial vector velocity $= \left|\frac{dx}{dt}\right| + \left|\frac{dy}{dt}\right| + \left|\frac{dz}{dt}\right|$

Coincidence function $= \left|\frac{dx}{dt}\right| \cdot \left|\frac{dy}{dt}\right| \cdot \left|\frac{dz}{dt}\right|$

$| \quad |$: absolute value, signs removed

gram. This noise can be reduced by using shielded patient cables. If in spite of these precautions this noise does appear, the simplest way to remove it is to design a notch filter and use it in series with the electrocardiographic amplifier. A notch filter removes only the line frequency, i.e., it attenuates all frequencies in a narrow band around 60 Hz. In some systems, this is removed by attenuating frequencies above 59 Hz. This method of removing line-frequency noise causes waveform distortion and results in a system that does not meet AHA specifications. The most obvious manifestation of distortion caused by such filters is a decrease in R-wave amplitude.

Muscle noise is generated by the activation of muscle groups and is usually of high frequency. This noise along with other types of high-frequency noise can be reduced by signal averaging. Motion noise, another type of high-frequency noise, is caused by the movement of skin and the electrodes, which causes a change in the contact resistance. Respiration causes an undulation of the waveform amplitude, and the baseline varies with the respiratory cycle. Baseline wander can be reduced by low-frequency filtering, which is the monitor mode available in most coronary care unit monitoring systems. Low-frequency filtering, however, results in distortion of the ST-segment and can cause artifactual ST-segment depression. Other various approaches have been used, including the cubic spline technique that can smooth the baseline. Changes in waveform amplitude with respiration are physiologic in nature and may well prove to have clinical significance; however, they can be reduced by signal averaging. This method can result in some problems when comparing average beats from rest and from exercise, because the ratio of inspiratory to expiratory beats is greater during exercise than at rest.

Contact noise appears as low-frequency noise or sometimes as step discontinuity baseline drift. It can be caused by either poor skin preparation, resulting in high skin impedance, or by air bubble entrapment in the electrode gel. It is reduced by meticulous skin preparation and by rejecting beats that show large baseline drift. Also, by using the median rather than the mean for signal averaging, drift can be reduced. Continuity noise caused by intermittent breaks in the electrocardiographic cables is almost obsolete now because of technologic advances in cables. NDM is an electrode company that markets exceptional cables.

Most of the sources of noise other than line-frequency noise require beat averaging as a means of noise removal. Two types of noise or artifact that can be caused by averaging are due to (1) the introduction of beats that are morphologically different in the average and (2) the misalignment of beats during averaging. As the number of beats included in the average increases, the level of noise reduction is greater. Electrocardiographic waveforms change in morphology over time, however, and consequently averaging time and the number of beats has to be compromised.

Averaging is performed after beats are aligned by a fiducial point specified in a mathematical construct derived from the electrocardiogram. After alignment, each time index referenced to the fiducial point has a series of values from each of the beats included in the alignment. These values can then be averaged in two ways. The easiest way is to sum the values and divide them by the number of beats included in the alignment array, yielding the mean. The second approach is to determine the median. The median requires calculation of the 50th percentile value at each time-index point. Because of its characteristics, the median has a greater central tendency and is less affected by discrepant values. When the median is used, however, the level of random noise is not reduced as much as when the mean is used. If a few premature ventricular contractions (PVCs) or aberrancies are included in beats used to generate an average, the median beat will not be affected, even though the mean beat will be distorted. Thus, the median beat appears to be a better estimate of the so-called true complex, although it is slightly higher in random noise. Calculation of median requires larger computer memory and execution time requirements. Median averaging has recently been applied in microprocessor-assisted electrocardiographic machines.

Many researchers have utilized approximately ten seconds of sampling time rather than a specific number of beats. This sample usually includes sufficient beats for averaging techniques and lessens the chances of physiologic changes occurring and disturbing the average. The resting electrocardiogram usually does not require averaging for noise reduction so that the duration of sampling is not critical. However, noise level increases with exercise as does the heart rate so that at increased levels of exercise the number of beats included in a time window increases. We have found 10 to 20 beats to be a reasonable sample size for noise reduction. At a heart rate of 60 beats/min, only six beats will be included, but at a heart rate of 180 beats/min approximately 30 beats will be included and this amount is more than adequate. Thus, ten seconds appears to be a reasonable sampling time for the exercise electrocardiogram. The effects of respiration on averaging and of changes in heart rate have not been adequately studied. Perhaps averaging should only lump together beats from inspiration and expiration and utilize a threshold for changes in RR intervals.

More work is needed to determine which algorithms best identify the offset and onset points of the QRS complex, P wave, and T wave. Offset of the T wave becomes especially difficult during high heart rates when T and P overlap. As previously stated, a three-dimensional approach seems most accurate because electrical forces perpendicular to one lead appear stopped but can be seen in a lead perpendicular to the first lead. We have found validation of offset and onset points with hand measurements to be quite difficult. Hand and eye measurements themselves are poorly reproducible. However, we have found good agreement with semiautomated measurements made by hand adjustment of a cursor on the screen of a computer system that expands the electrocardiographic amplitude and time scale. The onset and offset points are crucial to computerized measurements, and perhaps consistency will only be obtained by the use of standardized algorithms.

Computerized exercise electrocardiography will become ubiquitous in the next decade because of the current revolution in computer hardware. Miniaturization and reduction in cost have made computers very accessible and convenient. It is important to look to past research to understand the limitations as well as the potential of computer processing. Key technical questions remain in regard to the application of signal processing, and these should be resolved by research before computer analysis is accepted without human overreading. The next step will then be to determine the optimal criteria for application in different populations that will best discriminate those with disease from those without disease.

INTERPRETATION

When interpreting the exercise test, it is important to consider each of its facets separately. Each type of response has a different value in making a diagnostic or a clinical decision. A test should not be called abnormal (positive) or normal (negative), rather the interpretation should specify which responses were abnormal or normal and each should be given a weighted value. Certain objective responses to exercise testing (e.g., functional capacity, heart rate, blood pressure, electrocardiographic changes, and dysrhythmias) and subjective responses (symptoms, patient appearance, and the results of physical examination) require interpretation and will be discussed below. As with all test interpretation, the written summary should be directed to the level of understanding of the physician who ordered the test and who will receive the report.

Functional Capacity. Maximal oxygen uptake ($\dot{V}O_2$ max) is the greatest amount of oxygen that a person can extract from inspired air while performing dynamic exercise requiring a large part of the total muscle mass. Since maximal oxygen uptake is equal to the product of cardiac output and arterial venous oxygen difference, it is a measure of the functional limits of the cardiovascular system. Maximal arterial venous oxygen difference is physiologically limited to 15 to 17 vol%. Thus, maximal AV O_2 difference behaves as a constant, making maximal oxygen uptake an indirect estimate of maximal cardiac output. Maximal oxygen uptake is dependent on many factors, including natural physical endowment, activity status, age, and sex, but it is the best index of functional capacity and maximal cardiovascular function. The maximal oxygen uptake of the normal sedentary individual is approximately 30 ml O_2/kg-min, and the minimal level for physical fitness is 40 ml O_2/kg-min. Aerobic training can increase maximal oxygen uptake by approximately 25%. This increase is dependent on the initial level of fitness and the age of the trainee, as well as the intensity, frequency, and length of training sessions. Individuals performing aerobic training such as distance running can have maximal oxygen uptakes as high as 60 to 90 ml O_2/kg-min. A mongrel dog easily exceeds these values, however. There is some convenience in measuring oxygen consumption in multiples of basal resting requirements. The MET is a unit of basal oxygen consumption, or approximately 3.5 ml O_2/kg-min. This value is the oxygen requirement to maintain life in the resting state.

Figure 8 illustrates the relationship of maximal oxygen uptake to exercise habits and age. Though the three activity levels have regression lines that appropriately fit the data, there is much scatter around the lines and the correlation coefficients are poor. This finding demonstrates the inaccuracy involved with trying to predict maximal oxygen uptake from age and habitual physical activity. As previously discussed, it is preferable to estimate an individual's maximal oxygen uptake from the work load reached while performing a treadmill test, which avoids the problems of comparing the same time performed on different treadmill protocols and of assuming that the same work load has been performed.

There are few objective data available to establish the diagnostic value of maximal cardiac output or maximal oxygen uptake. These are the best measurements of functional capacity of the cardiovascular system, but they require techniques and equipment that make them impractical to measure in most clinical situations. Also, there is a wide biologic scatter of these parameters in healthy persons even when age, sex, and activity status are considered. Because both maximal cardiac output and maximal oxygen uptake decline with age, the effects of age and disease are usually difficult to separate.

McDonough and colleagues measured maximal cardiac output in cardiac patients and found a decline in maximal cardiac output to be the major hemodynamic consequence of symptomatic coronary artery disease and one that

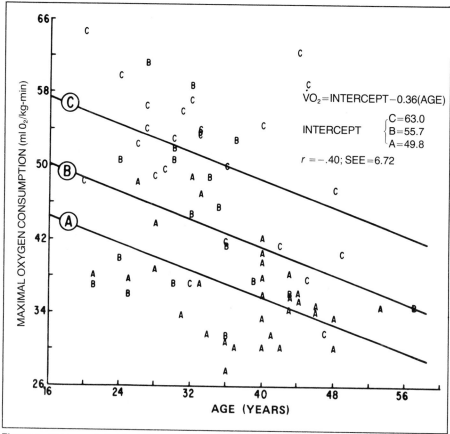

Figure 8. Data are plotted for VO$_2$, regressed against age for 77 men exercise tested with expired air analyzed. Activity status is indicated as A (sedentary), B (moderate exerciser), and C (heavy exerciser). Though the regression lines are as would be predicted, there is considerable individual scatter.

resulted in functional impairment. Acute reduction in left ventricle perform-ance, manifested by decreasing stroke volume and increasing pulmonary artery pressure, appeared to be the mechanism limiting cardiac output. As in other studies, maximal oxygen uptake was linearly related to maximal cardi-ac output. Hossack and colleagues measured cardiac output during treadmill exercise in 10 normal men and 77 patients with coronary heart disease using invasive techniques. These data were used to estimate limits of maximal cardiac output and stroke volume in normal subjects, and these normal stan-dards were then used to evaluate the results in the patients. Patients with an ejection fraction of less than 50% had significantly impaired age adjusted cardiac output and stroke volume.

Patterson and colleagues studied 43 patients with cardiac disease and compared their functional classification by maximal oxygen uptake and by clinical assessment. When a discrepancy occurred, the hemodynamic data from cardiac catheterization usually indicated that maximal oxygen uptake more accurately reflected the degree of impairment. Patients began to experience limiting symptoms when maximal oxygen uptake was less than 22 ml O_2/kg-min (7 METs) and considered themselves severely limited when maximal oxygen uptake was 16 ml O_2/kg-min (4 METs) or less. When a patient's functional capacity is estimated from testing at less than 4 METs, prognosis is guarded. When technologic advances make the measurement of maximal oxygen uptake and even noninvasive measurement of cardiac output convenient and practical, it should be possible to determine limits, or discriminant values, for these measurements depending on age, activity status, and sex. The findings of inadequate maximal oxygen uptake and maximal cardiac output should have a prognostic implication similar to that of ejection fraction and left ventricular end-diastolic pressure, whereas ST-segment changes should more closely predict the degree of angiographic coronary artery disease in areas of viable myocardium. Left ventricular performance and angiographic disease can be both discordant and have an impact on prognosis.

Heart Rate and Blood Pressure Response. Heart rate is influenced by age, body position, physical fitness, state of health, blood volume, and environment. During low levels of exercise and at a constant work load, heart rate will rise and reach a plateau or steady state within several minutes. At higher work loads, it takes progressively longer to reach a steady state heart rate. Heart rate during exercise increases linearly with work load and oxygen uptake. In fact, there is a definite linear relationship between percent maximal heart rate and percent maximal oxygen uptake. This relationship is very useful in writing an individualized exercise prescription. Relatively elevated heart rates during submaximal exercise or recovery could be due to vasoregulatory asthenia, any condition decreasing vascular volume or peripheral resistance, prolonged bed rest, anemia, or metabolic disorders. Relatively low heart rate at any point during submaximal exercise could be due to exercise training, enhanced stroke volume, or drugs. The common use of beta blockers, which lower heart rate, has complicated the interpretation of the heart rate response to exercise.

Maximal heart rate, which is the value achieved at fatigue, is inversely related to age. This decline with increased age is partially due to a reluctance to encourage older individuals to maximal effort and physical disability. It occurs also in rats, however, and appears to be due to intrinsic cardiac changes rather than to neural influences. There have been numerous population studies deriving linear regression equations relating maximal heart rate to age. These studies have reported different intercepts and slopes because of differences in technique and population. Since abrupt changes in heart rate can occur, a 10-second interval should be measured immediately prior to stopping exercise and not include the drop in heart rate caused by hanging on the handrails; in this way proper measurement of maximal heart rate can be ensured. Recorder paper speed or cardiotachometers should be properly calibrated. Motivated participants will exert a greater effort and on the average achieve a higher maximal heart rate. There is controversy as to whether trained individuals have lower maximal heart rates than do untrained individuals for any age group. All the studies have found a wide scatter around the declining regression line. A correlation coefficient of approximately −.4 has usually been obtained, and the standard deviation around the regression line is 10 to 12 beats/min. This relationship has not been improved by considering height or weight. Thus, at any age, two thirds of normal individuals will have maximal heart rates varying around the regression line by plus or minus 10 to 12 beats. So when the end point of an exercise test is 90% of the maximal age-predicted heart rate, the end point can be maximal for some and clearly submaximal for others.

Ellestad defined chronotropic incompetence as a heart rate response to his treadmill protocol below the 95% confidence limits for age and sex determined for patients referred to his exercise laboratory. Conditioned individuals were excluded. In a follow-up study, patients with chronotropic incompetence had the same incidence of coronary artery disease as did patients with ST-segment depression. The mechanism of chronotropic incompetence is poorly understood, but many of these patients have poor left ventricular function and most have multivessel coronary artery disease. Bruce uses the term heart rate impairment and measures it in a manner similar to measuring functional impairment.

Systolic blood pressure should rise with increasing treadmill work load. Diastolic blood pressure usually remains about the same, but Korotkoff sounds can sometimes be heard all the way to zero in healthy young subjects. One group of investigators has suggested that a rising diastolic blood pressure is a sign of coronary heart disease. More likely, it is a marker for labile hypertension, which leads to coronary disease. The highest systolic blood pressure should be achieved at maximal work load. When exercise is stopped, approximately 10% of the people tested will drop their systolic blood pressure owing to peripheral pooling. To avoid fainting, patients should not be left standing for very long. The systolic blood pressure that is elevated on resuming the supine position gradually returns to normal during recovery and then often drops below normal for several hours after the test. In spite of studies showing discrepancies between noninvasively and invasively measured blood pressure, the product of heart rate and systolic blood pressure, determined by cuff and auscultation, correlates excellently with measured myocardial oxygen consumption during exercise. Usually, an individual patient's angina pectoris will be precipitated at the same double product (systolic blood pressure times heart rate) when a standardized exercise test is used. This product is also an estimate of the maximal work load that the left ventricle can perform.

Systolic blood pressure can rise above 280 mm Hg with no reported clinical implications or complications. An inadequate systolic blood pressure rise can be due to aortic outflow obstruction or left ventricular dysfunction. Thomson and Kelemen reported that serious coronary artery disease was found in all their patients who developed hypotension along with angina during exercise testing. Six patients who had coronary artery bypass surgery had normal blood pressure responses to exercise testing without angina or ST-segment depression after their surgery. Morris and McHenry also support the diagnostic value of exercise-induced hypotension. This phenomenon also identifies patients at increased risk for the initiation of ventricular fibrillation in the exercise laboratory.

The early emphasis placed on the exercise electrocardiogram tended to deemphasize other exercise responses. Measurements of these responses may improve the diagnostic value of exercise testing and may be useful for identifying the presence or the severity of coronary artery disease. The value of any measurement in providing diagnostic information from exercise testing depends on (1) the accuracy and completeness with which a measurement has been made in healthy individuals (reference values) and (2) the effectiveness with which certain limits of the measurement (discriminant values) separate healthy individuals from those subgroups with disease. It is to be hoped that the complete set of reference values presented in Figure 9 will encourage investigators to determine discriminant values for separating patient groups. Using these discriminant values, sensitivity and specificity can be determined in a manner similar to that used for an abnormal ST-segment response. Many exercise test responses do not have a Gaussian distribution and require that nonparametric statistical tests be used. Therefore, discriminant values should be determined as percentiles rather than as standard deviations or confidence limits.

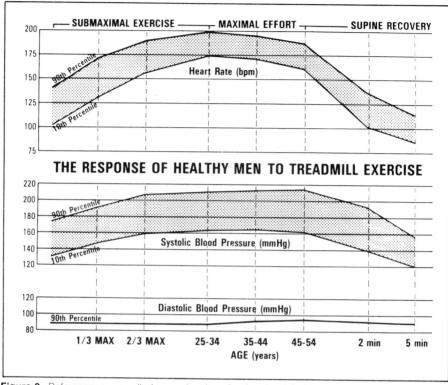

Figure 9. Reference, or so-called normal, values for the physiologic response to submaximal and maximal treadmill exercise based on testing apparently healthy men 24 to 54 years of age are shown. The bands represent the 10th and 90th percentile limits, that is, 10% of normal individuals could lie above or below the bands so that outliers are not necessarily abnormal but are at increased risk of being abnormal.

Though heart rate and stroke volume are important determinants of both maximal oxygen uptake and myocardial oxygen consumption, myocardial oxygen consumption has other independent determinants. It has been demonstrated that the relative metabolic loads of the entire body and those of the heart are determined separately and may not change in parallel with a given intervention. Although the heart receives only 4% of cardiac output at rest, it utilizes 10% of systemic oxygen uptake. The wide arteriovenous oxygen difference of 10 to 12 vol% at rest reflects the fact that oxygen in the blood passing through the coronary circulation is nearly maximally extracted. This value can be compared with the 4 vol% difference across the systemic circulation. When the myocardium requires a greater oxygen supply, coronary blood flow must be increased by coronary dilatation. During exercise, coronary blood flow can increase through normal coronary arteries up to five times the normal resting flow.

The increased demand for myocardial oxygen consumption required for dynamic exercise is the key to the use of exercise testing as a diagnostic tool for coronary artery disease. Myocardial oxygen consumption cannot be directly measured in a practical manner, but its relative demand can be estimated from its determinants, such as heart rate, wall tension (left ventricular pressure and diastolic volume), contractility, and cardiac work. Though all of these factors increase during exercise, increased heart rate is especially detrimental in patients who have obstructive coronary disease. Increased heart rate results in a shortening of the diastolic filling period, the time during which coronary blood flow is the greatest. In normal coronary arteries, dilatation occurs. In obstructed vessels, however, dilatation is limited and flow is decreased by the shortening of the diastolic filling period. This situation results in both inadequate blood flow and oxygen delivery.

The Electrocardiographic Response to Exercise. The first attempt to evaluate the response of the electrocardiogram to exercise was performed by Einthoven. In 1908, he made a number of accurate observations in a postexercise electrocardiogram, including an increase in the amplitude of the P and T waves and depression of the J junction. In 1953, Simonson studied the electrocardiographic response to treadmill testing of a wide age range of normal subjects but did not have the benefit of computer analysis. In 1965, Blomqvist reported his classic description of the response of the Frank vectorcardiographic leads to bicycle exercise using computer techniques. Rautaharju and colleagues analyzed P-, ST-, and T-vector functions in the Frank leads at rest and during exercise. All P-wave vector functions increased during exercise and were compatible with right atrial overload, whereas T-wave vectors decreased slightly. The ST-segment vector shifted clockwise, to the right, and upward. This esoteric paper did not deal with basic waveform analyses but presented an extensive vectorial approach.

Simoons and Hugenholtz reported Frank lead waveform changes during exercise in normal subjects. The direction and magnitudes of time-normalized P, QRS, and ST vectors and other QRS parameters were analyzed during and after exercise in 56 apparently healthy men, 23 to 62 years of age. The PR interval and the P-wave amplitude increased during exercise. Direction of the P vectors did not change consistently with right atrial overload. Surprisingly no significant change in QRS magnitude was observed, and the magnitude in spatial orientation and the maximum QRS vectors remained constant. QRS onset to T-wave peak shortened. The terminal QRS vectors and the initial ST vectors gradually shortened and shifted to the right and superiorly. The T-wave amplitude lessened during exercise. In the first minute of recovery, the P and T magnitudes markedly increased and then all measurements gradually returned to the resting level. There was an increase in S-wave duration in leads X and Y (14 to 24 msec). QRS right-axis shift was heart rate dependent. The ST segment shifted toward the right superiorly and posteriorly, and T-wave magnitude increased markedly in the first minute of recovery. Shortening of the QRS complex (3 msec) was found in some young individuals during exercise.

Laciga and Koller made quantitative electrocardiographic measurements on 30 young healthy subjects at rest and during the stress of moderately acute stepwise exposure to a simulated altitude of 7,000 m. A complete 12-lead electrocardiogram was recorded during ascent and descent. With increasing altitude, P-wave amplitude became significantly increased inferiorly. The duration of the P-wave and PQ interval shortened. In the inferior leads, the amplitude of the R wave decreased progressively with altitude by about 10%, whereas the S wave decreased and the R wave in V_5 increased by about 10%. The T-wave amplitude decreased with increasing altitude. Nonspecific ST-segment depression was noted on occasion in both the limb and lateral precordial leads.

Riff and Carleton demonstrated in patients with atrioventricular (AV) dissociation that the duration of atrial repolarization (the T_a wave) can extend all the way through the QRS complex and into the ST segment. Thus, the T_a wave can play a role in the normal rate-related depression of the J junction in inferior leads and can increase S-wave amplitude. The effect of atrial repolarization on the ST segments in the lateral leads may be less important, but it affects a bipolar lead such as CM_5, which contains anterior and inferior forces.

Using vectorcardiographic analysis after exercise testing, Kilpatrick found a higher sensitivity and specificity for coronary heart disease by using QRS criteria, including transient infarct patterns, rather than ST-segment changes. Such changes must be secondary to conduction abnormalities and not due to a loss of electrically active tissue. A recent study found exercise-induced Q waves to be of little diagnostic value.

Morales-Ballejo, Ellestad, and colleagues analyzed the response of Q waves in lead CM_5 in 50 patients with coronary artery disease and in 50 normal subjects before and immediately after exercise. The septal Q wave in lead CM_5 was smaller in patients with coronary disease than it was in normal subjects at rest and immediately after exercise. Disappearance of the Q wave in lead CM_5 along with ST-segment depression after exercise was 100% specific for coronary artery disease. They felt that low Q-wave voltage and its failure to increase after exercise indicated abnormal septal activation and reflected loss of contraction due to ischemia.

Exercise-induced R-wave amplitude changes were studied by Kentala and colleagues in healthy individuals and in patients with known coronary disease. Physically active normal subjects and patients with coronary disease who responded well to an exercise program demonstrated an increased R-wave amplitude in lead V_5 relative to preexercise supine rest measurements both on assumption of an upright posture and in response to exercise. The R-wave amplitude then decreased in the supine position postexercise. Such changes were not found in patients who did not benefit from physical conditioning. The significance of an R-wave index is thus unclear.

At rest, R-wave amplitude and spatial QRS measurements have been found to correlate with ventricular volume and with myocardial mass. When R waves occur over areas of asynergy they usually are reversible. The sum of the R waves in the vector leads at rest correlate with ejection fraction. Spatial QRS changes, including spatial vector length and velocity, can be used to estimate myocardial hypertrophy and damage.

Bonoris and colleagues suggested that an R-wave amplitude increase during exercise testing was diagnostic of severe coronary artery disease. More likely, this effect can be explained by the fact that most such patients perform submaximal tests and are subject to the normal variability in R-wave response, as has been demonstrated. It appears that many normal subjects increase R-wave amplitude during submaximal exercise, and then it drops at maximal and at one-minute recovery. Since good clinical judgment often limits cardiac patients to submaximal end points, they often have R-wave increases at the end of an exercise test—probably a physiologic phenomenon related to sympathetic influences. If changes were due to alterations in left ventricular volume, certainly all normal subjects would respond in the same direction with standing.

During exercise there is an increase in the S wave in the lateral precordial leads. Katzeff and Edwards hypothesized that this increase in the S wave reflects the normal increase in cardiac contractility during exercise and that its absence is indicative of ventricular dysfunction. It is more likely, however, that the increase in S wave is caused by exercise-induced axis shifts and conduction alterations.

Mirvis and colleagues studied junctional depression during exercise using left precordial isopotential mapping. During exercise, junctional depression was maximal along the left lower sternal border. In the early portion of the ST segment, they found a minimum isopotential along the lower left sternal border that was continuous with terminal QRS forces in both intensity and location. The late portion of the ST segment had a minimum isopotential located in the same areas as that observed at rest (i.e., the upper left sternal border). These observations suggested that junctional depression was the result of competition between normal repolarization and delayed terminal depolarization forces. Junctional depression was most marked along the left lower sternal border; most subjects did not exhibit these changes in only V_5 and V_6. Also, the slope of the ST segment varied from site to site and was directly correlated to magnitude and direction of the J-point deviation. Thus, junctional depression is the result of the presence of negative potentials over the left lower sternal border during early repolarization. These negative potentials responsible for physiologic junctional depression could be caused by delayed activation of basal areas of the left and right ventricles, which leads to accentuated depolarization-repolarization overlap. The numerous studies applying computer techniques to study the ST-segment response to exercise in normal subjects and in patients with coronary disease have been summarized elsewhere.

DeLanne and colleagues demonstrated that during exercise there are elevations in plasma osmolality, potassium, sodium, calcium, phosphate, lactate, and proteinase. There is a constant and gradual increase for both males and females in these measurements regardless of environmental conditions. Sodium and potassium rapidly return to normal after exercise. During respiratory acidosis, there is a loss of potassium from the musculoskeletal system that is increased by muscular activity. In contrast, Lade and Brown demonstrated that potassium enters the myocardium during acidosis and exits after exercise. The mechanism for this variance between myocardial and skeletal muscle is not known. Rose and co-workers noted an increase in serum potassium immediately postexercise and felt that this increase was related to postexercise T-wave changes. What they failed to relate is the increase in potassium during exercise along with the decrease in T waves during exercise. There is no explanation why there should be a postexertional T-wave peak due to hyperkalemia when there is no T-wave peak during exercise.

Coester and colleagues drew arterial samples for blood gases and electrolytes at rest, during the last minute of maximal bicycle exercise, and at recovery. Amplitude of T and P waves increased in bipolar lead CH_5 and reached a maximum in the first two minutes after exercise. All electrolytes measured were increased at the end of exercise, with potassium up 60% and phosphorus up 53%. Potassium dropped the most rapidly below resting values, along with plasma bicarbonate. Electrocardiographic changes were not closely related in time with any one factor such as potassium, but they appeared to reflect an interaction of the changes in mineral balance.

The normal right-axis and posterior-axis deviation of the QRS complex and decreasing R-wave amplitude could be due to right ventricular overload, respiratory-induced descent of the diaphragm, changes in thoracic impedance, or changes in ventricular blood volume. A patient has been reported who developed left anterior hemiblock during exercise that responded in a normal rightward fashion after coronary artery bypass surgery. The decreased T-wave amplitude may be related to decreased end-systolic volume, changes in sympathetic tone, electrolyte concentration changes, or shifts in the T-wave vector. Other factors may also contribute to the changes in the exercise electrocardiogram, such as positional changes in the electrodes, changes in action potentials, electrolyte or hematocrit changes, changes in intracardiac blood volume, and augmentation of the atrial repolarization wave. The effect of age must be considered because there is extensive normal variation related to age, for example, greater ST-segment depression and greater right-axis deviation in older persons.

Using computer techniques, we analyzed data from 40 low-risk normal subjects utilizing measurements of amplitude, intervals, and slope, which were then processed and analyzed for treadmill times on the basis of electrocardiographic component and lead.

Figures 10 to 15 show the waveforms measured using median values for leads V_5, Y, and Z. These figures demonstrate the specific waveform alterations that occur in response to maximal treadmill exercise. These visual diagrams help to conceptualize the normal exercise-induced changes. Supine, exercise to HR 120, maximal exercise, one-minute recovery, and five-minute recovery were chosen as representative times for presentation of these median-based simulated waveforms.

Depression of the J junction and the tall peaked T waves at maximal exercise and at one-minute recovery can be an early sign of ischemia but is seen here in normal subjects. Along with the J-junction depression, marked ST upsloping is seen. J-junction depression did not occur in our Z lead (which is equivalent to and of the same polarity as V_2). As the R wave decreases in amplitude, the S wave increases in depth. The QS duration shortens minimally, but the RT duration decreases in a larger amount.

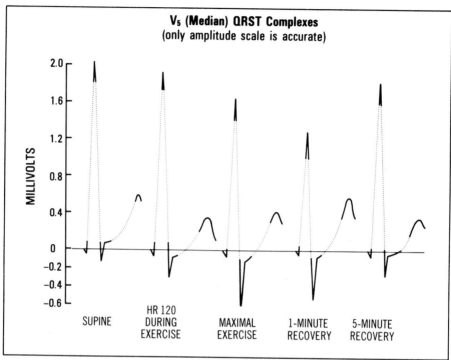

Figure 10. An illustration shows the median values for 40 low-risk normal men whose three electrocardiographic leads were computer-analyzed during maximal treadmill testing. Displayed are the median amplitude values for the QRS and T waves during supine rest, during exercise at a heart rate of 120 beats/min, at maximal exercise, at one-minute recovery, and five-minute recovery. These measurements were taken from analysis of the standard V_5 lead, and only the amplitude scale is accurate.

Q-Wave, R-Wave, and S-Wave Amplitudes. In leads CM_5, V_5, CC_5, and Y, the Q wave shows very small changes from the resting values; however, it does become slightly more negative at maximal exercise. Measurable Q-wave changes were not noted in the Z lead. Changes in median R-wave amplitude are not detected until near-maximal and maximal effort are approached. At maximal exercise and on into one-minute recovery, a sharp decrease in R-wave amplitude is observed in CM_5, V_5, and CC_5. These changes are not seen in the Z lead. The lowest median R-wave value in Y occurred at maximal exercise, with R-wave amplitude increasing by one-minute recovery. In leads CM_5, V_5, and CC_5 the lowest R-wave amplitude was seen at one-minute recovery. This quite different temporal response in R waves in the lateral versus inferior leads is unexplained. There is little change in S-wave amplitude in Z. In the other leads, however, the S wave became greater in depth or

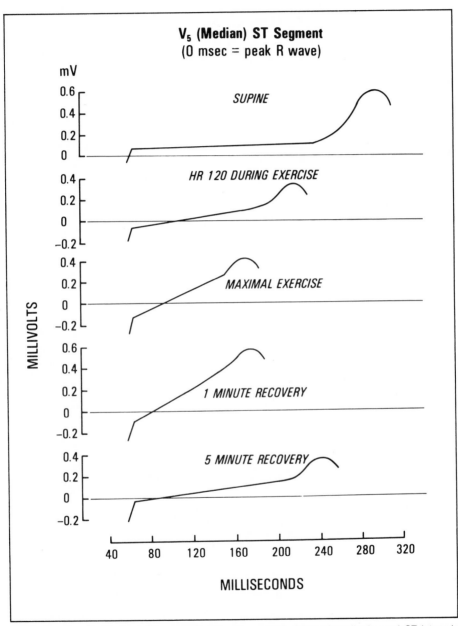

Figure 11. Graphs illustrate ST-segment depression, slope, T-wave amplitude, and ST intervals based on median values from 40 low-risk normal men. These data are based on a computer analysis of lead V_5. They are displayed to show the change over time of the ST-segment slope, depression, and intervals. HR = heart rate.

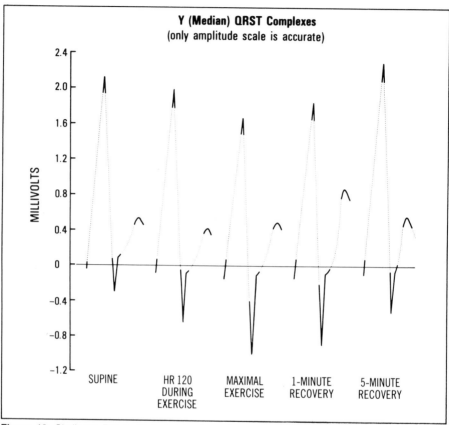

Figure 12. Similar to Figure 10, but data shown here are based on analysis of a bipolar Y lead (electrodes on the forehead and on the lower edge of the rib cage at the left mid-clavicular line). HR = heart rate.

more negative, showing a greater deflection at maximal exercise, and then gradually returning to resting values in recovery.

A decrease in the QS interval occurred and it was shortest at maximal exercise. By three-minute recovery, QS interval returned to normal. A steadily decreasing RT-interval duration was observed as exercise increased. The shortest interval was seen at maximal exercise and one-minute recovery. Changes in this interval followed changes in heart rate.

ST Slope, J-Junction Depression, and T-Wave Amplitude. The amplitude of the J junction in lead Z was very little changed through exercise but

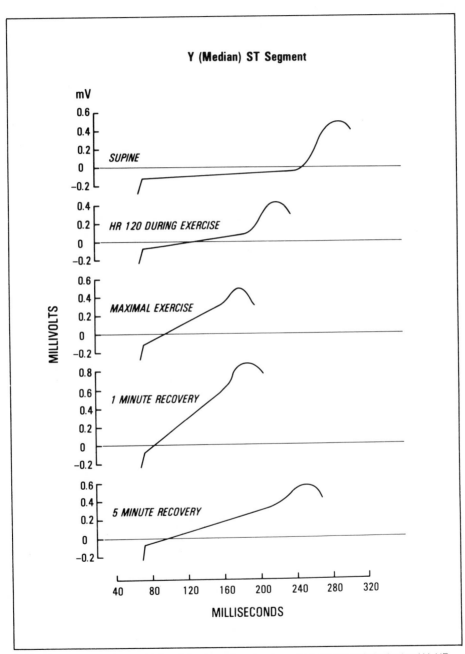

Figure 13. Similar to Figure 11, but data shown here are based on analysis of bipolar lead Y. HR = heart rate.

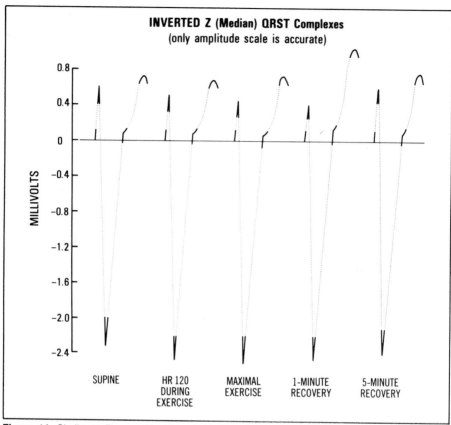

Figure 14. Similar to Figures 10, 11, and 12, but data shown here are based on analysis of a bipolar Z (electrodes on the sternum and on the spine) with the same polarity as V_1-V_2. HR = heart rate.

elevated slightly in recovery. The location of the J junction (QRS end) in Z was determined by using the Z-lead signal alone, rather by a three-dimensional method, so it is relatively inaccurate. Careful studies applying spatial determination of QRS end are needed to see whether the J-junction shifts anteriorly or posteriorly. The J junction was depressed in all other leads to a maximum depression at maximal exercise, then it gradually returned toward but not to preexercise values slowly in recovery. There was very little difference between the three left precordial leads. A dramatic increase in ST-segment slope was observed in all leads and was greatest at one-minute recovery. These changes return toward pretest values during later recovery. The greatest or steepest slopes were seen in lead CM_5, which did not show the

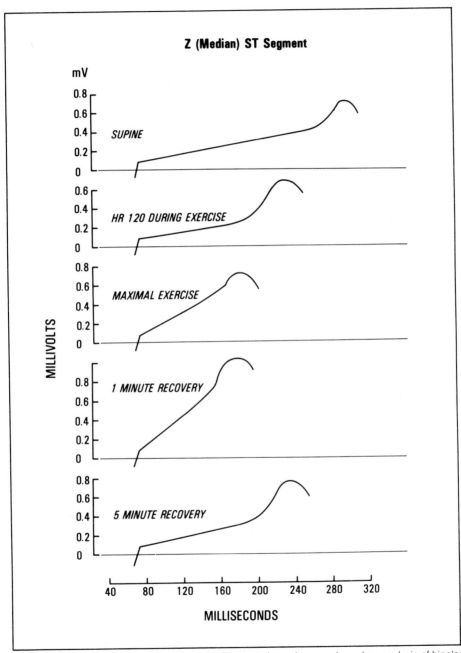

Figure 15. Similar to Figures 11, 12, and 13, but data shown here are based on analysis of bipolar lead Z. HR = heart rate.

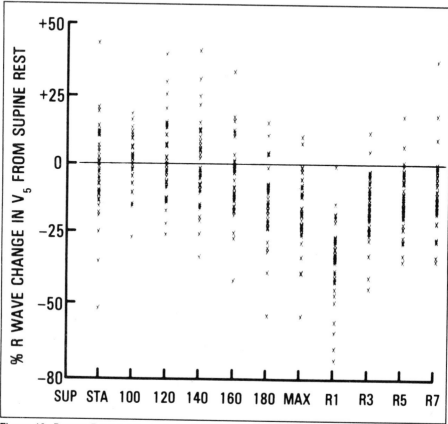

Figure 16. Percent R-wave change in leads V5 is compared with values measured supine before testing. Each cross represents the average R-wave amplitude value for one subject at the indicated time period and heart rate during the exercise testing protocol. SUP = supine; STA = standing; MAX = maximal heart rate.

greatest ST-segment depression. A gradual decrease in T-wave amplitude was observed in all leads during early exercise. At maximal exercise the T wave began to increase, and at one-minute recovery the amplitude was equivalent to resting values, except in leads Y and Z where they were greater than at rest. However, there was a great deal of overlap.

Percent R-Wave Changes. Figure 16 illustrates the percent change of R-wave amplitude for each individual compared with his R wave at supine rest in V_5. At lower exercise heart rates, the great variability of R-wave response was apparent and many normal individuals had significant increases in R-wave amplitude. Though most showed a decline at maximum exercise, some normal subjects had an increase, whereas others showed very little decrease. At one-minute recovery there was a greater tendency toward a decline in lead V_5 but not in Y. Further into recovery, R-wave amplitude remained decreased in lead V_5 but increased in Y.

We have safely exercised most of our patients with severe coronary heart disease to high exercise levels and have found declines in R-wave amplitude. If changes were due to left ventricular volume alterations, certainly all normal individuals would respond in the same direction with standing.

Abnormal Segment Changes. Epicardial electrode mapping usually records ST-segment elevation over areas of severe ischemia and ST-segment depression over areas of lesser ischemia. ST-segment depression is the reciprocal of the injury effect occurring in the endocardium as viewed from an electrode overlying normal epicardium. ST-segment elevation seen from the same electrode reflects transmural injury or, less frequently, epicardial injury. On the surface ECG, exercise-induced myocardial ischemia can result in one of three ST-segment manifestations: elevation, normalization, or depression.

ST-Segment Elevation. ST-segment elevation appears to be related to severe myocardial ischemia. In response to exercise, it has been associated with dyskinesia and it occurs frequently in patients in the early postmyocardial infarction period. ST-segment elevation is an insensitive indicator of exercise-induced ischemia, but it is relatively specific.

Fortuin and Friesinger reported the angiographic and clinical findings and two-year follow-up of 12 patients with 0.1 mV or more ST-segment elevation during or after exercise. These patients were selected from 400 patients who had ungone coronary angiography and exercise testing. Seven of them had previous myocardial infarctions, and 9 of the 10 with angina developed it during the exercise test. One patient with atypical chest pain had normal coronary arteries and improved during the follow-up. Seven of eight with exercise-induced ST-segment elevation in lead V_3 had left anterior descending coronary disease. All four with inferior elevation had right coronary disease. None had ST-segment elevation at rest, but many had Q-wave or T-wave inversion or both. Within two years, four of the patients had died suddenly, one had a documented myocardial infarction, and two had increasing symptoms. Bobba and associates presented four similar patients with exercise-induced ST-segment elevation. They noted an increase in R-wave amplitude in the leads with ST-segment elevation and ST-segment depression in other leads.

Hegge and co-workers found 11% of the patients they studied with maximal treadmill testing and coronary angiography to have exercise-induced ST-segment elevation in the postexercise 12-lead electrocardiogram. This relatively high incidence of ST-segment elevation is probably explained by inclusion of V_1 and V_2, leads not monitored in other studies. The ST-segment elevation was present in precordial leads only in 12 patients, in the inferior leads only in five patients, and in both in one patient. Seventeen patients had severe coronary artery disease in the arteries supplying the appropriate area, and the remaining patient had a normal coronary angiogram. Chahine and colleagues reported the incidence of exercise-induced ST-segment elevation in 840 consecutive patients to be 3.5%. CM_5 and CM_6 were the only leads monitored, so lateral wall ST-segment elevation was all that could be detected. Only about 20% of those who had coronary artery disease showed ST-segment elevation. Sixty-four percent of the patients with left ventricle dyskinesia displayed ST-segment elevation. Manvi and Ellestad presented results in 29 patients with coronary artery disease who had abnormal left ventriculograms. ST-segment elevation occurred in 48%, 33% developed ST-segment depression, and the remaining 19% had no changes. ST-segment elevation occurred in 1.3% of 2,000 exercise tests.

Simoons and colleagues investigated the spatial orientation of exercise-induced ST-segment changes in relation to the presence of dyskinetic areas, as demonstrated by left ventriculography. In patients with an anterior infarct, the ST vectors were widely scattered but were most often directed to the left, anterior, and superior. Patients with an inferior myocardial infarction had ST-segment vectors rightward and anterior and also inferiorly if inferior dyskinesia was present. Anteriorly orientated ST-segment changes were associated with anterior or apical scars in patients with anterior infarcts. Thus, ST-segment vector shifts associated with dyskinesia resulted in ST-segment elevation over the dyskinetic area. In patients with dyskinetic areas, the direction of the ST-segment changes varied so widely that only the magnitude of the changes could be used as a criterion for exercise-induced ischemia.

Sriwattanakomen and colleagues reviewed 1,620 exercise tests and found 3.8% to have ST-segment elevation when all leads except aVR were evaluated. They then correlated exercise-induced ST-elevation with the coronary arteriography and left ventriculograms of 38 patients, 37 of whom had significant coronary disease. In 27 patients with Q waves, 25 had significant disease and ventricular aneurysms, whereas among 11 patients with no Q waves and who had significant disease, only two had ventricular aneurysms. One patient had a ventricular aneurysm but no coronary disease. The sites of

ST elevation correctly localized the area of ventricular aneurysm in 30 of 33 instances and determined the diseased vessels in 38 of 40 instances. They concluded that ST elevation during exercise in the absence of Q waves indicates significant proximal disease without ventricular aneurysm, whereas with Q waves, ST elevation is indicative of ventricular aneurysm in addition to significant proximal disease. Ischemia and abnormal wall motion may independently or additively underlie the mechanism for ST-segment elevation during exercise.

Longhurst and Kraus reviewed 6,040 consecutive exercise tests and found 106 patients (1.8%) without previous myocardial infarctions who had exercise-induced ST-segment elevation. Their criterion was 0.5 mm elevation in a 15-electrode array. Forty-six of these patients with ST-segment elevation had left ventriculography and coronary angiography. Coronary disease was detected in 40 of 46, with nearly equal numbers having one-, two-, and three-vessel disease. Ventriculograms were normal in 36 of 40 patients. Of 21 patients with anterior ST-segment elevation, 86% had left anterior descending obstruction. There was no anatomic correlation in those with lateral or inferior-posterior exercise-induced elevation.

Dunn and colleagues performed exercise thallium scans on 35 patients with exercise-induced ST-segment elevation and coronary artery obstruction. Ten patients developed exercise ST-segment elevation in leads that showed no Q waves on the resting electrocardiogram. The site of elevation corresponded to a reversible perfusion defect and a severely obstructed coronary artery. Associated ST-segment depression in other leads occurred in seven patients, but only one had a second perfusion defect at the site of depression. Three of the 10 patients had a wall motion abnormality at the same site. Twenty-five patients developed exercise ST-segment elevation in leads with Q waves. The site of the elevation corresponded to a severe stenosis and a thallium perfusion defect that persisted on the four-hour redistribution scan. Associated ST-segment depression in other leads occurred in 11 patients, and eight had a second perfusion defect at the site of the depression. In all 25 patients, there was a wall motion abnormality at the site of the Q wave. Therefore, without a previous infarct, ST-segment elevation indicates the site of severe transient ischemia; associated ST-segment depression is usually reciprocal. In patients with Q waves, exercise-induced ST-segment elevation may be due to ischemia around the infarct, abnormal wall motion, or both. Associated ST-segment depression may be due to a second area of ischemia rather than being reciprocal. Chaitman has shown that exercise-induced coronary artery spasm can cause ST elevation. Figures 17 and 18 show examples of ST-segment elevation in a normal resting electrocardiogram and over Q waves, respectively.

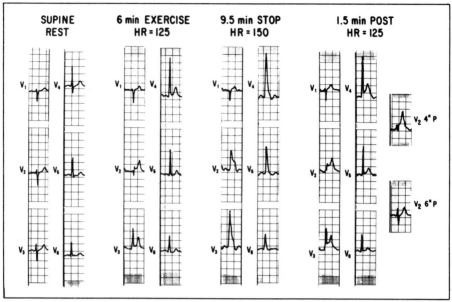

Figure 17. Example of ST-segment elevation is shown for a patient with a normal electrocardiogram, which is consistent with severe ischemia under the area of elevation. The patient had a 70% fixed obstruction in his left anterior descending coronary artery. A thallium exercise scan showed no uptake in the septum, but it filled in one hour later. HR = heart rate.

ST-Segment Normalization or Absence of Change. Another manifestation of ischemia can be no change or normalization of the ST segment due to cancellation effects. Electrocardiographic abnormalities at rest, including T-wave inversion and ST-segment depression, have been reported to return to normal during attacks of angina and during exercise in some patients with ischemic heart disease. This cancellation effect is a rare occurrence, but it should be kept in mind. The ST segment and T wave represent the uncancelled portion of ventricular repolarization. Since ventricular geometry can be roughly approximated by a hollow ellipsoid open at one end, the widespread cancellation of the relatively slowly dispersing electrical forces during repolarization is understandable. Patients with severe coronary artery disease would be most likely to have cancellation occur, yet they have the highest prevalence of abnormal tests. Manvi and Ellestad reported that 20% of the patients with dyskinesia and coronary artery disease had normal tests, and Chahine and co-workers reported that about 25% of their patients with dyskinesia and coronary artery disease normalized or minimally elevated their ST segments during exercise. Nobel and colleagues reported normalization of both inverted T waves and depressed ST segments in 11 patients

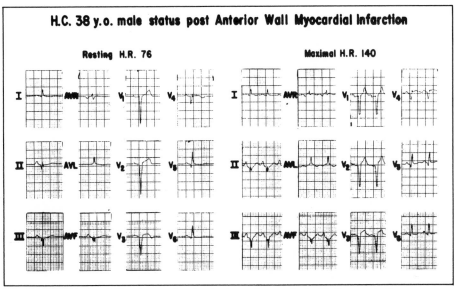

Figure 18. Example of ST-segment elevation is shown for a patient with Q waves in the same area, which is consistent with a severe wall motion abnormality and not necessarily ischemia. The patient had recovered from a large anterior infarct. A thallium scan showed only scarring and no ischemia.

during exercise-induced angina. When exercise testing fails to produce ST-segment depression or elevation in a patient with known coronary artery disease, this could be due to two or more severely ischemic myocardial segments causing cancellation of ST-segment vectors. Sweet and Sheffield reported a patient with minor ST-segment depression and T-wave inversion in lead V_5 who normalized, or "improved," his electrocardiogram during treadmill testing only to have an acute infarction 10 minutes after the test. This normalization of ST-segment depression should thus be considered ST-segment elevation.

The prevalence of the cancelling of surface ST-segment changes by multiple ischemic ST vectors is not known. Chronotropic incompetence and the inability of patients to give an adequate effort are more likely explanations for the majority of false-negative exercise tests in patients with multivessel coronary artery disease. In those with single-vessel disease, the decreased sensitivity of exercise testing is most likely due to insufficient myocardial ischemia to cause surface electrocardiographic changes.

ST-Segment Depression. The most common manifestation of exercise-induced myocardial ischemia is ST-segment depression. The standard criterion

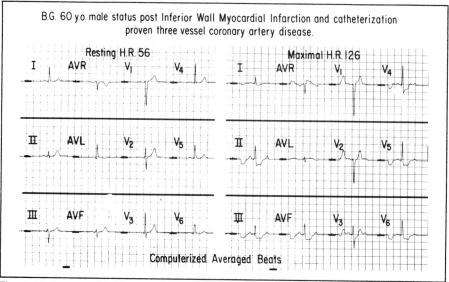

Figure 19. An example of the exercise response of a patient with triple-vessel disease showing ST-segment depression in multiple leads. Surprisingly, he does not get angina, just dyspnea.

for this type of abnormal response is horizontal or downsloping ST-segment depression of 0.1 mV or more for 80 msec. It appears to be due to generalized subendocardial ischemia. A "steal" phenomena is likely from ischemic areas because of the effect of extensive collateralization in the subendocardium. ST depression does not localize the area of ischemia as does ST elevation or help to indicate which coronary artery is occluded. The normal ST-segment vector response to tachycardia and to exercise is a shift rightward and upward. The degree of this shift appears to have a fair amount of biologic variation. Most normal individuals will have early repolarization at rest, which will shift to the isoelectric PR-segment line in the inferior, lateral, and anterior leads with exercise. This shift can be further influenced by ischemia and myocardial scars. When the later portions of the ST segment are effected, flattening or downward depression can be recorded. Both local effects and the direction of the spatial changes during repolarization cause the ST segment to have a different appearance at the many surface sites that can be monitored. Weiner demonstrated that the more leads with these apparent ischemic shifts, the greater the severity of disease. Figure 19 shows ST-segment depression in multiple leads in a patient with triple-vessel disease.

The probability and severity of coronary artery disease are directly related to the amount of J-junction depression and are inversely related to the

TABLE IV
CONDITIONS AND CIRCUMSTANCES THAT CAN CAUSE A FALSE-POSITIVE EXERCISE TEST

Valvular heart disease	Left ventricular hypertrophy
Congenital heart disease	Wolff-Parkinson-White syndrome
Cardiomyopathies	Preexcitation variants
Pericardial disorders	Mitral valve prolapse syndrome
Drug administration	Vasoregulatory abnormality
Electrolyte abnormalities	Hyperventilation repolarization
Nonfasting state	abnormalities
Anemia	Hypertension
Sudden excessive exercise	Excessive double product
Inadequate recording equipment	Improper lead systems
Bundle branch block	Incorrect criteria
Improper interpretation	

slope of the ST segment. Because of these related factors, computer measurements such as the ST index and the ST integral, which take into account both slope and depression, should prove to be superior to classic criteria. Downsloping ST-segment depression is more serious than is horizontal depression, and both are more serious than upsloping depression. However, patients with upsloping ST-segment depression, especially when the slope is less than 1 mV/sec, probably are at increased risk. If a slowly ascending slope is utilized as a criterion for abnormal, the specificity of exercise testing will be decreased (more false positives), although the test may become more sensitive. One electrode can show upsloping ST depression, while an adjacent electrode shows horizontal or downsloping depression. If an apparently borderline ST segment with an inadequate slope is recorded in a single precordial lead in a patient highly suspected of having coronary artery disease, multiple precordial leads should be scanned before the exercise test is called normal. An upsloping depressed ST segment may be the precursor to abnormal ST-segment depression in the recovery period or at higher heart rates during greater work loads. It is preferable to call tests with an inadequate ST-segment slope but with ST-segment depression borderline responses, but added emphasis should be placed on other clinical and exercise parameters. Examples of the different criteria for ischemic ST depression are shown in Figure 4.

Exercise-Induced ST-Segment Depression not due to Coronary Artery Disease. Table IV lists some of the conditions that can possibly result in false-positive responses. Simonson has suggested that in a population with a high prevalence of heart disease other than coronary artery disease, an abnormal exercise test would be as diagnostic for that disease as it would be for coronary artery disease in populations with a high prevalence of coronary artery disease. Digitalis and other drugs can cause exercise-induced repolarization abnormalities in normal individuals. Patients who have had abnormal responses and who have anemia, electrolyte abnormalities, or who are on medications should be retested when these conditions are altered. Meals and even glucose ingestion can alter the ST segment and T wave in the resting electrocardiogram and can potentially cause a false-positive response. To avoid this problem, all electrocardiographic studies should be performed after at least a four-hour fast. This requirement is also important because of the hemodynamic stress put on the cardiovascular system by eating; after eating, functional capacity is decreased and angina occurs sooner.

Whinnery and associates reported 31 asymptomatic men who serially developed left bundle branch block and who were studied with both maximal treadmill testing and coronary angiography. They demonstrated that there can be a marked degree of exercise-induced ST-segment depression in addition to that found at rest in healthy men with left bundle branch block. No difference was found between the ST-segment response to exercise in those with or those without significant coronary artery disease. Thus, the ST-segment response to exercise testing cannot be used to make diagnostic decisions on patients with left bundle branch block. In a second study, these investigators reported the response to maximal treadmill testing of 40 asymptomatic men with acquired right bundle branch block. There was no exercise-induced ST-segment depression in the inferior or lateral leads in either those with or those without significant coronary artery disease. Subsequently, two patients were seen with symptomatic coronary disease and right bundle branch block who developed exercise-induced ST-segment depression in inferior and lateral leads. Friedman and associates reported exercise-induced ST-segment depression in the anterior precordial leads in patients with right bundle branch block. This is most apparent in the right precordial leads with an rSR' or a notched R wave; these leads often show a downsloping ST segment at rest, and such a finding is thus not indicative of myocardial ischemia (Figure 20).

Individuals with the left ventricular hypertrophy and strain pattern on their resting electrocardiogram are at high risk for coronary artery disease. However, this can cause exercise-induced ST depression without coronary artery disease. Healthy individuals with the Wolff-Parkinson-White syndrome can have exercise-induced ST-segment depression. Some individuals

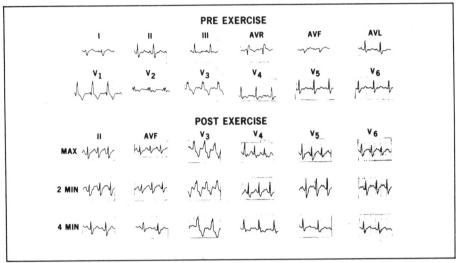

PRE EXERCISE

I   II   III   AVR   AVF   AVL

V₁   V₂   V₃   V₄   V₅   V₆

POST EXERCISE

II   AVF   V₃   V₄   V₅   V₆

MAX

2 MIN

4 MIN

Figure 20. Example of anterior ST-segment depression is shown for a normal subject with right bundle branch block. (With permission of Chest.)

with preexcitation, a short PR interval, and a normal QRS complex may have a false-positive exercise test. A group of patients with the prolapsing mitral valve syndrome were reported to have abnormal exercise tests but normal coronary angiograms. In individuals with this syndrome false-positive responses are apparently more common, occurring in approximately 25%.

Individuals with vasoregulatory asthenia and orthostatic or vasoregulatory abnormalities can have abnormal exercise-induced ST-segment changes without coronary artery disease. The same can be said for those with hyperventilation repolarization abnormalities. These conditions, however, can occur in the presence of coronary artery disease, and moreover, hyperventilation can precipitate true angina or pseudoangina. Patients can be screened for orthostatic and hyperventilation repolarization changes prior to treadmill testing, or these maneuvers can be reserved only for patients who have an abnormal response. Such changes are unusual and have rarely been responsible for false-positive tests. Orthostatic and hyperventilation changes have been associated with the mitral valve prolapse syndrome. When they do occur with exercise-induced changes, the interpretation of ischemia should be avoided and the clinician must rely on other parameters to make a diagnosis.

Persons with hypertension or an excessive blood pressure–heart rate product during exercise could hypothetically have a physiologic imbalance between myocardial oxygen supply and demand. An excessive number of false positives were not found, however, in one reported population of mild hypertensives. Barnard and co-workers demonstrated that a sudden high work load of treadmill exercise can yield ST-segment depression in healthy individuals on this basis. Recently, Foster and associates could not reproduce the ST-segment depression with sudden strenuous bicycle exercise, even though ejection fraction dropped in their normal subjects. A recorder with an inadequate frequency response can either artifactually induce ST-segment depression in normal subjects or show upsloping depression when horizontal depression is actually present. Use of the proper equipment should avoid this type of distortion. In conclusion, the conditions discussed above can be avoided and should not be the major causes of false-positive responses in a good exercise testing laboratory. The most common cause of a false-positive test should be the normal variant in a patient who has a physiologic ST-segment vector that is similar to that produced by ischemia.

ST-segment depression occurring at low heart rates and other patterns may be highly predictive of coronary disease. McHenry has suggested, though, that depression only occurring during recovery is indicative of a false-positive. Careful analysis of the time-occurrence patterns in two studies has failed to confirm this or to identify any pattern indicative of a false-positive response (Table V).

Exercise-Induced Ventricular Dysrhythmias. Since exercise increases myocardial oxygen consumption, myocardial ischemia in the presence of coronary artery disease could predispose to ectopic activity during exercise. Exercise-induced supraventricular dysrhythmias are unusual and have not been related to coronary artery disease. Of major concern are exercise-induced premature ventricular contractions. Premature ventricular contractions occur in approximately one third of asymptomatic men who perform a maximal treadmill test, and the prevalence is directly related to age. Premature ventricular contractions occur most frequently at maximal exercise and often are not reproducible on repeat testing. A subgroup of healthy men (approximately 2%) will have severe exercise-induced ventricular dysrhythmias. This group will have three times the normal risk of developing coronary artery disease, but only about 10% of them will actually do so. Only 7% of those who develop coronary artery disease will have had so-called ominous ventricular dysrhythmias. Coronary artery disease patients usually have a higher prevalence of serious ventricular dysrhythmias, and their premature ventricular contractions often occur at lower heart rates than they do in healthy subjects. Dysrhythmias suppressed by acute exercise do not rule out the presence of coronary artery disease. An exercise program may be able to

TABLE V
ANALYSIS OF TIME OCCURRENCE PATTERNS OF ST-SEGMENT DEPRESSION IN
TWO STUDIES SCREENING ASYMPTOMATIC MEN (ONE USING INCIDENCE END POINTS
AND THE OTHER ANGIOGRAPHY)*

Occurrence Time	140 Men with Abnormal Treadmill Response in a Follow-up Study			111 Men with Abnormal Treadmill Response in an Angiographic Study	
	Occurrence Rate (%)	Risk Ratio†	Predictive Value (%)	Occurrence Rate (%)	Predictive Value (%)
Exercise only	9	7.4	23	11	8
Recovery only	36	4	12	42	28
Exercise and recovery	55	12	25	47	39
All abnormal responders	100	14.3	20	100	30.6

*Froelicher et al.
†Times that for normal subjects.

reduce exercise-induced dysrhythmias. Ambulatory monitoring and isometric exercise can identify premature ventricular contractions in more people than can dynamic exercise testing. The demonstration of the prognostic significance of exercise-induced ventricular dysrhythmias in coronary artery disease and the value of medical suppression will require careful follow-up studies. Studies have shown, however, that serious premature ventricular contractions detected by ambulatory monitoring performed three weeks after a myocardial infarction will identify patients at high risk. Ventricular dysrhythmias induced by exercise testing may be as predictive but more specific in these patients. In addition, the total information from an exercise test may be more helpful in patient management and more cost effective than is ambulatory monitoring. When possible, though, it is advantageous to perform both procedures.

Subjective Responses. Careful observation of the patient's appearance is necessary for the safe performance of an exercise test and is helpful in the clinical assessment of a patient. Patients who exaggerate their limitations or symptoms and those unwilling to cooperate are usually easy to identify. A drop in skin temperature during exercise can indicate an inadequate cardiac output with secondary vasoconstriction and can be an indication for not encouraging a patient to a higher work load. Neurologic manifestations such as light-headedness or vertigo can also be indications of an inadequate cardiac output.

Findings on physical examination can be helpful, but their sensitivity and specificity have not been demonstrated. Gallop sounds, a mitral regurgitant murmur, or a precordial bulge could be due to left ventricular dysfunction. The physical findings of congestive heart failure, including rales and neck vein distention, should be encountered rarely in patients referred for exercise testing. However, some exercise testing laboratories use the sitting position for the recovery period to avoid problems with the patient who develops orthopnea. It is preferable to have patients lie supine after exercise testing and allow those who develop orthopnea to sit up. Also, severe angina or ominous dysrhythmias following exercise can be lessened by allowing the patient to sit up. Attempts to make the findings of the physical examination less subjective include the use of phonocardiography, apexcardiography, and cardiokymography. Left ventricular ejection time can be determined by the ear densitigram and its first derivative more easily than by trying to obtain a carotid pulse tracing. This measurement may have diagnostic value at four minutes after exercise.

Weiner and co-workers reported 281 consecutive patients studied with treadmill testing and coronary angiography with the following responses: (1) 76 patients with ST-segment depression and treadmill test–induced chest pain, (2) 85 patients with ST-segment depression and no chest pain, (3) 40 patients with treadmill test induced–chest pain who had no ST-segment changes, and (4) 80 patients with neither chest pain nor ST-segment changes. They found that 91% of the first group, 65% of the second group, 72% of the third group, and only 35% of the fourth group had significant angiographically determined coronary artery diseases. Cole and Ellestad followed 95 patients with abnormal treadmill tests. At five-year follow-up, the incidence of coronary artery disease was 73% in those with both chest pain and an abnormal ST-segment response compared with 43% in those who only had an abnormal ST-segment response. Mortality was also twice as high in those with both ST-segment changes and chest pain induced by the treadmill test. The results of these studies suggest that ischemic chest pain induced by the exercise test predicts the presence of coronary artery disease as well as ST-segment depression, and when they occur together, they are of even more predictive of coronary artery disease than of either alone. It is important, though, that a careful description of the pain be obtained from the patient to ascertain that it is typical rather than atypical angina.

Observer Agreement in Interpretation. The complexity of not only the human body but also the human mind has created in medicine science measurements, which when applied to medical diagnosis, lead to observations with large variability, i.e., ST-segment displacement. The inherent subjective nature of these medical observations require questioning of the results of most diagnostic methods—not only in regard to accuracy or validity but also agreement (among different interpreters for a given test). Attempts at describing or assessing agreement have been complex and variable as evidenced in the literature by the numerous terms used: agreement, variability, consistency, within-observer correlation coefficients of disagreement, and many others. Agreement has two subgroupings: intraobserver, referring to agreement of the individual observer with himself on two separate occasions; and interobserver, referring to agreement among two or more individuals. Nearly all diagnostic areas of cardiology have been scrutinized for agreement, including the clinical examination, electrocardiography, the exercise electrocardiography, echocardiography, and nuclear cardiology. Even the gold standard, coronary angiography, has been examined for observer variability.

In one of the few studies of agreement concerning the cardiac physical examination, Raftery and Holland found that two cardiologists had excellent agreement on heart size and murmurs (greater than 94% agreement), but agreement on extra sounds was in a range of 72% to 92%. They found best agreement between cardiologists, as opposed to three nonspecialists. In a study assessing agreement of three physicians as to the presence or absence of tibial or dorsalis pedis artery pulses, Meade and colleagues found an interobserver agreement in approximately 70% and 80%, respectively, and intraobserver agreement ranging from 73% to 87%, respectively.

The echocardiogram has been criticized not only for problems in technical reproducibility (the ability to give the same image on a second study) but also for its observer agreement in interpretation. Schieken and colleagues evaluated the echocardiogram as a possible tool for studying large groups in long-term studies and considered interobserver and intraobserver agreements for measuring left heart dimensions using standard criteria. Using correlation coefficients, they found a within-observer intraclass correlation coefficient (another method of describing intraobserver agreement) range of .87 to .98 for various dimensions. They found an interobserver coefficient range of .86 to .98, except for the left ventricular posterior wall measurement, which had a coefficient of .57. They attributed their relatively high intraobserver and interobserver agreements to the use of standardized measurement criteria, which defined technically acceptable interfaces and standard measurement techniques. Crawford and colleagues compared their methods with the standards recommended by the American Society of Echocardiography and found their own standards more accurate. Their study not only supports the use of standard reporting forms for increased precision but also stresses the importance of finding a standard that will give the greatest precision and agreement. Unfortunately, they did not address the problem of interinstitutional agreement.

Felner and associates evaluated experimental factors, both in interpretation and in testing protocol (subject gender, day and time of testing, and subject position) that might be involved in the variability of echocardiographic measurements. Using a variance component model, they determined the relative contribution of various factors to the total variability in measurement. As expected, the subject variance was a major component in all measurements, but technician, subject position, and day-to-day variance were minimal except for heart rate and right ventricular internal dimension. The interpreter variance component, however, was significant, particularly in measuring interventricular septal and posterior left ventricular wall thicknesses. Also of note is that intrainterpreter variability in measurement was as large or larger than was interinterpreter variability. To ensure greater agreement, they stressed the necessity of reading echocardiograms either using one interpreter on two separate occasions or by using two interpreters.

The electrocardiogram and vectorcardiogram have been noted to have a low level of observer agreement (or high reader variability). Segall had a group of physicians interpret 100 electrocardiograms as normal, old myocardial infarction, or nonspecifically abnormal. Although only paired interobserver correlation was calculated, he did note that 70% or more of the 20 readers were only able to agree on 77 of the 100 electrocardiograms. Using the same reporting categories, Davies and nine experienced electrocardiographers interpreted 100 electrocardiograms on two separate occasions at two or more weeks apart. He found that at least two thirds of his readers agreed on 78% of the electrocardiograms and that complete agreement occurred in only 29% of the cases. Interobserver correlations of readings were not calculated, but intraobserver consistency or agreement was done on each of the experienced nine readers and showed an intraobserver agreement with a range of 81% to 93%. In another study, Acheson noted a 90% intraobserver agreement in one reader and an overall agreement of 60%.

Simonson evaluated 10 observers in their interpretation of 114 vectorcardiograms and 105 electrocardiograms. In addition to an excellent review of the literature comparing the diagnostic value of the vectorcardiogram and electrocardiogram, he and his colleagues looked at many areas of interpretation, such as diagnostic accuracy of various myocardial conditions and comparisons between the vectorcardiogram and electrocardiogram. They also addressed interobserver and intraobserver variation (another form of agreement, but more in terms of lack of agreement than agreement). Among the observers, he found a wide variation in making the correct interpretation for five conditions, as evidenced by wide standard deviations for the average correct or incorrect diagnoses.

Blackburn had 14 observers (from seven separate institutions) interpret 38 individual exercise electrocardiographic tests as to normal, abnormal, or borderline. Five readers repeated the readings. In only nine of the 38 (24%) exercise electrocardiograms was there complete agreement among the 14 readers, and only 22 electrocardiograms (58%) were read in agreement. This low value may be due to the fact that Blackburn's study did not allow a dichotomous decision because there was the third interpretation of borderline. In terms of intraobserver agreement there was a wide range from 58% to 92% and an average still less than ours for a dichotomous decision. Blackburn attributed this wide variation in both interobserver and intraobserver agreement to: (1) the absence of defined criteria, (2) technical problems such as noise, and (3) differences in opinion as to ST-segment upsloping. Strict criteria such as the Minnesota code and computer analysis have been recommended as a means to increase agreement in electrocardiography.

Detre and colleagues studied observer agreement in detecting a lesion with 50% or or more diameter occlusion in 13 coronary angiograms. These angiograms were reviewed by 22 readers on two separate occasions. Interobserver variability (observer disagreement) was measured in terms of both standard deviation, agreement index, and pairwise disagreement index. Detre found results midway between chance expectation and 100% agreement. This study demonstrated considerable interobserver and intraobserver variability (low agreement) and found the lowest interobserver agreement among those who were least consistent, even with themselves (intraobserver agreement). There was also a strong correlation between observer experience and intraobserver consistency, that is, experienced observers usually agreed on two readings.

Zir and colleagues had four readers, two radiologists and two cardiologists, assess coronary artery stenoses and wall motion abnormalities in 20 patients. He found a striking degree of interobserver variability, particularly in the interpretation of arterial or ventricular wall segments with the highest percentage of positive findings. Galbraith and associates also correlated interobserver variability in the evaluation of coronary angiograms with postmortem pathologic findings. They found that in spite of the presence of coronary artery disease, angiographic interpretations of significant lesions (50% or more angiographic diameter occlusion) were noted in only approximately

80% of the arteries with such occlusions on pathologic examination. In addition, they found that when the majority opinion of angiographic interpretation was used, it added little to accuracy. This result was attributed to the large influence of a dominant, persistent, or senior reader on consensus interpretation and would suggest perhaps that, first, individual reader assessment may give a less biased interpretation and, second, that accuracy may be more a function of the reader than of the angiogram.

The measurement of wall motion and ejection fraction using both contrast angiography and radionuclides have been investigated for observer agreement. Chaitman and colleagues looked at both subjective evaluations (estimations) and objective evaluations (measurements from frame tracings) of angiographic film for volume, ejection fraction, and wall motion. Less interobserver variability (greater agreement) was demonstrated between the objective observers than between the subjective observers, particularly with respect to volume measurements. There was even less agreement when comparing objective observer measurements to those of the subjective observers in all areas. Best interobserver and intraobserver agreement occurred in ejection fraction measurements, especially in the objective intraobserver measurement of ejection fraction in which a .99 correlation was noted. Unfortunately, only one observer was tested for intraobserver agreement.

Slutsky and co-workers assessed reproducibility of ejection fraction and ventricular volumes by gated radionuclide angiography and included a small study on interobserver and intraobserver agreement. They found minimal variations of $.02 \pm .02$ and $.03 \pm .02$ ejection fraction units for intraobserver and interobserver variabililty. Okada and colleagues studied observer agreement (called variance) by comparing radionuclide with contrast angiographic assessment of left ventricular wall motion and ejection fraction. They found similar or superior interobserver variance for wall motion by radionuclide than by contrast angiography, except for the septal wall motion in which contrast angiography was superior. In determining radionuclide gated blood-pool ejection fraction both at exercise and rest, higher interobserver and intraobserver variance of ejection fraction was noted than was reported by Slutsky and co-workers, but they found it to be similar to contrast ventriculography.

McLaughlin and colleagues studied reproducibility of the thallium-201 technique, testing a group of individuals twice. They found only six nonreproducible segments out of 76. In terms of observer agreement, they noted total agreement of three observers in 60 of 76 studies but did not find intraobserver agreement when defect location was correlated with coronary artery stenoses. Only once was the defect seen in the absence of a significant lesion in the arteries supplying the area. In studies concerned with interpretation or reading of thallium scans, evaluation of agreement has considered primarily interobserver and not intraobserver agreement. Trobaugh and colleagues have reported an interinstitutional study of observer variability—another term describing interobserver agreement or reliability. Two readers from two different institutions interpreted a total of 100 resting electrocardiogram studies (50 from each institution) as normal, borderline, and abnormal. Exact agreement of all four observers occurred in 44% of the studies and in an additional 35% of the studies; three of the four observers agreed and the fourth observer differed by one grade of abnormality. Hence, in 79% of the studies, at least three of four observers agreed. The percentage of interobserver agreement is very similar to ours and to other studies (Bailey 90% agreement; Verani 82%; Blood 90%; Ritchie 80%; and Lenaers 80%).

In our study of thallium-201 images, the greatest intraobserver agreement occurred when the interpreters were asked for only an abnormal or normal response (a dichotomous interpretation). Intraobserver agreement averaged 91%, and interobserver agreement among at least three readers of abnormal scintigrams occurred in 77% of the studies. This increased consistency in dichotomous judgments is encouraging and has been found in other studies, but chance may well contribute to this phenomenon.

The poorest intraobserver or interobserver agreement was noted in the location of an abnormality. Part of the lack of observer agreement may also be due to inadequate definitions of terms as well as to normal variation. It appears that a reporting form that not only contains the usual written description and location of a lesion but also requires a shaded area or other drawing of a lesion on schematic representations would be very helpful.

Observer agreement is best when using dichotomous interpretations and the worst (most variability) when using more complex descriptions such as are involved in specifying location or overlapping areas. Several possible modes for improvement include: (1) simple dichotomous decisions, (2) standardized report forms such as the one used in this study, (3) multiple observers or one very experienced reader, (4) multiple blinded or unbiased interpretations, and (5) computer analysis. We have found computer analysis of the exercise electrocardiogram to be highly reproducible when modern algorithms are used. As long as human judgment with all its complexities remains the basis for the final interpretation, some minimum variation will always have to be accepted. The human element is, needless to say, what keeps medical diagnosis an art.

Summary. The interpretation of the exercise test is not a simple skill but requires the understanding of physiology and pathophysiology. One should not accept that all medical professionals can adequately interpret an exercise test. Training and experience are required as they are in other diagnostic procedures. Each objective and subjective result of the test must be considered. Attempts should be made to make the interpretation reliable by using good methods and following the above suggestions. When properly interpreted, the exercise test is one of the most important diagnostic and clinically helpful tests in medicine.

It appears that ST-segment depression is a global subendocardial phenomenon, with a direction determined largely by the placement of the heart in the chest. Since most of the electrical energy of the heart exists on a plane in space, it would seem best to make measurements along this plane. Severe transmural ischemia, resulting in wall motion abnormalities, causes a shift of the vector in the direction of the wall motion abnormalities. Again, spatial analysis should be able to differentiate these changes and determine whether the vector shift is occurring alone or in conjunction with subendocardial ischemia. Spatial techniques can best be applied by computer analysis, and this has the potential for improving the diagnostic value of exercise electrocardiography.

Preliminary radionuclide studies suggest that these techniques offer the opportunity to calibrate the exercise electrocardiogram and vectorcardiogram as has never before been possible. Simoons and colleagues have shown that there is no relationship between the ST-vector orientation and location of thallium perfusion defects during exercise. Dunn and colleagues studied exercise-induced ST-segment elevation using thallium. They found that when the resting electrocardiogram shows Q waves of an old infarction, ST elevation is due to ischemia or wall motion abnormalities or both, whereas accompanying ST depression is due to a second area of ischemia. When the electrocardiogram is normal, however, ST elevation is due to severe ischemia (spasm or a critical lesion), though accompanying ST depression is reciprocal. Battler and colleagues used radionuclide gated blood-pool angiography to study the relation of QRS amplitudes to function and volume changes during exercise. They found that R-wave and S-wave amplitude changes did not correlate with changes in left ventricular volume or in ejection fraction.

APPLICATIONS

Exercise can be considered the true test of the heart, because it is the most common everyday stress that humans undertake. The exercise test therefore may well be the most practical and useful procedure in the clinical evaluation of a person's cardiovascular status. The common clinical applications of exercise testing are diagnosis and prognosis, determination of functional capacity, use in treatment of dysrhythmias, exercise prescription, management of the early postmyocardial infarction period, and screening. A discussion of these concerns follows.

Diagnosis of Chest Pain and Other Cardiac Findings. To evaluate a test for a disease, one must demonstrate how well the test distinguishes between those individuals with and those without the disease. Evaluation of exercise testing as a diagnostic test for coronary artery disease depends on the population tested, which must be divided into those with and those without coronary artery disease by independent techniques. Coronary angiography and clinical follow-up for coronary events are two methods of separating a population into those with and those without coronary disease.

Coronary angiography has certain limitations. It has been demonstrated in studies comparing angiographic with pathologic findings that coronary angiography usually underestimates the pathologic severity of coronary artery disease. Coronary angiography can be interpreted as normal when severe coronary artery disease is present. This result can be due to total cut-off of an artery at its origin, by diffuse atherosclerotic narrowing of an artery, and by failure to use axial views to visualize proximal left coronary artery lesions. Another limitation of coronary angiography is that coronary artery spasm as a cause of ischemia may be missed because it is often transient. Also, coronary angiographic interpretation is subject to variability owing to observer error, as has been previously described.

There are some important limitations of using clinical events and pathologic end points to separate coronary artery disease patients and disease-free groups. Coronary artery disease events and symptoms can be due to relatively minor lesions. Hemorrhage into nonobstructive plaques can cause symptoms or even death. Spasm has been demonstrated to occur proximal to relatively minor lesions. Pathologic studies have shown that approximately 7% of people dying from a clinically diagnosed myocardial infarction have insignificant or no coronary artery disease. Coronary angiographic studies have shown that some patients with classic angina pectoris and myocardial infarction can have normal coronary angiograms. In spite of these limitations, coronary angiography and the observation of clinical symptoms or events are at present the most practical end points that distinguish those people with and those without coronary artery disease.

TABLE VI
DEFINITIONS AND CALCULATION OF TERMS USED TO DEMONSTRATE
THE DIAGNOSTIC VALUE OF A TEST

$$\text{Sensitivity} = \frac{TP}{TP + FN} \times 100$$

$$\text{Relative risk} = \frac{\dfrac{TP}{TP + FP}}{\dfrac{FN}{TN + FN}}$$

$$\text{Specificity} = \frac{TN}{FP + TN} \times 100 \qquad \text{Predictive value of abnormal test} = \frac{TP}{TP + FP} \times 100$$

TP = true positives or those with abnormal test and disease; FN = false negatives or those with normal test and with disease; TN = true negatives or those with normal test and no disease; FP = false positives or those with abnormal test and no disease.

Predictive value of an abnormal response is the percentage of individuals with an abnormal test who have disease.

Relative risk, or risk ratio, is the relative rate of occurrence of a disease in the group with an abnormal test compared to those with a normal test.

Sensitivity and specificity are the terms used to define how reliably a test distinguishes diseased from nondiseased individuals. Sensitivity is the percentage of total times that a test gives an abnormal result when those with the disease are tested. Specificity is the percentage of times that a test gives a normal result when those without the disease are tested. This is quite different from the colloquial use of the word specific. The method of calculating these terms is shown in Table VI.

A basic step in applying any testing procedure for the separation of normal subjects from patients with a disease is to determine a value measured by the test that best separates the two groups. A problem is that there is usually a considerable overlap of measurement values of a test in the groups with and without disease. Consider two bell-shaped normal distribution curves, one representing a normal population and the other representing a population with disease, with a certain amount of overlap of the two curves. Along the vertical axis is the number of patients and along the horizontal axis could be the value for such measurements as Q-wave size, exercise-induced ST-segment depression, or CPK. The optimal test would be able to achieve the most marked separation of these two bell-shaped curves minimizing the overlap. Unfortunately, most of the tests currently used for the diagnosis of coronary artery disease, including the exercise test, have a considerable overlap of the range of measurements for the normal population and for those with heart disease. Therefore, problems arise when a certain value is used to separate these two groups (i.e., 1 mm of ST-segment depression, a 10 mm Hg drop in systolic blood pressure, less than 5 METs of functional capacity, 3 beats of ventricular tachycardia). If the value is set far to the right (i.e., 2 mm of ST-segment depression) in order to identify nearly all the normal subjects as being free of disease, giving the test a high specificity, then a substantial number of those with disease are called normal. If a value is chosen far to the left (i.e., 0.5 mm ST-segment depression) that identifies nearly all those with disease as being abnormal, giving the test a high sensitivity, then many normal subjects are identified as abnormal. If a value is chosen that equally mislabels the normal subjects and those with disease, the test will have its highest predictive accuracy. However, there may be reasons for wanting to adjust a test to have a relatively higher sensitivity or relatively higher specificity than possible when predictive accuracy is optimal. But remember that sensitivity and specificity are inversely related. That is, when sensitivity is the highest, specificity is the lowest and vice versa. Any test has a range of inversely related sensitivities and specificities that can be chosen by specifying a certain discriminant or diagnostic value.

Further complicating the choice of a discriminant value is that many diagnostic procedures do not have values established that best separate normal subjects from those with disease. For instance, exercise radionuclide ventriculography does not have demonstrated values for the ejection fraction response or volume change that are normal or abnormal. Also, the identification of regional wall motion abnormalities and how to quantitate them has not been resolved. Even regarding the Q wave on the standard resting electrocardiogram or exercise-induced ST-segment depression, uncertainty remains regarding what measurement gives the best discriminant value and what the sensitivity and specificity of the currently used criteria are.

Once a discriminant value is chosen that determines a test's specificity and sensitivity, then the population tested must be considered. If the population is skewed toward individuals with a greater severity of disease, then the test will have a higher sensitivity. For instance, the exercise test has a higher sensitivity in individuals with triple-vessel disease than in those with single-vessel disease. Also, a test can have a lower specificity if it is used in individuals more likely to have false-positive results. For instance, the exercise test has a lower specificity in individuals with mitral valve prolapse and in women. However, these factors are usually relatively minor in influencing sensitivity and specificity as compared with the effects of prevalence on predictive value.

TABLE VII
DIAGNOSTIC VALUE OF ELECTROCARDIOGRAPHIC RESPONSE TO EXERCISE, WITH
CORONARY ANGIOGRAPHY AS THE END POINT FOR CORONARY DISEASE AND THE
NUMBER OF OBSTRUCTED ARTERIES SPECIFIED

Study	N	Specificity	Sensitivity*			
			1 Vessel	2 Vessel	3 Vessel	Total
Kassebaum	68	97%	25%	38%	85%	53%
Martin	100	89%	35%	67%	86%	62%
McHenry	166	95%	61%	91%	100%	81%
Helfant	63	83%	60%	83%	91%	79%
Bartel	609	94%	39%	62%	73%	63%
Goldschlager	410	93%	40%	63%	79%	64%
Average	—	90%	43%	67%	86%	70%

*Expressed in terms of number of obstructed arteries.

The sensitivity and specificity of exercise-induced ST-segment depression can be demonstrated by analyzing the results obtained when exercise testing and coronary angiography have been used to evaluate patients. From these studies (summarized in Table VII), it can be seen that the exercise test has approximately a 90% specificity for angiographically significant coronary artery disease; that is, 90% of those without significant angiographic disease had a normal exercise test.

These studies demonstrated a mean 70% sensitivity of exercise testing for angiographic coronary artery disease with a range from 43% for one-vessel disease to 86% for three-vessel disease. Most of these studies, however, used only the criterion of 0.1 mV horizontal or downsloping ST-segment depression to indicate an abnormal exercise test, and in many of them only a single lead was recorded. In studies that took into account the number of coronary arteries involved, all found increasing sensitivity of the test as more vessels were involved. The most false negatives were found among patients with single-vessel disease, particularly if the vessel was not the left anterior descending artery. Sensitivity decreased for the milder degrees of coronary artery disease, but it is likely that some patients with single-vessel coronary disease do not have myocardial ischemia. If ST-segment elevation, heart rate and blood pressure response, functional capacity, and symptomatology are considered, the sensitivity of the exercise test will certainly be higher. Yet case reports of individuals who have died or have had heart attacks immediately following a normal maximal treadmill test emphasize the limitations of sensitivity in exercise testing.

Two additional terms that help to define the diagnostic value of a test are its relative risk and its predictive value. Table VI also shows how these terms are calculated. The relative risk is the relative chance of having disease if the test is abnormal as compared with the chance of having disease if the test is normal. The predictive value of an abnormal test is the percentage of those persons with an abnormal test who have disease. Subtracting the predictive value from 100% yields the false-positive rate. Neither the predictive value nor the false-positive rate can be estimated directly from a test's demonstrated specificity or sensitivity. Predictive value and the false-positive rate are dependent on the prevalence of disease in the population tested. Table VIII illustrates how a test with a 70% sensitivity and a 90% specificity (comparable to the exercise ECG) performs in a population with a 5% prevalence of disease. As previously demonstrated, these values approximate the sensitivity and specificity of maximal or near-maximal exercise testing. Since 5% of 10,000 men have disease, 500 men have disease. In the middle column are the number of men with abnormal tests and in the far right column are the number with normal tests. Since the test is 70% sensitive, 350 of those with disease will have abnormal tests and are true positives. The remaining 150 have normal tests and are false negatives. Since the test is 90% specific, 90% of the 9,500 without disease are true negatives, whereas the remainder are false positives. To calculate the predictive value, the number of true positives is divided by the number of those with an abnormal test. Table VIII also shows the performance of a test with the same 70% sensitivity and 90% specificity in a population with a 50% prevalence of disease. The predictive value of an abnormal response is directly related to the prevalence of the disease in the population tested. There are more false-positive responses when exercise testing is used in a population with a low prevalence of disease than when it is used in a population with a high prevalence of disease. This fact explains the greater number of false positives found when using the test as a screening procedure in an asymptomatic group as opposed to when using it as a diagnostic procedure in patients with symptoms most likely due to coronary artery disease. Also, in Table VIII are the calculations for a test with a sensitivity and specificity of 90% (comparable to a thallium treadmill test) and for a test with a sensitivity of 90% and a specificity of 70% (comparable to exercise radionuclide ventriculography).

No matter what techniques are used, there is a reciprocal relationship between sensitivity and specificity. The more specific a test is (i.e., the more able it is to determine who is disease free), the less sensitive it is. The values for sensitivity and specificity can be altered by adjusting the criterion used

TABLE VIII
TEST PERFORMANCE VERSUS PREDICTIVE VALUE AND
RISK RATIO: A MODEL IN A POPULATION OF 10,000

Disease Prevalence	Subjects	Number with Abnormal Test	Test Performance	Number with Normal Test
5%	500 diseased	450 (TP)	90% sensitivity	50 (FN)
		350 (TP)	70% sensitivity	150 (FN)
	9,500 nondiseased	2,850 (FP)	70% specificity	6,650 (TN)
		950 (FP)	90% specificity	8,550 (TN)
50%	5,000 diseased	4,500 (TP)	90% sensitivity	500 (FN)
		3,500 (TP)	70% sensitivity	1,500 (FN)
	5,000 nondiseased	1,500 (FP)	70% specificity	3,500 (TN)
		500 (FP)	90% specificity	4,500 (TN)

	Predictive Value of Abnormal Test		Risk Ratio*	
Disease Prevalence	5	50	5	50
Sensitivity/Specificity				
70%/90%	27%	88%	27	3
90%/70%	14%	75%	14	5
90%/90%	32%	90%	64	9

*Times that for normal subjects.
TP = true-positive test result; FP = false-negative test result;
FN = false-negative test result; TN = true-negative test result.

for abnormal. For instance, when the criterion for an abnormal exercise-induced ST-segment response is altered to 0.2 mV depression, making it more
specific for coronary artery disease, the sensitivity of the test can be reduced
by half. For unknown reasons, the specificity of the ST-segment response is
decreased when the test is used in women and in patients who have ST-segment depression at rest, left ventricular hypertrophy, vasoregulatory abnormality, or mitral valve prolapse.

The information most important to a clinician attempting to make a diagnosis is the probability of the patient having the disease once the test result
is known. Such a probability cannot be accurately estimated from the test

result and the diagnostic characteristics of the test alone. It also requires knowledge of the probability of the patient having the disease before the test administration. Bayes's theorem states that the odds of a patient having the disease after a test will be the product of the odds before the test and the odds that the test provided a true result.

The odds of a test result being true can be shown as the likelihood ratio, which is the ratio of true results to false results. In the case of an abnormal test result, the positive likelihood ratio equals

$$\frac{\text{Percent with disease with abnormal test}}{\text{Percent without disease with abnormal test}} \quad \text{or} \quad \frac{\text{Sensitivity}}{1 - \text{Specificity}}$$

In the case of a normal test result, the negative likelihood ratio equals

$$\frac{\text{Percent without disease with normal test}}{\text{Percent with disease with normal test}} \quad \text{or} \quad \frac{\text{Specificity}}{1 - \text{Sensitivity}}$$

By analyzing the statements in the equations on the left side, it can be seen that they are equivalent to the numerators and denominators in the equations on the right.

The likelihood ratio is an indicator of the diagnosticity of a test; the higher it is, the greater the diagnostic impact of the test. Using conventional techniques of analyzing ST-segment depression, the maximal or near-maximal exercise test has a sensitivity of approximately 70% and a specificity of 90%. Therefore, the likelihood ratio for an abnormal test result equals

$$\text{Positive likelihood ratio} = \frac{0.7}{1 - 0.9} = 7.0$$

and the likelihood ratio for a normal test result equals

$$\text{Negative likelihood ratio} = \frac{0.9}{1 - 0.7} = 3.0$$

Bayes's theorem may be expressed in the following fashion:

$$\begin{matrix}\text{Posttest} \\ \text{odds} \\ \text{of disease}\end{matrix} = \begin{matrix}\text{Pretest odds} \\ \text{of disease}\end{matrix} \times \begin{matrix}\text{Likelihood ratio} \\ \text{of the results}\end{matrix}$$

The clinician often makes this calculation intuitively when he suspects as a false result the abnormal exercise test of a 30-year-old woman with chest pain (low prior odds or probability). The same abnormal response would be accepted as a true result in a 60-year-old man with angina who had a previous myocardial infarction (high prior odds or probability).

Angiographic studies have been used to investigate the prevalence of significant coronary artery disease in patients with different chest pain syndromes. Because chest pain is the presenting complaint in the majority of patients referred for a diagnostic exercise test, the nature of the pain would seem a practical basis for estimating the prior probability of coronary artery disease. Approximately 90% of the patients with true angina pectoris have been found to have significant angiographic coronary disease. In patients presenting with atypical angina pectoris, approximately 50% have been found to have significant angiographic coronary disease. Atypical angina refers to pain that has an unusual location, prolonged duration, or inconsistent precipitating factors or that is unresponsive to nitroglycerin. Figure 21 demonstrates the calculation of the probability of coronary artery disease in such patients.

The patient with typical angina pectoris has a 90% or 9:1 chance of having significant coronary artery disease. An abnormal exercise test increases these odds from 9:1 to 63:1. Such an impressive change in odds represents a relatively small increase in the probability of disease from 90% to 98%. Because such a patient still has a 75% probability of disease after a negative test, coronary angiography may yet be required to definitely rule out coronary disease. The greatest diagnostic impact of such a circumstance would be in patients with atypical angina. An abnormal test result would increase the odds from 1:1 to 7:1, the probability of disease to 88% and, for practical purposes, establish the diagnosis. With a normal test, the probability of coronary disease would be reduced to 25%.

Even though a test may not have an important impact on disease probability in a patient, the test can be used for other purposes, such as demonstrating the severity or prognosis of a disease or the result of a therapeutic intervention. In addition, we should remember that any test only gives a probability statement and how this affects an individual patient is greatly dependent on the art of medicine.

Determination of Prognosis and Severity. Exercise testing can be used to determine the prognosis for patients with coronary artery disease. The results of an exercise test can help to establish the risk of mortality and morbidity after an acute myocardial infarction and in patients with angina pectoris. Numerous studies have supported the hypothesis that the severity of angiographic coronary artery disease is directly related to the work load that can be performed; however, there are exceptions. Exercise-induced hypotension, extremely limited functional capacity, chronotropic incompetence, marked ST-segment depression, downsloping ST-segment depression,

CALCULATION OF PROBABILITY OF CAD

	PRE-TEST ODDS	LIKELIHOOD RATIO	POST-TEST ODDS	POST-TEST PROBABILITY
ANGINAL	9 : 1	ABNORMAL TEST (×7)	63 : 1	(63/64) = 98%
		NORMAL TEST (×3)	9 : 3	(9/12) = 75%
ATYPICAL ANGINA	1 : 1	ABNORMAL TEST (×7)	7 : 1	(7/8) = 88%
		NORMAL TEST (×3)	1 : 3	(1/4) = 25%
NON-ANGINAL	1 : 9	ABNORMAL TEST (×7)	7 : 9	(7/16) = 44%
		NORMAL TEST (×3)	1 : 27	(1/28) = 4%
ASYMPTOMATIC	1 : 19	ABNORMAL TEST (×7)	7 : 19	(7/26) = 27%
		NORMAL TEST (×3)	1 : 57	(1/58) = 2%

Figure 21. Illustration of the practical clinical application of Baye's theorem shows a calculation of the probabilities of coronary artery disease. The pretest odds were determined from angiographic and epidemiologic data, and the likelihood ratios are based on a sensitivity of 70% and a specificity of 90% for the electrocardiographic response to the exercise test.

an increased number of leads with ischemic depression, ST-segment depression beginning at a low heart rate, systolic blood pressure drop, and inverted U waves are more predictive of severe coronary artery disease and left ventricular dysfunction than is 0.1 mV of horizontal ST-segment depression only at maximal exercise. Patients who can achieve a normal work load, a normal maximal heart rate, and a normal maximal systolic blood pressure during treadmill testing appear to have better ventricular function and a better prognosis than do those unable to do the same. Patients without chest pain during exercise testing also appear to do better.

McNeer and colleagues demonstrated that a combination of exercise test parameters was both diagnostically and prognostically important. Their study involved 1,472 patients who underwent exercise testing and coronary angiography and were then followed for at least one year. Ninety-seven percent of the patients who had abnormal ST-segment depression in the first or second stage of the Bruce protocol had significant coronary artery disease. More than 60% had three-vessel disease, and more than 25% had significant narrowing of the left main coronary artery. Those who achieved the fourth stage and did not have abnormal ST-segment responses had less than 15% incidence of three-vessel disease and less than 1% incidence of left main coronary disease. Patients able to exercise to or beyond stage 4 and able to achieve a maximal heart rate of 160 beats/min or greater or with a normal ST-segment response or both had a one-year survival of almost 100%. Patients forced to stop exercising in stages 1 or 2 with a low heart rate response and with abnormal ST-segment depression had a one-year survival of 85%.

In some situations, identifying which patients could attain greater longevity from coronary artery bypass surgery is helpful in clinical decision making. From current information, it appears that patients with left main or triple-vessel disease will have improved survival if treated surgically. However, this expectation is most realizable in those patients with moderately reduced resting left ventricular ejection fractions (less than 50% to greater than 30%). The two studies of exercise testing discussed below have addressed the problem of identifying that subset of patients most likely to benefit with greater longevity from coronary artery bypass surgery.

Weiner and colleagues reported a study of 436 consecutive patients referred for suspected or known coronary artery disease who were able to undergo both exercise testing and coronary angiography. All patients underwent treadmill testing using the Bruce protocol, and 12-lead electrocardiograms were obtained during exercise. A lesion of the left main coronary artery was considered significant if it had greater than 50% diameter narrowing; this criterion was 70% in other vessels. Fifty-five patients were excluded because of left ventricular hypertrophy, digoxin therapy, left bundle branch block, and for the attainment of less than 85% maximal predictive heart rate (of these 55, two had left main coronary artery disease and four had three-vessel disease; therefore, the predictive value of being excluded was about 10%). Four patient groups were defined by angiographic findings: (1) 35 with left main disease, (2) 89 with three-vessel disease without left main disease, (3) 188 patients with either one- or two-vessel disease, and (4) 124 patients with no significant coronary disease. Of the 35 patients with left main disease, most had disease of other coronary arteries and nearly half had three-vessel disease. Exercise test responses that were considered included the amount of ST-segment depression, configuration, onset, and duration and the number of leads in which it occurred. Hemodynamic responses included treadmill time, systolic blood pressure, and maximal heart rate. Other measurements included angina, premature ventricular contractions, and abnormal R-wave response in lead V_5.

Ninety-seven percent of patients with left main disease had at least 0.1 mV of ST depression and 91% had 0.2 mV or more of ST-segment depression. Patients with left main disease as a group were distinguished from patients with three-vessel disease by an early onset and longer persistence of ST-segment depression, as well as by a greater number of leads in which the depression occurred. A fall in systolic blood pressure occurred in 23% of the patients with left main disease versus 17% of those with triple-vessel disease and 6% of those with single- or double-vessel disease. As an indicator of either left main or three-vessel disease this variable had a predictive value of 66% and a sensitivity of 19%. The criterion of 0.3 mV or more of ST-segment depression occurred in 44% of such patients and had only a slightly lower predictive value (64%). Combined analysis of test variables disclosed that the development of 0.2 mV or more of downsloping ST-segment depression beginning in stage 1, persisting for at least six minutes into recovery and involving at least five electrocardiographic leads had the greatest sensitivity (74%) and predictive value (32%) for left main coronary disease. This abnormal pattern identified either left main or three-vessel disease with a sensitivity of 49% and a predictive value of 74%.

It appears that individual clinical or exercise test variables are unable to detect left main coronary disease because of their low sensitivity or predictive value. However, a combination of the amount, pattern, and duration of ST-segment response was highly predictive and reasonably sensitive for left main or three-vessel coronary disease. The question still remains of how to identify those with abnormal resting ejection fractions, i.e., those who will benefit the most with prolonged survival after coronary artery bypass surgery. Perhaps those with a normal resting electrocardiogram will not need surgery for improvement of their prognosis because of the high probability that they have good ventricular function.

Bruce and colleagues demonstrated noninvasive screening criteria for patients who had improved four-year survival after coronary artery bypass surgery. Their data have come from 2,000 men with coronary heart disease enrolled in the Seattle Heart Watch who had a symptom-limited maximal

TABLE IX
NONRANDOMIZED STUDY OF THE RELATIONSHIP OF TREADMILL EXERCISE
AND CLINICAL FINDINGS TO SURGICAL AND MEDICAL OUTCOME
(THE SEATTLE HEART WATCH)

	Group III Left Ventricular Dysfunction	Group II* Ischemia	Group I Neither
Annual cardiac mortality	5.6%	2.2%	1.2%
Annual cardiac morbidity	7.1%	6.8%	3.8%
Coronary artery bypass surgery (16%) annual mortality	2.1%÷	2.2%	—
Unoperated annual mortality	7.0%	2.2%	—

*4.6% death rate due to surgery.
÷Only 34% had improved survival.

Group I	No left ventricular dysfunction, no ischemia, no cardiomegaly
Group II	Only ischemia (i.e., angina or ST shifts up or down)
Group III	Left ventricular dysfunction (i.e., cardiomegaly or an exercise test response of less than 4 METs functional capacity or with systolic blood pressure less than 130 mm Hg)

treadmill test; these subjects received usual community care, which resulted in 16% of them having coronary artery bypass surgery in nonrandomized fashion. The diagnosis of coronary heart disease was based on a history of angina, myocardial infarction, or cardiac arrest. Cardiomegaly was determined by physical and chest x-ray examinations. The patients were divided into three groups. One group had only myocardial ischemia manifested by exercise test–induced normal ST-segment elevation or depression and/or angina. The second group could have myocardial ischemia but had to have left ventricular dysfunction manifested by at least two of the following: cardiomegaly, less than 4-MET exercise capacity, and less than 130 mm Hg maximal systolic blood pressure. A third group had none of the above. Comparisons were then made within each group between the operated and unoperated patients and surprisingly little difference was found. However, life table analysis showed a significantly higher survival rate of 94% at four years among the operated patients, as compared with the 68% survival of the unoperated patients in the group with left ventricular dysfunction (summarized in Table IX). If the 4.6% death rate due to surgery in those with ischemia only was reduced, perhaps the patients who were operated on in that group would have had a significantly improved survival as well. This is most likely the case since the European randomized trial of coronary artery bypass surgery demonstrated that patients with 0.2 mV of exercise-induced ST-segment depression had improved mortality in the surgical cohort.

Tubau and colleagues evaluated different electrocardiographic lead systems for the detection of multivessel disease in 118 male survivors of transmural myocardial infarction. They were classified according to anterior or inferior location and anginal class, and the test results were correlated with angiographic findings. Only ST-segment depression was considered an abnormal response and this included a slow upsloping segment. Sensitivity of the test for multivessel disease was greater using 14 electrocardiographic leads (72%) or CC_5, CM_5, and V_5 (64%) than it was using lead V_5 alone (50%). Sensitivity was less for anterior infarction (64%) versus inferior infarction (77%). The predictive value was clearly dependent on the class of angina. The test was of greatest value in patients with minimal angina in whom an abnormal test increased the likelihood of multivessel disease from 50% to 90%, and a negative test reduced the risk of three-vessel disease to less than 10%. ST-segment depression greater than 0.2 mV or a treadmill performance of less than stage 4 of the Bruce protocol increased the likelihood of extensive disease.

The recent study by Podrid and colleagues has placed some doubt on the use of exercise testing to identify high-risk patients. They were reacting to the current practice of often referring patients with severe ST-segment depression to coronary angiography. They contend that the prevailing view is that such patients have far-advanced multivessel disease and that coronary artery bypass surgery is the only way to improve their outlook. In their select group of patients referred because of profound ST-segment depression, they did not find a bad prognosis. In 142 patients with CAD and severe ST-segment depression with a mean follow-up of 59 months, there was only 1.4% mortality and only 1.3% had coronary artery bypass surgery per year. Sixty-six percent of these patients had a prior myocardial infarction and 70% had angina. This low mortality suggests an unusual selection process resulting from the referral patterns to this group of physicians. This study points out that it is necessary to consider multiple variables when predicting the risk of ischemic heart disease. A relatively low-risk group can be found in any population identified using one risk predictor, such as the ECG response to an exercise test, by excluding other risk predictors.

Evaluation of Functional Capacity. The exercise test can be used to evaluate the functional capacity of asymptomatic individuals or of patients with various forms of heart disease. Patients who exaggerate their symptoms or who mainly have a psychologic impairment often can be identified. Exercise testing can more accurately measure the degree of cardiac impairment than can a physician's assessment of functional capacity. As previously described, maximal oxygen uptake, either directly measured or estimated, is the best noninvasive measurement of the functional capacity of the cardiovascular system. Being unable to complete the first stage of the Bruce test (a maximal oxygen consumption below 18 ml O_2/kg-min) has been found to have a poor prognosis in several studies in spite of either medical or surgical treatment. The determination of patient's functional capacity affords an objective measurement of the degree of cardiac impairment and can be useful in patient management. Exercise testing can also be used to evaluate the effects of training, whether it be part of an athletic program, a fitness program, or a rehabilitation program. A maximal oxygen uptake of 40 ml O_2/kg-min is the lowest level of fitness, and measurements of up to 80 ml O_2/kg-min can be found in Olympic-class long-distance runners. Following a trainee's progress in an exercise program with serial exercise testing can optimize the training program and it is often a good way to encourage adherence.

Evaluation of Treatment. The exercise test can be used to evaluate the effects of both medical and surgical treatment. Recently, there have been reports of the use of submaximal exercise testing as part of a program to mobilize patients while still hospitalized with an acute myocardial infarction. Exercise tests are now widely used as part of rehabilitation after an acute myocardial infarction, in programs that begin as soon as three weeks after the infarction. The test is usually done just prior to discharge and certainly seems a safer and more scientific way to make recommendations regarding activities after discharge. The effects of various medications including nitrates, digitalis, and antihypertensive agents have been evaluated by exercise testing. Though exercise testing has been used to evaluate patients before and after coronary artery bypass surgery, the reported studies have not given a definitive answer mainly because of alterations in medications after surgery. One problem with using treadmill time or work load rather than measuring maximal oxygen uptake in serial studies is that people learn to perform treadmill walking more efficiently. Treadmill time or work load can increase during serial studies without any improvement in cardiovascular function. Thus, it is probably important to include the measurement of maximal oxygen uptake when the effects of medical or surgical treatment are being evaluated by treadmill testing.

Evaluation of Dysrhythmias. An exercise test can be used to evaluate patients with dysrhythmias or to induce dysrhythmias in patients with the ap-

propriate symptoms. The dysrhythmias that can be evaluated include premature ventricular contractions, sick sinus syndrome, and various degrees of
heart block. When used in the same population, ambulatory monitoring or
isometric exercise detects a higher prevalence of dysrhythmias, including
serious dysrhythmias, than does dynamic exercise testing. The findings in
each of these tests, however, may have different significances. The diagnostic value of exercise-induced premature ventricular contractions has been
previously discussed.

Evaluation for an Individualized Exercise Program. The exercise test can
be used to evaluate the safety of participating in an exercise program and
can help formulate an exercise prescription. Because of the wide scatter of
maximal heart rate when plotted against age, it is much better to determine
an individual's maximal rate, in order to assign a target for training, rather
than give a predicted value. In certain individuals, it would be advantageous
to evaluate objectively their response to exercise in a monitored situation
prior to embarking on an exercise program. In adult fitness or cardiac rehabilitation programs, an exercise test can be used to progress an individual
safely to a higher level of performance. Also, the improvement in functional
performance secondary to training demonstrated by an exercise test can be
an effective incentive and encouragement to people in such programs.

Exercise Testing soon after Myocardial Infarction. Submitting patients
with a recent acute infarction to an exercise test to optimize their progression through hospitalization and discharge is desirable. The test can be performed to determine the possible risk the patient may incur during physical
activities. It is certainly better that adverse reactions be observed in controlled circumstances. The exercise test can be used to demonstrate the patient's reactions to exercise so that work capacity and limiting factors are
known at the time of discharge. This provides a safer basis for advising a
patient's activity level and return to work. The test can demonstrate to the
patient, as well as to his relatives and employer, how capacity for physical
performance was affected by infarction. It can also have a therapeutic effect
by making a patient less anxious about daily physical activities. The exercise
test can thus be the first step in cardiac rehabilitation.

The benefit-risk ratio of this procedure can be improved by a number of
considerations. Although maximal testing has been reported, we still feel
that until two months after an infarction a heart rate–limited test is indicated. Arbitrarily, a heart rate limit of 140 beats/min is used for patients under
40 and 130 beats/min for patients over 40. Also, we use conservative clinical
indications for stopping the test. The exercise test should not be ordered

without the patient's primary physician involved in its performance. It is important that the physician who knows the patient be there during the test and interact with the patient.

Cain and colleagues reported their use of a graded activity program in 335 patients who had an uncomplicated myocardial infarction and were at least 15 days postinfarct. The patients had been restricted to bed, chair, and commode. The electrocardiogram was monitored after the patient performed activities such as climbing stairs and walking up a grade. They concluded that electrocardiographic monitoring of early activity was a more reliable means of ascertaining the presence of coronary insufficiency than were physical signs or symptoms. Torkelson reported results of ten patients with uncomplicated myocardial infarctions. During the sixth week of an in-hospital rehabilitation program, a low-level treadmill test was performed using 1.7 mph at a 10% grade. He concluded that the treadmill test was a valuable procedure for the discernment of specific exercise responses of patients recovering from an acute myocardial infarction. Atterhog and colleagues reported the electrocardiographic response to exercise at varying periods after an anterior myocardial infarction. Three weeks after the infarction, 10 of their 12 patients exhibited an exercise-induced rise in ST segments in anterior precordial leads over the infarcted area. This electrocardiographic response decreased over the follow-up months and some subjects had exercise-induced ST-segment depression. The ST-segment elevation was interpreted as a sign of ischemia in the infarcted zone, and the rate at which this resolved was thought to have prognostic significance. In their hospital, a submaximal bicycle test was performed three weeks after an acute myocardial infarction as a routine procedure.

Ericsson and colleagues reported their results of treadmill testing on 100 patients three weeks after an acute infarction. Premature ventricular contractions were recorded in three patients immediately before the test and in 19 patients during or after the test. It was concluded that the treadmill test proved to be a sensitive method for demonstrating dysrhythmias in patients with recent infarctions. Ibsen and colleagues reported the results of a maximal bicycle test in the third week after an acute myocardial infarction in 209 patients. They concluded that an exercise test was safe in such patients, that it was an objective measure of physical work capacity, and that it described the reaction to physical activity. They felt that because it was a maximal test, it gave a better basis for advising return to a normal life and was of great psychologic importance to the patient. Granath and colleagues performed exercise tests at three and nine weeks after an acute myocardial infarction in 205 patients and followed them for two to five years. The appearance of tachycardia at low work loads, major ventricular dysrhythmias, or anginal complaints during these early exercise tests was followed by a significantly increased mortality during the observation period. Exercise-induced premature ventricular contractions proved to be of greater prognostic significance than those recorded at rest. They found that early exercise tests were valuable for evaluating the response to antidysrhythmic agents.

Sivarajan and colleagues evaluated 12 patients with acute myocardial infarction. They assessed symptoms, signs, and hemodynamic and electrocardiographic responses during and after three activities: sitting upright, walking to an adjacent toilet, and walking on a treadmill. These activities were studied at three, six, and ten days, respectively, after infarction. They concluded that successful performance of these three activities provided useful criteria for discharge of a patient with a myocardial infarction. Wohl and colleagues studied 50 patients after an acute myocardial infarction. They found that in stable patients, there was an early improvement of the relationship between myocardial oxygen supply and demand, as detected by ST-segment changes. There was a delayed improvement of functional capacity associated with increased stroke volume and cardiac output. The early improvement was noted in a study done at three weeks, and the later studies were done between three and six months. Markiewicz and colleagues studied 46 men under the age of 70 using treadmill testing at 3, 5, 7, 9, and 11 weeks after a myocardial infarction. They concluded that two tests, the one at 3 to 5 weeks and the one at 7 to 11 weeks, appeared to provide most of the information obtained in all five tests performed. In selected low-risk patients, they performed maximal treadmill testing at three weeks after infarction and found that a low heart rate response indicated a poor prognosis.

Sami and colleagues studied the prognostic value of treadmill testing in 200 males who were tested serially from 3 to 52 weeks after a myocardial infarction. There were approximately five tests per patient, and the patients had a mean age of 53 years. None of these patients had congestive heart failure or angina, and they were a relatively low-risk group of postmyocardial infarction patients since only 2% died over the two years of follow-up. A Naughton protocol was used and 12-lead electrocardiograms were obtained during testing. At three weeks, 100% of those who subsequently had an episode of cardiopulmonary resuscitation and 60% of those who required coronary artery bypass surgery had 0.2 mV of ST-segment depression during treadmill testing. Only 35% of those without an event had a similar amount of ST-segment depression. At five weeks and beyond, recurrent premature ventricular contractions during serial treadmill testing occurred in 90% of those who had a recurrent myocardial infarction and in only 47% of those without an event. Exercise-induced ventricular ectopy or ischemic ST-segment depression 11 weeks after infarction identifies patients with an increased risk of subsequent coronary event, whereas the absence of either identifies a group of patients with an excellent prognosis.

Theroux and colleagues from the Montreal Heart Institute studied the prognostic value of a limited treadmill test performed one day before hospital discharge after a myocardial infarction in 210 consecutive patients. These patients were followed for end points of heart disease for one year. The test was ended at 5 METs, or at 70% maximal heart rate. CM_5 was the only lead monitored, and a Naughton protocol was followed. Sixty-five percent (28 of 43) who had angina during treadmill testing reported it later, versus 36% of those without chest pain during exercise testing. In those with a normal electrocardiographic response to exercise testing, there was a 2% mortality and a 0.7% sudden death rate; in those with ST-segment depression, there was a 27% mortality (17 of 64) and a sudden death rate of 16%.

Smith and colleagues did treadmill tests on 62 patients 18 days after admission for acute myocardial infarction. The test was done to 60% maximal heart rate, and leads V_{4-6} were monitored. The patients were followed for two years. Thirty percent (6 of 20) of the patients who developed ST-segment depression either died or had another myocardial infarction after discharge from the hospital. This finding is in contrast to the occurrence of death or reinfarction in only two (5%) of the 42 patients who did not have ST-segment depression during exercise.

Davidson and DeBusk reported results of treadmill testing in 195 men tested three weeks after acute myocardial infarction. Multiple logistic analysis showed ST-segment depression equal or greater than 0.2 mV, angina, and a work capacity of less than 4 METs to be risk markers. These patients were followed for a median of two years and had a 19% event rate. More than half of these end point events, however, were coronary artery bypass surgery. The exercise test clearly could have biased this group of patients toward angiography and surgery. Ventricular ectopy on a single treadmill test three weeks after infarction had no independent prognostic value.

Haskell and DeBusk reported the cardiovascular responses to repeated treadmill testing at 3, 7, and 11 weeks after acute MI. Two symptom-limited tests were performed on 24 males (mean age 54) several days apart. All test variables measured at maximum increased significantly between 3 and 11 weeks, whereas within-week findings were reproducible. Thus, tolerance increases after infarction, even in nonexercised patients.

Weld and colleagues reported the results of low-level exercise testing on 236 of 250 patients who had diagnosed acute myocardial infarctions. Only 14 patients were excluded from this study because of contraindications. A progressive protocol of 3 stages, each lasting 3 minutes, with a maximal work load of 4 METs was performed just prior to hospital discharge (mean hospital stay was 16 days). Forty-three percent had ventricular dysrhythmias and 51% had less than a 4-MET exercise capacity. Twenty-two percent had exercise-induced ST-segment depression in V_5, but of the total population one half were on digoxin. A one-year follow-up was performed for recurrent infarction and death. There was a 12% cardiac death rate during the one-year follow-up. Surprisingly, the exercise test variables of duration, premature ventricular contractions, and ST-segment depression ranked ahead of the clinical variables of x-ray vascular congestion, prior myocardial infarction, and x-ray cardiomegaly in predictive value. This is the first study that has used standard clinical risk predictors in the same population in which the exercise test was used, and it clearly shows that the exercise test outperforms the clinical variables. The exercise test variables ranked as follows: (1) exercise duration, (2) premature ventricular contraction, (3) ST-segment depression. Patients unable to reach an exercise capacity of 4 METs had a relative risk of 15 versus being able to reach a 4-MET exercise capacity.

Though the use of electrocardiographic monitoring of activities after an acute infarction requires additional time and an interested staff, it would appear to be the ideal way of prescribing a safe level of physical activity. An exercise test prior to discharge is important for giving a patient guidelines for exercise at home, reassuring him of his physical status, and determining his risk of complications. An exercise test approximately two months after an infarct may be the best way to determine a patient's prognosis. From the results, decisions regarding cardiac rehabilitation, medications, angiography, or possibly cardiac surgery could be made. An interesting question is whether the predischarge exercise test is therapeutic. The psychologic impact of a good performance on the exercise test is impressive. Many patients increase their activity and actually rehabilitate themselves after being encouraged and reassured by their response to this test.

Recent studies demonstrated the prognostic value of exercise testing in the first two months after myocardial infarction. A high-risk group of patients can be identified who should have coronary angiography and be considered for coronary artery bypass surgery after myocardial infarction.

Screening Apparently Healthy Individuals. Since it will be some time before the primary prevention of coronary heart disease is a reality, it is advisable to evaluate screening methods for detection prior to death or disability. Risk factor screening and resting techniques have limited sensitivity, and so exercise testing, which brings out abnormalities not present at rest, deserves consideration. The varying predictive value is due to its use in populations with different prevalences of disease. Various techniques have been recommended to improve the sensitivity and specificity of exercise testing such as new computerized and noncomputerized electrocardiographic criteria, non-electrocardiographic exercise test responses, cardiac radionuclide procedures, systolic time intervals, cardiokymography, cardiac fluoroscopy, and the computerized application of Bayesian statistics using risk factors and risk markers. These techniques may improve attempts to screen for latent coronary heart disease. Limited data suggest that angiographically documented asymptomatic coronary disease has a relatively good prognosis compared with symptomatic disease and rarely should lead to coronary artery bypass surgery. Individuals so identified should be prime targets for behavior modification with the hope of avoiding the usual course of this disease.

Breslow and Somers suggested eight criteria for the selection of a screening procedure. They are: (1) the procedure is appropriate and acceptable, (2) the procedure is directed to primary or secondary prevention of a disease or condition, (3) the results of the procedure and intervention outweigh any adverse effects, (4) the disease or condition has an asymptomatic period in which detection and treatment are effective, (5) acceptable methods of effective treatment are available, (6) the prevalence and seriousness of the disease or condition justify the cost of intervention, (7) the procedure is relatively easy and cost-effective to administer, and (8) resources are generally available for diagnostic or therapeutic intervention if required. With respect to exercise testing as a screening tool for coronary heart disease, criteria 4 and 5 have yet to be fulfilled.

Exercise Testing as a Screening Tool. Exercise testing has been used to evaluate asymptomatic individuals in whom sudden incapacitation could compromise public safety. Such individuals include pilots, firemen, and policemen. Others who possibly should be screened in this manner are railroad engineers, air traffic controllers, and drivers of large commercial vehicles. Because an exercise program does present a risk to sedentary, coronary prone middle-aged men, it may be prudent to evaluate such individuals with exercise testing prior to prescribing an exercise program.

Hartley and colleagues reported an exercise testing program designed to examine large numbers of people effectively, conveniently, and inexpensively. This study was designed to evaluate the possible future application of exercise testing as a routine screening tool. A bicycle ergometer was used, and multilead testing was performed. More than 1,800 subjects were examined in three years. As many as 55 tests per day were performed at a cost of $60 to $70 each. Abnormalities uncovered were similar to those observed in other studies. The program was considered successful for rendering services conveniently, at low cost, and with accuracy.

Maximal or near-maximal exercise tests are superior screening techniques compared with submaximal exercise tests. One shortcoming of submaximal testing is its relatively low sensitivity. Other shortcomings, specifically of a step test like the double Master's test, are that it cannot be used to evaluate functional capacity and that the electrocardiogram is not monitored during exercise. There is a physiologic fallacy in adjusting the number of steps as determined by Master according to body weight. Rowell and colleagues have shown that the oxygen consumption per kilogram is much greater for light individuals than it is for heavy individuals when the number of steps performed is in accord with the Master's step tables. The work load can be near maximal for light persons, whereas it is minimal for heavy subjects. A danger of the Master's test is that it is usually performed with the electrocardiogram monitored only in the postexercise period. There have been numerous anecdotal reports of patients who fibrillated during a double Master's test, and there is at least one case reported in the literature.

The advantages of a progressive, continuous exercise test with electrocardiographic and blood pressure monitoring during the test have been discussed elsewhere. Numerous studies using such a test to screen asymptomatic individuals have been reported without subsequent follow-up data. Nevertheless, these studies have demonstrated that maximal testing is more sensitive and that abnormal responses correlate directly with other risk factors. These studies also show that women tend to have more false-positive electrocardiographic responses than do men.

Table X summarizes seven follow-up studies that utilized maximal or near-maximal exercise testing to screen asymptomatic individuals for latent coronary heart disease and one that evaluated men and women with atypical chest pain. The populations in these studies were tested and followed for the coronary heart disease end points of angina, acute myocardial infarction, and sudden death. Angiographic findings were not used as end points in these studies.

Bruce and colleagues studied 221 clinically normal men in Seattle who were 35 to 82 years of age. A CB_5 bipolar lead was used, and 0.1 mV or more

TABLE X

RESULTS OF EXERCISE ELECTROCARDIOGRAPHIC TESTING IN 7 PROSPECTIVE STUDIES SCREENING ASYMPTOMATIC MEN FOR LATENT CORONARY ARTERY DISEASE AND IN 1 STUDY EVALUATING MEN AND WOMEN WITH ATYPICAL CHEST PAIN (MANCA), WITH ST- SEGMENT DEPRESSION AS THE ONLY CRITERION FOR ABNORMAL

Principal Investigator	N	Age Range (mean)	Incidence of Coronary Heart Disease	Years Follow-up	% with Abnormal Exercise Test	Sensitivity	Specificity	Predictive Value	Relative Risk of an Abnormal Response
Bruce	221	35–82	2.3%	5.0	11%	60%	91%	14%	14
Aronow	100	38–64 (51)	9.0%	5.0	13%	67%	92%	46%	14
Cumming	510	40–65	4.7%	3.0	13%	58%	90%	25%	10
Froelicher	1390	20–54	3.3%	6.3	10%	61%	92%	20%	14
Allen	356	>40	9.6%	5.0	23%	41%	79%	17%	2
Bruce	2365	>25 (44)	2.0%	6.0	11%	30%	89%	5%	3
MacIntyre	548	47–57 (52)	6.9%	8.0	4%	16%	97%	26%	4
Manca	947 (men)	>30 (48)	5.0%	5.2	18%	67%	84%	18%	10
	508 (women)	>30 (49)	1.6%	5.2	28%	88%	73%	5%	15
Average (men only)	—	—	—	—	13%	50%	89%	21%	10

of ST-segment depression was the criterion for an abnormal response. The patients were monitored in the sitting position postexercise. Ten percent of them had abnormal ST-segment responses to the symptom-limited maximal treadmill test. They were followed for five years. The sensitivity was 60%, that is, of those who developed coronary heart disease over the follow-up period, 60% had an abnormal treadmill test when they entered the study. The specificity was 91%, that is, of those without coronary heart disease, 91% had a normal treadmill test. The probability of developing coronary artery disease for those with an abnormal treadmill test (the predictive value of an abnormal response) was 13.6%. The relative risk of developing coronary heart disease over the follow-up period was 13.6 times greater for those who had an abnormal ST-segment response to treadmill testing than for those who had a normal response.

Aronow and colleagues tested 100 normal men in Los Angeles, age 38 to 64, and followed them for five years. Risk factor analysis was not performed, but all subjects were normotensive. A V_5 lead was used and 0.1 mV or more of ST-segment depression was the criterion for an abnormal response. Patients were monitored in the supine position after exercise. Thirteen percent had an abnormal ST-segment response to near-maximal treadmill testing. Sensitivity for an abnormal response was 67%, specificity was 92%, predictive value was 46%, and risk ratio was 13.6.

Cumming and colleagues reported their three-year follow-up for coronary heart disease end points in 510 asymptomatic men 40 to 65 years of age. Maximal or near-maximal effort was performed and a CM_5 lead was monitored. The criterion for abnormal was 0.2 mV or more of ST-segment depression, and the patients were monitored in the supine position postexercise. Twelve percent had an initial abnormal response to a bicycle exercise test. Subjects with an abnormal response had a higher prevalence of hypertension and hypercholesterolemia. The sensitivity of the test was 58%, the specificity was 90%, the predictive value was 25%, and the risk ratio was 10.

At USAFSAM, 1,390 asymptomatic men 20 to 54 years of age who did not have any of the known causes for false-positive treadmill tests were screened for latent coronary heart disease by maximal treadmill testing and followed for a mean of 6.3 years. A CC_5 lead was mainly used, but additional leads were obtained in the supine position postexercise. The criterion for abnormal was 0.1 mV or more horizontal or downsloping ST-segment depression. Ten percent of these men had abnormal treadmill tests. The sensitivity of the test was 61%, the specificity was 92%, the predictive value was 20%, and the risk ratio for an abnormal response was 14.3.

In Italy, Manca and colleagues studied 947 men and 508 women who were referred for exercise testing because of atypical chest pain. Those with typical symptoms of angina pectoris, valvular disease, hypertension, bundle branch block, dysrhythmias, Wolff-Parkinson-White syndrome, left ventricular hypertrophy with strain, significant resting repolarization abnormalities, and previous myocardial infarction were excluded. No patient received drugs such as digitalis, beta blockers, antidysrhythmics, or diuretics in the two weeks preceding exercise testing. Exercise was carried out after routine hyperventilation, using a supine bicycle, until at least 85% of the predicted maximal heart rate was reached. The conventional 12 electrocardiographic leads were recorded during and after the exercise test. The criterion for an abnormal response was 0.1 mV or more of horizontal or downsloping ST-segment depression. Eighteen percent of the men and 28% of the women had an abnormal electrocardiographic response. The end points for coronary disease were myocardial infarction or sudden death, and there was a mean follow-up of 5.2 years. The overall incidence of coronary disease was 5% in the men and 1.6% in the women. The sensitivity was 67% in the men versus 88% in the women. The specificity of the test in the men was 84% versus 73% in the women. The predictive value of a positive test was 18% in men but only 5% in women. Men with positive tests had a relative risk of 10 for developing clinical manifestations of coronary heart disease; the relative risk for women with positive tests was 15. This study clearly shows how predictive value is influenced by the prevalence of coronary heart disease in the population under study and that the specificity of the exercise test is lower in women.

Allen and colleagues recently reported a five-year follow-up of 888 a-symptomatic men and women without known coronary heart disease who had initially undergone maximal treadmill testing. When tested, none of the subjects was on medications that would affect the electrocardiogram. None had pathologic Q waves or other abnormalities. None had clinical evidence of pulmonary disease or vascular disease. No subject who was included developed serious dysrhythmias, conduction abnormalities, or chest pain in conjunction with the exercise test. Maximal treadmill testing was performed using the Ellestad protocol, and leads CM_5, V_1, and a bipolar vertical lead were recorded. Subjects were exercised until they reached 100% of predicted maximal heart rate, fatigue, or marked dyspnea. Flat ST-segment depression of 0.1 mV or greater and downsloping of the ST segment were considered a positive response. Subjects with major ST-segment changes at rest were excluded. If there were minor changes in the ST segment before exercise, an additional 0.15 mV of depression at 80 msec from the J point were required to indicate an abnormal exercise test. R-wave amplitude was measured for an average of six beats during a control period and immediately after exercise, and an increase or no change in the R wave immediately after exercise compared with control was defined as an abnormal response. A decrease in R-wave amplitude was defined as a normal response.

The original population included 1,077 subjects, 888 (82.5%) of whom were contacted for follow-up. Of the 113 subjects who initially had abnormal exercise tests, 105 were located (92.9%). There was a 1.1% incidence of coronary heart disease per year. End points for coronary heart disease were angina pectoris, myocardial infarction, or sudden cardiac death. Only 2 of 221 men 40 years of age or under developed heart disease end points, and neither of the two had ST-segment abnormalities, abnormal R-wave response, or exercise duration of five minutes or less. Hence, in this study, abnormal maximal treadmill test results did not correlate with subsequent coronary heart disease in asymptomatic men 40 years of age or younger. These results contrast with those of a similar study of 563 men 30 to 39 years of age that found a 1.4% incidence of coronary disease. The exercise electrocardiogram was found to have a 50% sensitivity, 95% specificity, 13% predictive value, and a risk ratio of 17, and thus it still had value in this age range (Table XI).

Allen and colleagues concluded that the exercise test was only of value in men older than 40 years of age. For these men, subsequent coronary heart disease within five years was predicted by an abnormal ST-segment response, an increase or no change in R wave, and an exercise duration of five minutes or less. The ST-segment, R-wave, and exercise duration criteria had sensitivities of 41%, 47%, and 26%, respectively. With the test results interpreted as abnormal when either ST- or R-wave criteria were present, sensitivity was 65%. Adding exercise duration of five minutes or less as a third alternative criterion for a positive test did not change sensitivity. The performance of the exercise test responses is summarized in Table XII. When all three criteria were present, a sensitivity of 29% with a specificity of 100% was achieved. In men older than 40 years of age, the ST-segment criteria had the above-mentioned sensitivity of 41%, specificity of 79%, predictive value of 17%, and risk ratio of 2.4. With the exception of predictive value, these values are strikingly lower than those found in earlier studies, including results previously presented by this group.

Of the 311 women whom Allen and colleagues followed, 10 developed coronary heart disease end points. The authors found that ST-segment depression and R-wave response did not correlate with subsequent development of coronary heart disease. Exercise duration of three minutes or less, however, proved to be a significant predictor of coronary heart disease. Four of 13 women with limited exercise tolerance developed coronary heart dis-

TABLE XI
EXERCISE ELECTROCARDIOGRAPHIC TEST PERFORMANCE IN
ASYMPTOMATIC MEN LESS THAN 40 YEARS OF AGE, WITH DIFFERING RESULTS

Principal Investigator	Age Range	N	Incidence of CHD	Years Follow-up	% with Abnormal Exercise Test	Sensitivity	Specificity	Predictive Value	Relative Risk*
Froelicher	30–39	563	1.4%	6.3	5.5	50%	95%	13%	17
Allen	<40	221	0.9%	5.0	3.6	0%	96%	0%	0

*Times that for normal subjects.
CHD = coronary heart disease.

TABLE XII
ABNORMAL EXERCISE TEST RESPONSES IN MEN OVER 40 YEARS OF AGE*

Abnormal Response	Sensitivity	Specificity	Predictive Value	Risk Ratio†
ST depression	41%	79%	17%	2
R-wave increase or no change	47%	78%	19%	3
Exercise duration	27%	96%	43%	6
ST & R wave	40%	86%	27%	5
ST & exercise duration	24%	99%	71%	11
R-wave & exercise duration	33%	99%	82%	12
All three criteria	29%	100%	100%	17

*Allen et al.
†Times that for normal subjects.

ease. When used as a criterion for abnormal, exercise duration of three minutes or less in asymptomatic women had a sensitivity of 40%, specificity of 97%, predictive value of 31%, and risk ratio of 15. Contrary to the conclusions of Allen and colleagues, we feel that maximal exercise tests may prove to be of value in screening asymptomatic women for coronary heart disease. Limited follow-up of 80% of the original population and the low incidence of coronary disease end points in women and in men younger than 40 years of age are limitations of this study.

Bruce and colleagues recently reported a six-year follow-up of 2,365 clinically healthy men (mean age 45 years) who were exercise tested as part of the Seattle Heart Watch. They underwent symptom-limited maximal treadmill testing using neither ST depression nor target heart rates as end points of maximal exercise. The Bruce protocol was used, and the electrocardiogram was monitored with a bipolar CB_5 lead. Conventional risk factors were assessed at the time of the initial examination in a subset of the population. Follow-up was obtained by questionnaire, with morbidity defined as hospital admission. Forty-seven men (2%) experienced coronary heart disease morbidity or mortality. Univariate analysis of the individual conventional risk factors (positive family history, hypertension, smoking, hypercholesterolemia) did not show a statistically significant increase in the five-year probability of primary coronary heart disease events. Only when the sum of risk factors in an individual were assessed did conventional risk factors become statistically significant in relation to the event rate. Four variables from treadmill testing were predictive: (1) exercise duration less than six minutes (which requires 6 to 7 METs, or multiples of resting oxygen requirement); (2) 0.1 mV ST depression during recovery; (3) greater than 10% heart rate impairment (defined as the percent reduction of age-adjusted maximal heart rate); and (4) chest pain during maximal exertion. The ST-segment criteria had a sensitivity of 30%, specificity of 89%, predictive value of 5.3%, and a risk ratio of 3.3. Angina and exercise duration each had sensitivities of about 6%. Heart rate impairment had a sensitivity of 19% and was comparable to ST-segment depression for the other parameters.

Table XIII summarizes the performance of the exercise test predictors. The presence of two or more of the exercise test predictors identified men in all age groups who were at increased risk. Furthermore, it was found that in the presence of one or more conventional risk factors and as the prevalence of exertional risk predictors rose from none to any three, the relative risk rose from 1 to 30. The group that had one or more conventional risk factors and two or more exertional risk predictors was found to have the highest five-year probability of primary coronary heart disease. In the absence of

TABLE XIII
PERFORMANCE OF THE ABNORMAL EXERCISE TEST RESULTS
IN THE SCREENING PORTION OF THE SEATTLE HEART WATCH

Abnormality	Sensitivity	Specificity	Predictive Value	Relative Risk*
ST depression	30%	91%	5%	3.5
Angina	6%	99%	15%	8
Duration	6%	99%	19%	10
Heart rate impairment	19%	93%	7%	4

*Times that for normal subjects.

conventional risk factors, however, exercise testing in this study failed to provide additional prognostic information in normal men.

MacIntyre and colleagues performed maximal exercise tests on 548 fit, healthy middle-aged former aviators at the Naval Aerospace Medical Laboratory. To be included, subjects had to have no clinical evidence of heart or lung disease as determined by history, physical examination, chest x-ray, and a completely normal resting electrocardiogram. Leads X, Y, Z, and V_5 were analyzed only after exercise for 0.1 mV or more of horizontal depression 80 msec after QRS end. Criteria for coronary disease after an eight-year follow-up were sudden death, myocardial infarction, coronary artery bypass surgery, and/or angina. The predictive value of the test was not significantly greater in those with the cardinal risk factors. An abnormal exercise electrocardiogram generated a higher risk ratio than the risk factors.

Maximal or Near-Maximal Exercise Testing and Coronary Angiography. Froelicher and colleagues used cardiac catheterization to evaluate 111 asymptomatic men with an abnormal treadmill test. Only one third of the subjects had at least one lesion equal to or greater than 50% luminal narrowing of a major coronary artery. Barnard and colleagues used near-maximal treadmill testing to screen randomly selected Los Angeles fire fighters. Ten percent showed an abnormal exercise-induced electrocardiographic response despite few risk factors for coronary heart disease. Six men with an abnormal exercise test elected to undergo cardiac catheterization. One had severe three-vessel disease, and another had a 50% obstruction of the left circumflex coronary artery. The other four men had normal studies. Borer and colleagues reported angiographic findings in 11 asymptomatic individuals with hyperlipidemia and an abnormal exercise test. Only 37% were found to

---

TABLE XIV
ANCILLARY TECHNIQUES USED WITH EXERCISE TESTING TO SCREEN FOR ASYMPTOMATIC CORONARY HEART DISEASE

Computerized and new noncomputerized electrocardiographic criteria

Thallium perfusion imaging

Radionuclide ventriculography during bicycle exercise and posttreadmill exercise

Cardiac fluoroscopy for coronary artery calcification

Cardiokymography

Total to high-density lipoprotein cholesterol ratio, conventional risk factors

Electrocardiographic gated chest x-ray preexercise and postexercise

Computerized multifactorial risk prediction using Bayesian statistics (CANDENZA
program, marketed by Cardiokinetics)

Systolic time intervals during and after exercise

---

have angiographically documented coronary heart disease. Erikssen and colleagues reported angiographic findings in 105 men aged 40 to 59 of a working population with one or more of the following criteria: (1) a questionnaire for angina pectoris positive on interview, (2) typical angina during a near-maximal bicycle test, and (3) an abnormal exercise electrocardiogram. The exercise test had a predictive value of 84% if a slowly ascending ST segment was included. The higher predictive value in this study may be due to the older age of the population and inclusion of men with angina.

Numerous techniques have been recommended to improve the sensitivity and specificity of exercise testing. Various computerized criteria for ischemia have been proposed, as well as new standard visual ST criteria. In addition, there are ancillary techniques that could possibly improve the discriminating power of the exercise test. These methods are listed in Table XIV.

New Electrocardiographic Criteria. Lozner and Morganroth studied 37 subjects (10 asymptomatic and 27 symptomatic) who had undergone maximal treadmill testing and coronary angiography to determine whether the predictive value of ST-segment depression could be enhanced. These investigators felt that the predictive value for coronary artery disease could not be enhanced by increasing the degree of ST-segment depression for qualification as abnormal. However, if ST changes that persisted for longer than two minutes were interpreted as a positive test, then a more accurate identification of an abnormal response was possible.

Chahine evaluated the predictive value of an abnormal response by considering different exercise-induced patterns of ST-segment depression. Fifty consecutive symptomatic patients with abnormal ST-segment depression who displayed an evolutionary ST-segment pattern were compared with 50 similar patients with simple ST-segment depression. Those with the evolutionary ST depression showed upsloping or horizontal ST-segment depression followed by a downsloping pattern with complete or partial inversion of the T wave and gradual return to its baseline. Those with simple ST-segment depression showed horizontal or downsloping ST-segment depression returning directly to baseline without any significant T-wave inversion. Correlation of ST depression with coronary angiography showed an overall predictive value of 90%, which improved to 94% after excluding 19 patients who were receiving digitalis. The predictive value improved to 98% when only the patients with evolutionary ST-segment depression were considered, in comparison with 82% in those with simple ST-segment depression.

Thallium-201 Exercise Testing. Caralis and colleagues used thallium-201 exercise testing and coronary angiography to evaluate asymptomatic individuals with abnormal ST-segment responses to exercise testing. Of 3,496 consecutive treadmill exercise tests performed primarily on asymptomatic individuals, 22 developed 0.2 mV or more of asymptomatic horizontal ST-segment depression. These individuals had physical examinations, routine laboratory studies, chest x-rays, and resting electrocardiograms, all of which were normal. Fifteen of these 22 patients agreed to be evaluated further with thallium and coronary angiography. These 15 included 14 men and one woman; the mean age was 52. Thallium-201 was administered intravenously for separate rest and exercise myocardial studies. Myocardial imaging began 10 minutes after administration, and imaging in each of the views required 8 to 12 minutes. The rest and subsequent exercise studies were performed one week apart, and all of the resting studies were normal. The thallium-201 was injected at peak bicycle exercise, and patients were encouraged to keep a constant level of exercise for an additional one minute. Rest and exercise studies were examined together and considered positive for ischemia only if a new perfusion defect involved more than 15% of the left ventricular circumference. Of the 15 asymptomatic individuals with horizontal ST-segment depression on exercise testing, 5 had normal scans with exercise, whereas 10 individuals developed new defects. The angiographic criterion for abnormal was based on 70% luminal narrowing. Four of the five individuals with normal exercise thallium images had normal coronary angiograms, and one had an abnormal angiogram. Of the ten with abnormal exercise scans, nine had significant narrowing of two or more major coronary arteries and one patient had essentially normal coronary vessels. Hence, once subjects were selected

on the basis of an abnormal exercise test, the thallium exercise scans classified 13 of 15 patients properly.

Nolewajka and colleagues performed thallium treadmill tests on 58 a-
symptomatic men as part of a screening study. The risk for coronary heart
disease was determined using the Framingham risk equation, based on age,
cholesterol, systolic blood pressure, cigarette-smoking history, left ventricular hypertrophy on the electrocardiogram, and glucose intolerance. The risk
calculation was greater in those with abnormal exercise studies compared
with those who had normal studies. Five of the subjects had electrocardiographic left ventricular hypertrophy, six had abnormal exercise-induced ST
depression, and six had abnormal thallium scans (five consistent with ischemia, one with scar). Three of the subjects with abnormal thallium studies
underwent coronary angiography, and all had normal coronary arteries. Surprisingly, two of these had left bundle branch block (one with exercise only,
the other at rest). The disappointment of these results was compounded by
the stresses to the individuals who were told they had "abnormal" results.

Uhl and colleagues performed thallium-201 exercise tests on 119 aircrewmen prior to undergoing coronary angiography because of abnormal
treadmill tests or serial ECG changes. Of these, 41 men had significant angiographic disease (equal or greater than 50% occlusion), for a predictive value
of the ECG screening procedures of 21%. The sensitivity of the computer-enhanced thallium exercise test was 95%, as compared with 68% for analog
Polaroid interpretation, and its specificity was 90%. There were mixed results in the 10 men who had minimal angiographic disease (less than 50%
occlusion); 10 had abnormal scans and 5 had normal scans. The high sensitivity and specificity of the computer-enhanced thallium exercise test in this
population of apparently healthy men is a strong support for its use as a
second-line screening procedure.

Radionuclide Left Ventricular Angiography During Exercise. Borer and
associates reported their study of ten men and one woman, all of whom had
coronary heart disease and normal resting left ventricular function confirmed by angiography. Fourteen normal subjects were also studied. Gated
radionuclide angiography was performed in the supine position at rest and
during exercise. Imaging was performed during exercise for at least two
minutes of near-maximal effort. From resting values, ejection fraction increased during exercise in all normal subjects, with the increase ranging
from 7% to 30%. In patients with coronary disease, ejection fraction during
exercise diminished in all but one patient, and in that patient it remained
unchanged. At least one new region of left ventricular dysfunction developed
during exercise in each of the patients with coronary heart disease.

Studies at the University of California, San Diego, have shown gated blood-pool radionuclide ejection fractions to be reproducible at rest and during symptom-limited maximal supine bicycle exercise. An overshoot response of ejection fraction during low levels of exercise and after exercise can occur, especially in physically fit individuals. In our laboratory, an ejection fraction of 0.50 or greater at rest is considered normal, whereas any lower values are abnormal. The normal response to exercise is a 10% increase over the resting value. Patients with coronary heart disease without angina usually have a flat ejection fraction response to exercise, and those with angina have a drop in ejection fraction. Regional wall motion abnormalities should be highly specific for coronary heart disease. We have not found such abnormalities during exercise to be very reproducible, however, and therefore we currently measure only the ejection fraction response to exercise.

The results of resting and exercise electrocardiograms, thallium-201 myocardial perfusion imaging, and equilibrium radionuclide angiography were analyzed in 71 consecutive patients referred to our laboratory for diagnosis or for evaluation of coronary heart disease. The overall sensitivity for the resting and exercise electrocardiogram was 66%; for thallium-201 scan, 74%; for both, 79%; and for the ejection fraction response to exercise, 97%. The specificity was lowest with supine bicycle radionuclide angiography, but all patients with false-positive results had cardiomyopathies. Thus, supine bicycle radionuclide angiography is highly specific for left ventricular dysfunction rather than for coronary heart disease alone. The following approach to evaluate patients with symptoms suggestive of coronary heart disease was proposed. Resting and exercise electrocardiogram remain the first step. The next step should be radionuclide angiography at rest and during exercise to assess left ventricular function. If normal, radionuclide angiography almost always excludes left ventricular dysfunction and hemodynamically significant coronary heart disease. If abnormal, the workup should then proceed to cardiac catheterization if clinically indicated.

At the University of California, San Diego, we have presented an approach using radionuclide angiography to increase the sensitivity and specificity of treadmill testing. Tagged technetium was administered intravenously in order to perform sequential left ventriculograms in ten coronary heart disease patients and eight normal subjects. All 18 subjects underwent maximal treadmill testing. Ejection fractions were measured at two to four, four to six, and eight to ten minutes of recovery. At eight to ten minutes of recovery, all normal subjects but none of the coronary heart disease patients had higher ejection fractions than they did at rest. The addition of regional wall motion analysis after treadmill testing could add further discriminant value. Posttreadmill analysis could be more sensitive than the supine bicycle technique because of the higher work load achieved, and an increase in specificity could possibly be obtained over standard ST-segment analysis by detecting regional wall motion abnormalities.

Cardiokymography. The cardiokymograph is an electronic device that produces noninvasively a representation of regional left ventricular wall motion. It generates an electromagnetic field, and motion within the field causes a change in the frequency of an oscillator. A change in frequency is converted into a change in voltage proportional to the motion. The cardiokymograph produces a recording similar to the apexcardiogram and the kinetocardiogram. The advantage of the cardiokymograph is that it records absolute cardiac motion without chest motion, thus eliminating the distortion problem inherent in both the apexcardiogram and the kinetocardiogram. There is considerable tissue penetration, so the cardiokymograph responds to deeper cardiac motion as well as precordial surface movement. Cardiokymographic recordings have been shown to be predictive of ventriculographic wall motion abnormalities.

Silverberg and colleagues reported their use of the cardiokymograph after exercise in 157 patients, including 27 apparently healthy volunteers and 130 patients with suspected coronary heart disease who underwent coronary angiography. The subjects performed a progressive symptom-limited maximal treadmill test. The cardiokymograph was recorded within two minutes of termination of exercise, and every minute thereafter for 10 minutes. Two sets of empiric criteria for an abnormal cardiokymographic pattern were defined in relation to known effects of ischemia on regional wall motion. The first abnormality was defined as paradoxic systolic outward motion. The second abnormality was defined as development of total absence of inward motion, a resultant holosystolic outward motion, or systolic outward motion occurring for less than the entire period of ejection but not preceded by inward motion. For detecting coronary heart disease in atypical chest pain patients, the cardiokymogram had a higher sensitivity, specificity, and predictive value than did the electrocardiogram. However, no statistical difference existed between the electrocardiogram and the cardiokymogram in asymptomatic patients. This may be explained by the distribution of disease in this study: patients with atypical chest pain had a 30% prevalence of disease, whereas asymptomatic patients had a 64% prevalence of angiographic coronary artery disease. Exercise-induced cardiokymographic abnormalities persisted longer during recovery than electrocardiographic changes. Although the cardiokymogram had higher sensitivity and specificity than the electrocardiogram for the detection of coronary disease in patients with atypical chest pain, the results could be owing to the patient population sample selected for this study.

Coronary Artery Calcification on Fluoroscopic Examination. Kelly and Langou reported the use of cardiac fluoroscopy as a prescreening tool in asymptomatic men prior to exercise tests. In one study, 129 healthy men (average age 49) were evaluated with cardiac fluoroscopy to detect coronary artery calcification, followed by a submaximal exercise test. Of the 108 subjects who completed the exercise test, 37, or 34%, had at least one fluoroscopically detected calcified coronary artery. Of this group of subjects with positive fluoroscopic findings, 13 (35%) had an abnormal ST-segment response to the exercise test. Of the 68 subjects with normal fluoroscopy, only 3 (4%) had an abnormal exercise response. Consequently, those with calcification of at least one coronary artery had a ninefold increased risk of having an abnormal exercise electrocardiographic test. Of the 16 subjects with an abnormal exercise test, 81% had calcification of at least one coronary artery. The location of the calcific deposit conferred greater risk for exercise-induced ischemic changes than did multivessel involvement. Forty-seven percent of men with calcification in the left anterior descending coronary artery had an abnormal exercise electrocardiogram versus 33% and 16% of persons with left circumflex and right coronary artery calcifications, respectively.

In a second study, the 13 men who had both coronary artery calcification and an abnormal exercise test had coronary angiography. They had a mean age of 44, none had any symptoms or signs of coronary disease, and all had a normal resting electrocardiogram. Coronary artery calcification was first detected by fluoroscopy in a single artery in 10 men, in two arteries in two men, and in three arteries in one man. On angiography, coronary artery disease was considered clinically significant if there was greater than 50% luminal narrowing in any major coronary branch. Coronary arteriography revealed 12 men with clinically significant coronary artery disease: single-vessel disease in four, double in five, and triple in three men. One man had only a minor lesion. On a three year follow-up in these 13 patients, 3 had developed typical angina and 1 had developed a transmural myocardial infarction. The results of this study suggest that the combination of coronary artery calcification and an abnormal exercise test is highly predictive of coronary heart disease. However, the sensitivity and specificity of the combination of these procedures remains to be clarified. Questions remaining are: Did the three subjects with an abnormal exercise test and no fluoroscopically detected coronary artery calcification have angiographic disease?, and What of the 24 individuals with coronary artery calcification and a normal exercise electrocardiogram?

Lipid Screening. Total cholesterol to high-density lipoprotein cholesterol (TC-HDL) ratios have been shown to be directly correlated with coronary heart disease risk. In a study by Williams and colleagues on 2,568 asymptomatic men, a TC-HDL ratio of four correlated with a very low coronary heart disease conventional risk factor rating, and a TC-HDL ratio of eight was correlated with very high risk for coronary heart disease.

Uhl and colleagues measured fasting total cholesterol and high-density lipoproteins in 572 asymptomatic aircrewmen. Of these, 132 had an abnormal treadmill test and underwent coronary angiography. Coronary disease defined as a lesion of 50% or greater diameter narrowing was found in 16, with the rest having minimal (N = 14) or no coronary artery disease (N = 102). The 14 men with minimal coronary artery disease had TC-HDL ratios that differed from the normals (*P* < .001). Two of the 16 with angiographic coronary artery disease had TC-HDL ratios of less than six, whereas four of the 102 angiographic normal subjects had a ratio of greater than six. Only 42 of 440 (9.5%) with a normal treadmill test had a total cholesterol to high-density liproprotein cholesterol ratio greater than six; 87% of those with coronary heart disease had TC-HDL ratios greater than six. This ratio generated a risk of 172. A limitation of this study is that true sensitivity cannot be determined because only those with an abnormal treadmill test underwent coronary angiography.

Gated Chest X-Rays. Dinsmore and colleagues reported the use of electrocardiographically-triggered chest x-rays to diagnose coronary heart disease. A bicycle ergometer was pedaled directly in front of an x-ray film cassette, and chest x-rays were taken at rest and at peak exercise. Wall motion abnormalities, volume change, and pulmonary hypertension were criteria for ischemia. They suggest that this procedure is suitable for screening the apparently healthy population, but no data are available yet.

Computer Probability Estimates. Diamond and Forrester have reviewed the literature to estimate pretest likelihood of disease by age, sex, symptoms, and the Framingham risk equation (based on blood pressure, smoking, glucose intolerance, resting electrocardiogram, and cholesterol). In addition, they have considered the sensitivity and specificity of four diagnostic tests (the exercise test, cardiokymography, thallium, and cardiac fluoroscopy) and applied Bayes's theorem. This information has been assimilated in a computer program written in Apple basic that can be used to determine probabilities of coronary disease for a given individual after entry of any of the above data. CADENZA is the acronym for this program and it is commercially available (Cardiokinetics, Seattle).

Systolic Time Intervals. Spodick and colleagues reported that systolic time intervals measured using ear densitography during exercise appeared to improve the sensitivity and specificity of the exercise test. These workers recorded ear densitograms using a photoelectric earpiece attached to the pinna of the ear that enables measurements of the preejection period (PEP) and left ventricular ejection time (LVET). Ten patients with coronary heart disease were compared with 17 normal men. Despite nearly identical heart rate and blood pressure responses, men with coronary heart disease had a significantly greater reduction of preejection period at one minute and four minutes during exercise as well as a greater decrease in the PEP-LVET ratio. The investigators felt that the early fall in the PEP-LVET ratio respresented limited functional reserve, and the subsequent increase was consistent with functional deterioration. Louis and colleagues noted prolongation of left ventricular ejection time postexercise and suggested that this enhanced the diagnostic power of the exercise test. These approaches need further evaluation to determine if they have additional value compared with standard exercise measurements.

Prognosis in Asymptomatic Coronary Disease. Hammermeister and colleagues reported the effects of coronary artery bypass surgery on functional class I and class II patients who were studied as part of the Seattle Heart Watch. The report was based on 227 medically treated and 392 surgically treated patients who were nonrandomly assigned to medical or surgical therapy. Cox's regression analysis was used to correct for the differences in baseline characteristics. Patients with three-vessel disease who underwent surgery had significantly improved survival, but surgically treated patients with one-vessel disease and two-vessel disease did not. The results of this study suggest that surgery may be indicated in the asymptomatic or mildly symptomatic patient with three-vessel disease, moderate impairment of left ventricular function (ejection fraction 31% to 50%), good distal vessels, and no other major medical illness. Asymptomatic patients with normal left ventricular function (ejection fraction greater than 51%) have an excellent prognosis regardless of the treatment.

Hickman and colleagues at USAFSAM followed for approximately five years 90 men aged 45 to 54 years with asymptomatic angiographically documented coronary heart disease without previous infarction. Sixteen patients developed angina, four had myocardial infarctions, and two died suddenly. The events were not significantly different in those with one-, two-, or three-vessel disease. They concluded that in asymptomatic patients with angiographic coronary heart disease, the five-year prognosis was good even in those with high-risk lesions. Conventional risk factors predicted risk more than the angiographic severity of disease did. Angina, as opposed to sudden death or myocardial infarction, was the most common initial event.

Summary. In screening for asymptomatic coronary heart disease, risk factor analysis alone has a sensitivity of only approximately 20%. In the studies reviewed here, sensitivity of the maximal exercise electrocardiogram ranged from 30% to 67%, or in other words, only 30% to 67% (average 55%) of those who developed end points for coronary heart disease had an abnormal electrocardiographic response when tested. The recent studies by Allen and colleagues and by the Seattle Heart Watch show markedly lower sensitivity and predictive value for the exercise electrocardiogram compared with prior investigations. In Allen's study, roughly 20% of the subjects were lost to follow-up; hence, the incidence of coronary heart disease may well have been underestimated. Furthermore, risk factor data were not given for abnormal responders or for those who developed coronary heart disease. The Seattle Heart Watch study is difficult to interpret in light of preceding studies done by Bruce and others. There was no predictive value for an abnormal exercise electrocardiogram in the subgroup that had no risk factors. Unfortunately, not all of the population had a serum cholesterol measurement, so the risk factor data were not complete. Early investigations paid less attention to risk factors. Had previous studies subdivided the population according to the presence and absence of risk factors, perhaps results similar to those of the Seattle Heart Watch would have been obtained. These latter two studies also took into consideration exercise test responses other than ST-segment depression, and thereby improved sensitivity and specificity. Future studies are needed to substantiate these findings.

Because an abnormal exercise electrocardiogram is neither 100% sensitive nor specific, an abnormal test does not absolutely predict the presence of coronary heart disease or its future development; nor does a normal test rule out disease or the future occurrence of coronary events. Some of those individuals who eventually develop coronary disease will change on retesting from a normal to an abnormal response, so possibly serial testing will increase sensitivity. However, McHenry has reported that a change from a negative to a positive test is no more predictive than is an initially abnormal test and an individual has been reported who changed from a normal to an abnormal test but was free of angiographically significant disease.

The predictive value of the abnormal maximal exercise electrocardiogram ranged from 5% to 46% in the studies reviewed. That is, 5% to 46% (average 21%) of the abnormal responders developed coronary heart disease over the follow-up period. Thus, more than one half of the abnormal responders were false positives. The possibility exists that some of these individuals have coronary disease that has yet to manifest itself, but angiographic studies have supported this high false-positive rate when using the exercise test in asymptomatic populations. This result is explained by the fact that the predictive value of an abnormal exercise test response is directly related to the prevalence of coronary heart disease in the population tested. Thus, the usefulness of the test is enhanced in populations with increased risk factors or markers for coronary heart disease.

Exercise testing may prove to have another value in asymptomatic populations in addition to its screening capabilities. Bruce and colleagues examined the motivational effects of maximal exercise testing for modifying risk factors and health habits. A questionnaire was sent to nearly 3,000 men 35 to 65 years of age who had undergone symptom-limited treadmill testing at least one year earlier. Individuals were asked if the treadmill test motivated them to stop smoking (if already a smoker), increase daily exercise, purposely lose weight, reduce the amount of dietary fat, or take medication for hypertension. There was a 69% response to this questionnaire, and 63% of the responders indicated that they had modified one or more risk factors and health habits and that they attributed this change to the exercise test. In fact, a greater percentage of patients with abnormal functional aerobic impairment, compared with normal subjects reported a modification of risk factors or health habits.

Various techniques have been recommended to improve the performance of a maximal exercise test as a screening tool. All of these techniques require further research to optimize methodologies and establish limitations, particularly in regard to their application in asymptomatic populations. Of particular interest is the fact that wall motion abnormalities can precede and can occur without electrocardiographic changes as shown by both animal and human studies. Development of a technique that accurately and reproducibly detects exercise-induced regional wall motion abnormalities could revolutionize identification of latent coronary heart disease.

When considering the use of procedures for a screening tool, one must ask if the procedure fulfills a number of criteria. Before we can recommend the routine application of maximal exercise testing or any other method to screen latent coronary heart disease, it must be demonstrated that acceptable methods of effective treatment are available and that detection and treatment can substantially reduce morbidity, mortality, or both. One study suggests that in asymptomatic patients with three-vessel disease, coronary artery bypass surgery confers improved survival. More research is necessary to demonstrate unequivocally that any form of secondary prevention, medical or surgical, may improve the prognosis for asymptomatic men with coronary heart disease.

Hypothetically, if a method of secondary prevention were proved and available today, we would offer the following three-step approach to screening for asymptomatic coronary heart disease in men over 35 years old. First, angina history, risk factor analysis (including HDL level), and a resting electrocardiogram should be obtained. It must be remembered that the sensitivity and predictive value of these resting techniques are low. If any data collected place the individual at risk, the second step should be a maximal exercise test. If this test is interpreted as abnormal, based on ST-segment shifts and perhaps other abnormal responses, the third step should be utilization of cardiac radionuclide imaging, cardiac fluoroscopy, or cardiokymography. The lack of data on the diagnostic value of these tools in asymptomatic individuals prevents strict recommendations at this time. Good clinical judgment must be exercised to avoid the iatrogenic complication of producing cardiac cripples by mislabeling healthy people.

The greatest advances in health care have been through prevention and not treatment. The physician's interest in expensive invasive testing and in maintaining patient dependency for medications and surgery could be taken as self-serving. The optimal methods for screening are those with the highest sensitivity and specificity available: routine exercise electrocardiography coupled with radionuclide testing procedures. Radionuclide ventriculography has too low a specificity but thallium scintigraphy has excellent sensitivity and specificity. Since there remains some doubt about the risk factor hypothesis, one key strategy would be to identify a high-risk population using the exercise ECG and thallium scintigraphy and design a randomized intervention trial to erase these doubts. Research is needed in applying these techniques to normal subjects, since specificity can only be tested in large numbers of normals. Also it is necessary to see if there is an overlap in calling false positives; i.e., the exercise electrocardiogram and thallium could be abnormal in women because of attenuation by breast tissue causing cold spots and the X phenomena causing ST-segment depression. Also, thallium may be falsely positive for unknown reasons in mitral valve prolapse, as is the exercise electrocardiogram. It must be remembered that a low specificity must be avoided in screening. A key to applying screening procedures is how the physician uses the information. There is no need to cause cardiac cripples, yet the patient should be allowed to know his true status. The severity of the abnormal response must be considered, and serial testing is often appropriate to follow a patient with an abnormal response.

CONCLUSION

Once the diagnosis of coronary heart disease is made, the exercise test still functions in an important way to demonstrate the severity of disease and to establish prognosis. There are two important considerations in evaluating the severity of coronary heart disease: (1) the amount of myocardium in jeopardy due to ischemia and (2) the amount of myocardium remaining or the mechanical reserve of the heart.

Signs of ischemia that can be brought out by the exercise test to judge the amount of ischemic myocardium include angina, ST-segment depression, ST-segment elevation when it occurs without Q waves, and dropping systolic blood pressure (probably only when accompanied by any of the above). When patients have ischemic end points during exercise testing it is nearly impossible to use the exercise test to quantitate the mechanical reserve of the heart. Severe ischemia can be present with an entirely intact, normal ventricle. This situation is suggested by the patient with ischemia who has an entirely normal resting electrocardiogram. Patients are seen often with marked ischemic responses to exercise testing due to an equivalent of left main disease who have both a normal resting electorcardiogram and completely normal resting ventricular function. The double product (systolic blood pressure times heart rate) is a good way of estimating the relative amount of myocardial blood flow at the time of ischemia; the higher or more normal the double product, the less severe the ischemia.

Evaluating the mechanical reserve or the amount of functional heart muscle is still difficult even in the patient without ischemia during exercise testing and even in those only with respiratory or fatigue as test end points. It has been assumed that cardiac function can be estimated by measuring or estimating total body oxygen consumption. But actually there are two reasons for obtaining maximal oxygen consumption: (1) to assess the total aerobic work capacity of the body and (2) to estimate the maximal performance of the heart as a pump. The classic method of measuring maximal oxygen consumption has been to collect expiratory air and use gas analyzers to measure the difference between inspiratory and expiratory oxygen content, and measure flow. A problem with this technique has been the difficulty in accurately measuring flow. This is still best done by collecting expired air in bags over a time interval and then measuring the gas volume. Flow meters are notoriously inaccurate. They are greatly affected by the phasic nature of respiration, moisture, and changes in flow rate. In addition to inaccuracies, the expense of the technical support and equipment necessary makes it even less desirable.

Several approaches have been recommended to estimate total body oxygen consumption ($\dot{V}O_2$) that do not require measurment. Bruce and colleagues have used the relationship between total treadmill time in a standard progressive protocol, and oxygen consumption. The longer the time exercising, the greater the work load achieved and the greater the oxygen consumption. They have used the relationship of oxygen consumption to age, sex, and activity status to estimate functional aerobic impairment. This estimation gives a percent expected aerobic capacity. However, there are difficulties with this approach. The relationship between treadmill time and oxygen consumption is poor (r values of .7 to .8). This makes estimating maximal oxygen consumption from treadmill time for a given individual rather tenuous. Also, the relationship between maximal oxygen consumption and age is weaker, even when sex and activity status are considered. This makes the concept of functional aerobic impairment a very gross estimate indeed. Further complicating this are the problems of (1) a subject hanging-on to the treadmill while walking or running and (2) the amount of treadmill experience. Hanging-on decreases the oxygen cost of a work load and running has a higher oxygen cost than walking at the same speed. Total treadmill time will increase with serial treadmill testing even though measured oxygen consumption stays the same.

Another approach is to keep treadmill time as close to 10 minutes or less as possible, in order to minimize the effects of endurance and maximize the effects of aerobic capacity. In this approach, only the treadmill work load achieved and the time in the final work load need to be considered. Because the mechanical efficiency of the body is roughly constant, the cost of performing any work load has been established. Therefore, the highest work load achieved can be used to estimate maximal oxygen consumption. However, cardiac patients often have a lower measured oxygen consumption than predicted for a given work load. Also, it has been shown that oxygen kinetics are slower in cardiac patients. Because of this, the question of when steady state is achieved is critical in testing such patients. The time in the work loads probably affects the difference between predicted and measured. For instance, at higher work loads (particularly those beyond the anaerobic threshold), it takes longer to narrow the difference between predicted and measured oxygen consumption. These problems are particularly striking in cardiac patients with extensive myocardial damage who can still reach high treadmill work loads. AV O_2 difference must be wider and cardiac output lower in such patients. Frequently, cardiac patients with poor ejection fractions can reach high work loads and the difference between their predicted and measured oxygen consumption is striking. In athletes, the rate of lactic acid production in muscle better correlates with distance running performance than does maximal oxygen consumption. Perhaps differences in the rate of lactic acid production partially explains the dissociation between predicted and measured oxygen consumption in cardiac patients. In addition, these patients often have a lower maximal heart rate, not due to ischemia, but due to a limitation intrinsic to the heart itself. This has been called chronotropic incompetence and heart rate impairment by Ellestad and Bruce, respectively.

Ejection fraction response to exercise has not explained the lower measured oxygen consumption for a work load seen in cardiac patients. A relationship between measured or predicted maximal oxygen consumption and rest or exercise-induced change in ejection fraction has not been demonstrated. Therefore, predicted oxygen consumption, treadmill time, functional aerobic impairment, treadmill work load, or even maximal measured oxygen consumption cannot predict intrinsic myocardial function or mechanical reserve. Perhaps a way to identify patients with poor myocardial reserve will be to consider the difference between predicted and measured oxygen consumption.

What is more important in predicting prognosis in coronary heart disease: resting ejection fraction or total body functional capacity? Both appear to be independent prognostic determinants, but at the present time it appears that total body work capacity is more important. This is rather surprising since ejection fraction approximates the amount of remaining myocardium and would seem to be more predictive for this reason. Treadmill time, functional aerobic impairment, treadmill work load, estimated oxygen consumption, or even measured oxygen consumption have not been found to correlate with intrinsic myocardial function or mechanical reserve as measured by both resting and exercise ejection fraction. Interestingly, poor ventricular function and poor external work capacity function are risk predictors, but possibly in independent fashion. Further work is needed to clarify the relationship of total body functional capacity and myocardial function. It is important to acknowledge the inaccuracies in measuring or estimating maximal oxygen consumption and the difficulties in estimating ventricular function from treadmill performance.

There are many applications of exercise testing that have been demonstrated to have clinical and epidemiologic value. Newer applications include its use as a motivational tool for behavior modification and as a therapeutic tool in cardiac rehabilitation. It is a practical tool that can be used in the office or hospital setting with readily available technology and technical expertise.

REFERENCES
CHAPTER I

METHODOLOGY

Safety Precautions

Atterhog JH, Jonsson B, Samuelsson R: Exercise testing: A prospective study of complication rates. Am Heart J 98:572, 1979.

Bruce RA, Hornstein TR, Blackman JR: Myocardial infarction after normal response to exercise. Circulation 38:552, 1968.

The Committee on Exercise Testing and Training (EM565): A Handbook for Physicians. New York American Heart Association, 1972 and 1975.

The Exercise Standard Book (70-041-A). Dallas American Heart Association, 1979.

Lintgen AB: Death from myocardial infarction after exercise test with normal result. JAMA 235:837, 1976.

McHenry P: Risks of graded exercise testing. Am J Cardiol 39:935, 1977.

Rochmis P, Blackburn H: Exercise tests: A survey of procedures, safety and litigation experience in approximately 170,000 tests. JAMA 217:1061, 1971.

Shepard RJ: Do risks of exercise justify costly caution? Physician and Sports Medicine 5:58, 1977.

Stuart RJ, Ellestad MH: National survey of exercise stress testing facilities. Chest 77:94, 1980.

Recording Instruments

Arbeit SR, Rubin IL, Gross H: Dangers in interpreting the electrocardiogram from the oscilloscope monitor. JAMA 211:453, 1970.

Berson AS, Pipberger HV: Electrocardiographic distortions caused by inadequate high frequency response of direct-writing electrocardiographs. Am Heart J 74:208, 1967.

Berson AS, Pipberger HV: The low-frequency response of electrocardiographs, a frequent source of recording errors. Am Heart J 71:779, 1966.

Bragg-Remschel DA, Anderson CM, Winkle RA: Frequency response characteristics of ambulatory ECG monitoring systems and their implications for ST segment analysis. Am Heart J 103:20, 1982.

Lategola MT, Busby DE, Lyne PJ: ST segment distortions by high-side frequency filtration in direct-writing ECG recorders. Aviat Space Environ Med 48:264, 1977.

Meyer JL: Some instrument induced errors in the ECG. JAMA 201:351, 1967.

Osborne D, Froelicher VF, Stoner DL: Digital storage and analog distortion of an ECG (abstract.) Annual Conference of Engineering in Medicine and Biology, Los Angeles, November 1977.

Pipberger HB, et al: Recommendations for standardization of leads and specifications of instruments and electrocardiography and vectorcardiography. Circulation 55:11, 1975.

Sheffield LT, Prineas R, Cohen H, et al: Task Force II: Quality of ECG records. l0th Bethesda Conference on Optimal Electrocardiography. Am J Cardiol 41:36, 1977.

Exercise Test Modalities

Astrand P, Rodahl K: Textbook of Work Physiology. New York, McGraw-Hill, 1977.

Keul J, Dickhuth HH, Simon G, et al: Effect of static and dynamic exercise on heart volume, contractility, and left ventricular dimensions. Circ Res 48:162, 1981.

Kilbom A, Persson J: Cardiovascular response to combined dynamic and static exercise. Circ Res 48:93, 1981.

Niederberger M, Kusumi BF, Whitkanack S: Disparities in ventilatory and circulatory responses to bicycle and treadmill exercise. Br Heart J 36:377, 1974.

Shepherd J, Blomqvist C, Lind A, et al: Static (isometric) exercise. Circ Res 48:179, 1981.

Wickes JR, Oldridge N, et al: Comparison of the electrocardiographic changes induced by maximum exercise testing with treadmill and cycle ergometer. Circulation 57:1066, 1978.

Supine Versus Erect Exercise Testing

Bevegard S, Holmgren A, Jonsson B: Circulatory studies in well trained athletes at rest and during heavy exercise, with special reference to stroke volume and the influence of body position. Acta Physiol Scand 57:26, 1963.

Epstein SE, Beiser GD, Stampfer M, et al: Characterization of the circulatory response to maximal upright exercise in normal subjects and patients with heart disease. Circulation 35:1049, 1967.

Jones WB, Finchum RN, Russel RO, et al: Transient cardiac output response to multiple levels of supine exercise. J Appl Physiol 28:183, 1970.

Lecerof H: Influence of body position on exercise tolerance, heart rate, blood pressure, and respiration rate in coronary insufficiency. Br Heart J 33:78, 1971.

Thadani U, West RO, Mathew TM, et al: Hemodynamics at rest and during supine and sitting bicycle exercise in patients with coronary artery disease. Am J Cardiol 39:776, 1977.

Thomas H, Gaos C, Reeves TJ: Resting AV O_2 difference and exercise cardiac output. J Appl Physiol 17:922, 1972.

Protocols

Froelicher VF, Brammel H, Davis G, et al: A comparison of the reproducibility and physiologic response to three maximal treadmill exercise protocols. Chest 65:512, 1974.

Froelicher VF, Thompson AJ, Noguera I, et al: Prediction of maximal oxygen consumption: Comparison of the Bruce and Balke treadmill protocols. Chest 68:331, 1975.

Pollock ML, Bohannon RL, Cooper KH, et al: A comparative analysis of four protocols for maximal treadmill stress testing. Am Heart J 92:39, 1976.

Wilmore JH, Norton AC: The Heart and Lungs at Work: A Primer of Exercise Physiology. Schiller Park, Ill, Beckman Instruments, Inc, 1974.

Wolthuis RA, Froelicher VF, Fischer J, et al: A new practical treadmill protocol for clinical use. Am J Cardiol 39:697, 1977.

Submaximal Versus Maximal Exercise Testing

Cumming GR: Yield of ischaemic exercise electrocardiograms in relation to exercise intensity in a normal population. Br Heart J 34:919, 1972.

Sheffield LT, Reeves TJ: Graded exercise in the diagnosis of angina pectoris. Mod Concepts Cardiovasc Dis 34:1, 1965.

Lead Systems

Berson A, Haisty R, Pipberger H: Electrode position effects on Frank lead ECGs. Am Heart J 95:463, 1978.

Blackburn H, Katigbak R: What electrocardiographic leads to take after exercise? Am Heart J 67:184, 1963.

Chaitman B, Hanson J: Comparative sensitivity and specificity of exercise electrocardiographic lead systems. Am J Cardiol 47:1335, 1981.

Froelicher VF, Wolthuis R, Keiser N, et al: A comparison of two bipolar electrocardiographic leads to lead V5. Chest 70:611, 1976.

Kleiner JP, Nelson WP, Boland MJ: The 12-lead electrocardiogram in exercise testing. Arch Intern Med 138:1572, 1978.

Mason RE, Likar I: A new system of multiple-lead electrocardiography. Am Heart J 71:196, 1966.

McHenry P, Morris S: Exercise electrocardiography, in Schlant R, Hurst JW (eds): Advances in Electrocardiography. New York, Grune & Stratton, 1976, p 263.

Rautaharju PM, Prineas RJ, Crow RS, et al: The effect of modified limb electrode positions on electrocardiographic wave amplitudes. J Electrocardiol 13:109, 1980.

Rautaharju PM, Wolf HK, Eifler WJ, et al: A simple procedure of positioning precordial ECG and VCG electrodes using an electrode locator. J Electrocardiol 9:35, 1976.

Robertson D, Kostuk WJ, Ahuja SP: The localization of coronary artery stenoses by 12 lead ECG response to graded exercise test: Support for intercoronary steal. Am Heart J 91:437, 1976.

Tucker SC, Kemp VE, Holland WE, et al: Multiple lead ECG submaximal treadmill exercise tests in angiographically documented coronary heart disease. Angiology 27:149, 1976.

Watanabe K, Bhargava V, Froelicher V: Computer analysis of the exercise ECG: A review. Prog Cardiovasc Dis 22:423, 1980.

Measurement or Estimation of Maximal Oxygen Uptake

Astrand P, Rodahl K: Textbook of Work Physiology, 2nd ed. New York, McGraw-Hill, 1977.

Bruce RA: Progress in exercise cardiology, in Yu P, Goodwin J (eds): Progress In Cardiology, vol 4. Philadelphia, Lea & Febiger, 1974, p 113.

Froelicher VF, Allen M, Lancaster MC: Maximal treadmill testing of normal USAF aircrewmen. Aerospace Medicine 45:310, 1974.

Froelicher VF, Brammel H, Davis, et al: A comparison of three maximal treadmill exercise protocols. J Appl Physiol 36:720, 1974.

Froelicher VF, Lancaster MC: The prediction of maximal oxygen consumption from a continuous exercise treadmill protocol. Am Heart J 87:445, 1974.

Froelicher VF, Thompson AJ, Noguero I, et al: Prediction of maximal oxygen consumption: Comparison of the Bruce and Balke treadmill protocols. Chest 68:331, 1975.

Froelicher VF, Thompson AJ, Yanowitz F, et al: Treadmill exercise testing at the USAF-SAM: Physiological responses in aircrewmen and the detection of latent coronary artery disease. Agardograph No. 210. Springfield, Va, NTIS, 1975.

Harrison M, Brown G, Cochrane L: Maximal oxygen uptake: Its measurement, application, and limitations. Aviat Space Environ Med 51:1123, 1980.

Postexercise Period

Gutman RA, Alexander ER, Li YT, et al: Delay of ST depression after maximal exercise by walking for 2 minutes. Circulation 42:229, 1970.

Froelicher VF, Thompson AJ, Longo MR, et al: Value of exercise testing for screening asymptomatic men for latent coronary artery disease. Prog Cardiovasc Dis 43:265, 1976.

Computerized Exercise Electrocardiographic Analysis

Blomqvist G: The Frank lead exercise electrocardiogram. Acta Med Scand 178(suppl 440):5, 1965.

Bruce RA, Detry JM, Early K, et al: Polarcardiographic responses to maximal exercise in healthy young adults. Am Heart J 83:206, 1972.

Bruce RA, Mazzarella JA, Jordan JR Jr, et al: Quantitation of QRS and ST segment responses to exercise. Am Heart J 71:455, 1966.

Crow RS, Campbell S, Prineas RJ: Accurate automatic measurement of ST-segment response in the exercise electrocardiogram. Comput Biomed Res 11:243, 1978.

Golden DP, Hoffler GW, Wolthuis RA, et al: Vectan II: A computer program for the spatial analysis of the vectorcardiogram. J Electrocardiol 8:217, 1975.

Hollenberg M, Budge WR, Wisneski JA, et al: Treadmill score quantifies electrocardiographic response to exercise and improves test accuracy and reproducibility. Circulation 61:276, 1980.

Hornstein TR, Bruce RA: Computed ST forces of Frank and bipolar exercise electrocardiograms. Am Heart J 78:346, 1969.

McHenry PL, Morris SN: Exercise electrocardiography—current state of the art, in Schlant RC, Hurst JW (eds): Advances In Electrocardiography, vol 2. New York, Grune & Stratton, 1976, p 265.

McHenry PL, Phillips JR, Knoebel SB: Correlation of computer-quantitated treadmill exercise electrocardiogram with arteriographic location of coronary artery disease. Am J Cardiol 30:747, 1972.

McHenry PL, Stowe DE, Lancaster MC: Computer quantitation of the ST-segment response during maximal treadmill exercise. Circulation 38:691, 1968.

Meyer C, Keiser N: Electrocardiogram baseline noise estimation and removal using cubic splines and state space computation techniques. Comput Biomed Res 10:459, 1977.

Mortara DW: A new pattern recognition approach to exercise analysis, in vanBemmel KJ, Williams JL (eds): Trends in Computer-Processed Electrocardiograms. Amsterdam, North-Holland Publishing, 1977, p 407.

Niederberger M, Bruce RA, Dower GE, et al: Influence of age and ischemic heart disease on spatial ST-T magnitudes at rest and after maximal exercise. J Electrocardiol 6:279, 1973.

Rautaharju PM, Punsar S, Blackburn H, et al: Waveform pattern in Frank-lead rest and exercise electrocardiograms of healthy elderly men. Circulation 43:541, 1973.

Sheffield LT, Holt TH, Lester FM, et al: On-line analysis of the exercise electrocardiogram. Circ 40:935, 1969.

Simoons ML: Optimal measurements for detection of coronary artery disease by exercise electrocardiography. Comput Biomed Res 10:483, 1977.

Simoons ML, Boom HD, Smallenburg E: On-line processing of orthogonal exercise electrocardiograms. Comput Biomed Res 8:105, 1975.

Simoons ML, Van Den Brand M, Hugenholtz PG: Quantitative analysis of exercise electrocardiograms and left ventricular angiograms in patients with abnormal QRS complexes at rest. Circulation 55:55, 1977.

Simoons M, Block P, Ascoop C, et al: Computer processing of exercise ECGs—A cooperative study, in vanBemmel KJ, Williams JL (eds): Trends in Computer-Processed Electrocardiograms. Amsterdam, North-Holland Publishing, 1977, p 383.

Sketch MH, Mohiuddin SM, Nair CK, et al: Automated and nomographic analysis of exercise tests. JAMA 243:1051, 1980.

Subramanian VB, Lahiri A, Paramasivan R, et al: Long-term verapamil in angina evaluated by computerized treadmill exercise. Am J Cardiol 48:529, 1981.

Taback L, Marden E, Mason HL, et al: Digital recording of electrocardiographic data for analysis by digital computer. IRE Transaction on Medical Electronics ME-6:167, 1959.

vanBemmel JH, Talmon JL, Duisterhout JS, et al: Template waveform recognition applied to ECG/VCG analysis. Comput Biomed Res 6:430, 1973.

Werner JO, Jansson L, Johansson K, et al: A system for computer-assisted ECG recording at rest and exercise. Scand J Clin Lab Invest 36:7, 1976.

Werner O, Johansson K, Jonson B: Computer classification of ST and T in averaged ECGs during rest and exercise. Scand J Clin Lab Invest 36:31, 1976.

Wolf HK, Stock MS, Helppi RK, et al: Computer analysis of rest and exercise electrocardiograms. Comput Biomed Res 5:329, 1972.

Wolthuis R, Hopkirk A, Keiser N, et al: T-waves in the exercise ECG: Their location and occurrence. IEEE Transactions on Biomedical Engineering 26:639, 1979.

Yanowitz F, Froelicher VF, Keiser N, et al: Quantitative exercise ECG in the evaluation of patients with early coronary artery disease. Aerospace Medicine 45:443, 1974.

INTERPRETATION

Functional Capacity

Astrand P: Quantification of exercise capability and evaluation of physical capacity in man. Prog Cardiovasc Dis 19:51, 1976.

Bruce RA: Exercise testing for evaluation of ventricular function. N Engl J Med 296:671, 1977.

Bruce R, Fischer LD, Cooper MN: Separation of effects of cardiovascular disease and age on ventricular function with maximal exercise. Am J Cardiol 34:758, 1974.

Bruce RA, Kusumi F, Niederberger M, et al: Cardiovascular mechanisms of functional aerobic impairment in patients with coronary heart disease. Circulation 49:696, 1974.

Hossack K, Bruce R, Green B, et al: Maximal cardiac output during upright exercise: Approximate normal standards and variations with coronary heart disease. Am J Cardiol 46:204, 1980.

McDonough JR, Danielson RA, Wills RE, et al: Maximal cardiac output during exercise in patients with coronary artery disease. Am J Cardiol 33:23, 1974.

McGraw BF, Hemberger, JA, Smith AL, et al: Variability of exercise performance during long-term placebo treatment. Clin Pharmacol Ther 30:321, 1981.

Mitchell JH, Blomqvist G: Maximal oxygen uptake. N Engl J Med 284:1018, 1971.

Patterson J, Naughton J, Pietras R, et al: Treadmill exercise in assessment of the functional capacity of patients with cardiac disease. Am J Cardiol 30:757, 1972.

Wasserman K, Whipp B: Exercise physiology in health and disease. Am Rev Respir Dis 112:219, 1975.

Heart Rate and Blood Pressure Response

Brunelli C, Lazzari M, Simonetti I, et al: Variable threshold of exertional angina: A clue to a vasospastic component. Eur Heart J 2:155, 1981.

Ellestad MH, Wan MK: Predictive implications of stress testing: Followup of 2700 subjects after maximal treadmill stress test. Circulation 51:363, 1975.

Irving JB, Bruce RA: Exertional hypotension and postexertional ventricular fibrillation in stress testing. Am J Cardiol 39:849, 1977.

Morris SN, McHenry PL: The incidence and significance of exercise-induced drop in systolic blood pressure. Am J Cardiol 41:221, 1978.

Nelson RR, Gobel FL, Jorgensen CR, et al: Hemodynamic predictors of myocardial oxygen consumption during static and dynamic exercise. Circulation 50:1179, 1974.

Rowell L: What signals govern the cardiovascular response to exercise? Med Sci Sports 12:307, 1980.

Schiffer F, Hartley L, Schulman C, et al: Evidence for emotionally induced coronary arterial spasm in patients with angina pectoris. Br Heart J 44:662, 1980.

Sheps DS, Ernst JC, Briese FW, et al: Exercise-induced increase in diastolic pressure: Indicator of severe coronary artery disease. Am J Cardiol 43:708, 1979.

Thomson PD, Kelemen MH: Hypotension accompanying the onset of exertional angina. Circulation 52:28, 1975.

Wolthuis RA, Froelicher VF, Fischer J, et al: The response of healthy men to treadmill exercise. Circulation 55:153, 1977.

The Electrocardiographic Response to Exercise

Battler A, Froelicher VF, Gallagher KP, et al: Effects of changes in ventricular size on regional and surface QRS amplitudes in the conscious dog. Circulation 62:735, 1980.

Battler A, Froelicher V, Slutsky R, et al: Relationship of QRS amplitude changes during exercise to left ventricular function, volumes, and the diagnosis of coronary artery disease. Circulation 60:1004, 1979.

Bonoris PE, Greenberg PS, Castellanet MJ, et al: Significance of changes in R-wave amplitude during treadmill stress testing: Angiographic correlation. Am J Cardiol 41:846, 1978.

Coester N, Elliott JC, Luft UC: Plasma electrolytes, pH, and ECG during and after exhaustive exercise. J Appl Physiol 34:677, 1973.

Cohen D, Kaufman LA: Magnetic determination of the relationship between the ST segment shift and the injury current produced by coronary artery occlusion. Circ Res 36:414, 1976.

DeLanne R, Barnes JR, Brouha L: Changes in osmotic pressure and ionic concentrations of plasma during muscular work and recovery. J Appl Physiol 14:804, 1959.

Dunn RF, Freedman B, Bailey IK, et al: Localization of coronary artery disease with exercise electrocardiography: Correlation with thallium-201 myocardial perfusion scanning. Am J Cardiol 48:837, 1981.

Einthoven W: Weiteres uber das Electrokardiogram. Archives Physiology 122:517, 1908.

Ekmekli A, Toyoshima I, Kwozynsei JK, et al: Angina pectoris: Clinical and experimental difference between ischemia with ST elevation and ischemia with ST depression. Am J Cardiol 7:412, 1961.

Gerson MC, Phillips JF, Morris SN, et al: Exercise induced U wave inversion as a marker of stenosis of the left anterior descending coronary artery. Circulation 60:1014, 1979.

Greenberg PS, Ellestad MH, Berge R, et al: Radionuclide angiographic correlation of the R wave, ejection fraction, and volume responses to upright bicycle exercise. Chest 80:459, 1981.

Greenspan M, Anderson GJ: The significance of exercise-induced Q waves. Am J Med 67:454, 1979.

Katzeff IE, Edwards H: Exercise testing: Does the S wave voltage change with increasing work rate? S Afr Med J 49:1088, 1974.

Kentala E, Heikkila J, Pyorala K: Variation of QRS amplitude in exercise ECG as an index predicting result of physical training in patients with coronary heart disease. Acta Med Scand 194:81, 1973.

Kilpatrick D: Exercise vectorcardiography in diagnosis of ischemic heart disease. Lancet 2:332, 1976.

Laciga P, Koller EA: Respiratory, circulatory, and ECG changes during acute exposure to high altitude. J Appl Physiol 41:159, 1976.

Lade R, Brown EB Jr: Movement of potassium between muscle and blood in response to respiratory acidosis. Am J Physiol 204:761, 1963.

Mirvis DM, Keller DW, Cox JW Jr, et al: Left precordial isopotential mapping during supine exercise. Circulation 56:245, 1977.

Morales-Ballejo H, Greenberg P, Ellestad M, et al: Septal Q wave in exercise testing: Angiographic correlation. Am J Cardiol 48:247, 1981.

Oliveros R, Seaworth J, Diabal P, et al: Electrocardiographic aspects of acute left anterior hemiblock induced by exercise. Aviat Space Environ Med 51:1144, 1980.

Rautaharju PM, Punsar S, Blackburn H, et al: Waveform patterns in Frank-lead rest and exercise electrocardiograms of healthy elderly men. Circulation 48:541, 1973.

Riff D, Carleton R: Effect of exercise on the atrial recovery wave. Am Heart J 82:759, 1971.

Rogers JH Jr, Hellerstein HK, Strong WB: The exercise electrocardiogram in trained and untrained adolescent males. Med Sci Sports 9:164, 1977.

Rose KD, Dunn FL, Bargen D: Serum electrolyte relationship to electrocardiographic change in exercising athletes. JAMA 195:155, 1966.

Ross J Jr: Electrocardiographic ST-segment analysis in the characterization of myocardial ischemia and infarction. Circulation 53:73, 1976.

Simonson E: Effect of moderate exercise on the electrocardiogram in healthy young and middle-aged men. J Appl Physiol 5:584, 1953.

Simoons ML, Hugenholtz PG: Gradual changes of ECG and waveform during and after exercise in normal subjects. Circulation 52:570, 1975.

Slutsky R, Froelicher VF: Electrocardiographic response to dynamic exercise, in Hutton R (ed): Exercise and Sports Reviews, vol 6. Philadelphia, Franklin Institute Press, 1979, p 105.

Vincent GM, Abildskov JA, Burgess MJ: Mechanisms of ST displacement in myocardial ischemia. Circulation 56:559, 1977.

Watanabe K, Bhargave V, Froelicher VF: The relationship between exercise-induced R wave amplitude changes and QRS vector loops. J Electrocardiol 14:129, 1981.

Wolthuis RA, Froelicher VF, Hopkirk A, et al: Normal electrocardiographic waveform characteristics during treadmill exercise testing. Circulation 60:1028, 1979.

Abnormal Segment Changes

ST-Segment Elevations

Bobba P, Vecchio C, DiGulieloma L, et al: Exercise induced RS T elevation. Cardiology 57:162, 1972.

Chahine RA, Raziner AE, Ishimori T: The clinical significance of exercise induced ST segment elevation. Circulation 54:209, 1976.

Chaitman B, Waters D, Theroux P, et al: ST segment elevation and coronary spasm in response to exercise. Am J Cardiol 47:1350, 1981.

De Feyter PJ, Majid PA, Van Eenige MJ, et al: Clinical significance of exercise-induced ST segment elevation. Br Heart J 46:84, 1981.

Dunn RF, Bailey IK, Uren R, et al: Exercise-induced ST-segment elevation: Correlation of thallium-201 myocardial perfusion scanning and coronary arteriography. Circulation 61:989, 1980.

Dunn RF, Freedman B, Kelly DT: Exercise-induced ST-segment elevation in leads V1 or aVL. Circulation 63:1357, 1981.

Fortuin NJ, Friesinger GC: Exercise induced ST segment elevation. Am J Med 49:459, 1970.

Guyton RA, McClenathan JH, Newman GE, et al: Significance of subendocardial ST segment elevation caused by coronary stenosis in the dog. Am J Cardiol 40:373, 1977.

Hegge FN, Tuna N, Churchill HB: Coronary arteriographic findings in patients with axis shifts or ST segment elevation on exercise stress testing. Am Heart J 86:63, 1973.

Holland R, Arnsdorf MB: Solid angle theory and the electrocardiogram: Physiologic and quantitative interpretations. Prog Cardiovasc Dis 19:431, 1977.

Lahiri A, Blasubrahanian V, Craig M, et al: Exercise-induced ST segment elevation— electrocardiographic, angiographic, and scintigraphic evaluation. Br Heart J 43:582, 1980.

Longhurst J, Kraus W: Exercise-induced ST elevation in patients without myocardial infarction. Circulation 60:616, 1979.

Manvi KN, Ellestad MH: Elevated ST segment with exercise in ventricular aneurysm. J Electrocardiol 5:317, 1972.

Servi S, Falcone C, Gavazzi G, et al: The exercise test in variant angina: Results in 114 patients. Circulation 64:684, 1981.

Simoons ML, Brand M, Hugenholtz PG: Quantitative analysis of exercise ECGs and left ventricular angiograms in patients with abnormal QRS complexes at rest. Circulation 55:55, 1977.

Simoons ML, Withagen A, Vinke R, et al: ST-vector orientation and location of myocardial perfusion defects during exercise. Nucl Med 17:154, 1978.

Sriwattanakomen S, Ticzon A, Zubritzky S, et al: ST elevation during exercise. Am J Cardiol 45:762, 1980.

Stiles G, Rosati R, Wallace A: Clinical relevance of exercise-induced S-T segment elevation. Am J Cardiol 46:931, 1980.

Vincent G, Abildskov JA, Burgess M: Mechanisms of ischemic ST segment displacement. Circulation 56:559, 1977.

ST-Segment Normalization or Absence of Change

Haiat R, Halpen C, Derrida JP, et al: Pseudonormalization of the repolarization during transient episodes of myocardial ischemia. Am Heart J 94:390, 1977.

Nobel RJ, Rothbaum DA, Knoebel SB, et al: Normalization of abnormal T waves in ischemia. Arch Intern Med 136:391, 1976.

Sweet RL, Sheffield LT: Myocardial infarction after exercise-induced electrocardiographic changes in a patient with variant angina pectoris. Am J Cardiol 33:813, 1974.

ST-Segment Depression

Goldman S, Tselos S, Cohn K: Marked depth of ST segment depression during treadmill exercise testing: Indicator of severe coronary artery disease. Chest 69:729, 1976.

Kurita A, Chaitman B, Bourassa M: Significance of exercise-induced junctional S-T depression in evaluation of coronary artery disease. Am J Cardiol 40:492, 1977.

Exercise-Induced ST-Segment Depression Not Due To Coronary Artery Disease

Adair RF, Hellerstein HK, White LW: Digoxin induced exercise ECG changes in young men: ST-T walk through phenomena above 80% maximal heart rate. Circulation 45:11, 1972.

Alvarez-Mena S, Frank M: Phenothiazine-induced T wave abnormalities. JAMA 224:1730, 1973.

Aronow WS, Harris CN: Treadmill exercise test in aortic stenosis and mitral stenosis. Chest 68:507, 1975.

Astrand I, Blomqvist G, Orinius E: ST changes at exercise in patients with short P-R interval. Acta Med Scand 185:205, 1969.

Barnard R, MacAlpin R, Kattus A, et al: Ischemic response to sudden strenuous exercise in healthy men. Circulation 48:936, 1973.

Bruce RA: The effects of digoxin on fatiguing static and dynamic exercise in man. Clin Sci 34:29, 1968.

Cumming GR, Dufresne C, Samm J: Exercise ECG changes in normal women. CMA Journal 109:108, 1973.

Evans DW, Lum LC: Hyperventilation: An important cause of pseudoangina. Lancet 1:155, 1977.

Friesinger G, Biern R, Likar I, et al: Exercise ECG and vasoregulatory abnormalities. Am J Cardiol 30:733, 1972.

Gazes PC: False positive exercise test in WPW. Am Heart J 78:13, 1969.

Georgopoulos A, Proudfit W, Page I: Effect of exercise on ECG of patients with low serum potassium. Circulation 23:567, 1961.

Goldstein RE, Redwood DR, Rosing DR, et al: Alterations in the circulatory response to exercise following a meal and their relationship to postprandial angina pectoris. Circulation 44:90, 1971.

Grant D, Crawford MH, O'Rourke RA: Effects of diazepam on the exercise electrocardiogram. Am Heart J 102:465, 1981.

Harris C, Aronow W, Parker D, et al: Treadmill stress test in left ventricular hypertrophy. Chest 63:353, 1973.

Hellerstein HK, Prozan GB, Liebow IM, et al: Two step exercise test as a test of cardiac function in chronic rheumatic heart disease and in arteriosclerotic heart disease with old myocardial infarction. Am J Cardiol 7:234, 1961.

Kansal S, Roitman D, Sheffield LT: Stress testing with ST-segment depression at rest: An angiographic correlation. Circulation 54:636, 1976.

Lachman A, Semler H, Gustafson R: Postural ST-T wave changes in the electrocardiogram simulating myocardial ischemia. Circulation 31:557, 1965.

Lary D, Goldschlager N: Electrocardiographic changes during hyperventilation resembling myocardial ischemia in patients with normal coronary arteriograms. Am Heart J 87:383, 1974.

Lobstein HP, Horwitz LD, Curry GC, et al: Electrocardiographic abnormalities and coronary arteriograms in the mitral click-murmur syndrome. N Engl J Med 289:127, 1973.

McHenry P, Cogan O, Elliott W, et al: False-positive ECG response to exercise secondary to hyperventilation: Cineangiographic correlation. Am Heart J 79:683, 1970.

Profant GR, Early RG, Nilson KL, et al: Responses to maximal exercise in healthy middle-aged women. J Appl Physiol 33:955, 1972.

Ramsey LH, Beeble J: Electrocardiographic response to exercise in patients with mitral stenosis. Circulation 19:424, 1959.

Riley C, Oberman A, Sheffield L: Electrocardiographic effects of glucose ingestion. Arch Intern Med 130:703, 1972.

Simonson E, Keys A: The effect of an ordinary meal on the electrocardiogram. Circulation 1:1000, 1950.

Sketch MH, Mohinddin SM, Lynch JD, et al: Significant sex differences in the correlation of electrocardiographic exercise testing and coronary arteriograms. Am J Cardiol 36:169, 1975.

Sketch MH, Moss AN, Butler ML, et al: Digoxin-induced positive exercise tests: Their clinical and prognostic significance. Am J Cardiol 48:655, 1981.

Soloff L, Fewell J: Abnormal ECG responses to exercise in subjects with hypokalemia. Am J Med Sci 242:724, 1961.

Tanaka T, Friedman M, Okada R, et al: Diagnostic value of exercise-induced S-T segment depression in patients with right bundle branch block. Am J Cardiol 41:670, 1978.

Whinnery JE, Froelicher VF: Acquired bundle branch block and its response to exercise testing in asymptomatic aircrewmen: A review with case reports. Aviat Space Environ Med 47:1217, 1976.

Whinnery JE, Froelicher VF, Stewart AJ, et al; The electrocardiographic response to maximal treadmill exercise of asymptomatic men with left bundle branch block. Am Heart J 94:316, 1977.

Whinnery JE, Froelicher VF, Stewart A, et al: The electrocardiographic response to maximal treadmill exercise of asymptomatic men with right bundle branch block. Chest 71:335, 1977.

Whinnery JE, Froelicher VF: Exercise testing in right bundle branch block. Chest 72:684, 1977.

Exercise-Induced Ventricular Dysrhythmias

Abbott JA, Hirschfeld DS, Kunkel FW, et al: Graded exercise testing in patients with sinus node dysfunction. Am J Med 62:330, 1972.

Blackburn H, Taylor HL, Hamrell B, et al: Premature ventricular complexes induced by stress testing. Am J Cardiol 31:441, 1973.

Codini MA, Sommerfeldt L, Eyel CE, et al: Clinical significance and characteristics of exercise-induced ventricular tachycardia. Cathet Cardiovasc Diagn 7:227, 1981.

Faris JV, McHenry PL, Jordan JW: The prevalence and reproducibility of exercise-induced PVCs during maximal exercise in normal men. Am J Cardiol 37:617, 1976.

Faris JV, Morris SN: Detection, prevalence, and significance of arrhythmias during exercise. Heart Lung 10:644, 1981.

Goldschlager N, Cake D, Cohn K: Exercise-induced ventricular arrhythmias in patients with coronary artery disease. Am J Cardiol 31:434, 1973.

Goldschlager N, Cohn K, Goldschlager A: Exercise-induced ventricular arrhythmias. Mod Concepts Cardiovasc Dis 48:67, 1979.

Josephson ME, Horowitz LN, Waxman HL, et al: Sustained ventricular tachycardia: Role of the 12-lead electrocardiogram in localizing site of origin. Circulation 64:257, 1981.

McHenry PL, Faris JV, Jordan JW, et al: Comparative study of cardiovascular function and ventricular premature complexes in smokers and nonsmokers during maximal treadmill exercise. Am J Cardiol 39:493, 1977.

McHenry PL, Morris SN, Kavalier M: Exercise-induced arrhythmias—recognition, classification, and clinical significance. Cardiovasc Clin 6:245, 1974.

McHenry PL, Morris SN, Kavalier M, et al: Comparative study of exercise-induced ventricular arrhythmias in normal subjects and patients with documented coronary artery disease. Am J Cardiol 37:609, 1976.

Moss A: Clinical significance of ventricular arrhythmias in patients with and without coronary artery disease. Prog Cardiovasc Dis 23:33, 1980.

Rozanski J, Castellanos A, Sheps D, et al: Paroxysmal second-degree atrioventricular block induced by exercise. Heart Lung 9:887, 1980.

Ryan M, Lown B, Horn H: Comparison of ventricular ectopic activity during 24 hour monitoring and exercise testing in patients with coronary artery disease. N Engl J Med 292:224, 1975.

Sheps DS, Ernst JC, Briese FR, et al: Decreased frequency of exercise-induced ventricular ectopic activity in the second of two consecutive treadmill tests. Circulation 55:892, 1977.

Udall JA, Ellestad MH: Predictive implications of ventricular premature contractions associated with treadmill stress testing. Circulation 56:985, 1977.

Subjective Responses

Cole J, Ellestad M: Significance of chest pain during treadmill exercise. Am J Cardiol 41:227, 1978.

Lown B: Verbal conditioning of angina pectoris during exercise testing. Am J Cardiol 40:630, 1977.

Weiner DM, McCabe C, Hueter D, et al: The predictive value of anginal chest pain as an indicator of coronary disease during exercise testing. Am Heart J 96:458, 1978.

Observer Agreement in Interpretation

Acheson RM: Observer error and variation in the interpretation of electrocardiograms in an epidemiological study of coronary heart disease. Br J Prev Soc Med 14:99, 1960.

Atwood JE, Jensen D, Froelicher V, et al: Agreement in human interpretation of analog thallium myocardial perfusion images. Circulation 64:601, 1981.

Blackburn H: The exercise electrocardiogram: Differences in interpretation. Am J Cardiol 21:871, 1968.

Botvinick EH, Dunn RF, Hattner RS, et al: A consideration of factors affecting the diagnostic accuracy of thallium-201 myocardial perfusion scintigraphy in detecting coronary artery disease. Semin Nucl Med 10:157, 1980.

Chaitman BR, DeMots H, Bristow JD, et al; Objective and subjective analysis of left ventricular angiograms. Circulation 52:420, 1975.

Crawford MH, Grant D, O'Rourke RA, et al: Accuracy and reproducibility of new M-mode echocardiographic recommendations for measuring left ventricular dimensions. Circulation 61:137, 1980.

Davies LG: Observer variation in reports on electrocardiograms. Br Heart J 20:153, 1958.

Detre KM, Wright E, Murphy ML, et al: Observer agreement in evaluating coronary angiograms. Circulation 52:979, 1975.

Felner JM, Blumenstein BA, Schlant RC, et al: Sources of variability in echocardiographic measurements. Am J Cardiol 45:995, 1980.

Galbraith JE, Murphy ML, de Soyza N: Coronary angiogram interpretation. JAMA 240:2053, 1978.

McLaughlin PR, Martin RP, Doherty P, et al: Reproducibility of thallium-201 myocardial imaging. Circulation 55:497, 1977.

Mason JW, Myers RW, Goris ML, et al: Reliability and reproducibility of interpretation of 99m technetium pyrophosphate myocardial scintigrams. Clin Cardiol 2:446, 1979.

Mead TW, Gardner MJ, Cannon P, et al: Observer variability in recording the peripheral pulses. Br Heart J 30:661, 1968.

Okada RD, Kirshenbaum HD, Kushner FG, et al: Observer variance in the qualitative evaluation of left ventricular wall motion and the quantitation of left ventricular ejection fraction using rest and exercise multigated blood pool imaging. Circulation 61:128, 1980.

Raftery EB, Holland WW: Examination of the heart: An investigation into variation. Am J Epidemiol 85:438, 1967.

Rose GA, Blackburn H: Minnesota code for resting electrocardiograms, in Cardiovascular Survey Methods. Brussels, World Health Organization, 1968, p 137.

Sahn DJ, DeMaria A, Kisslo J, et al: Recommendations regarding quantitation in M-mode echocardiography: Results of a survey of echocardiographic measurements. Circulation 58:1072, 1978.

Schieken RM, Clarke WR, Mahoney LT, et al: Measurement criteria for group echocardiographic studies. Am J Epidemiol 110:504, 1979.

Segall HN: The electrocardiogram and its interpretation: A study of reports by 20 physicians on a set of 100 electrocardiograms. Can Med Assoc J 82:2, 1960.

Simonson E, Tuna N, Okamoto N, et al: Diagnostic accuracy of the vectorcardiogram and electrocardiogram. Am J Cardiol 17:829, 1966.

Slutsky R, Karliner J, Battler A, et al: Reproducibility of ejection fraction and ventricular volume by gated radionuclide angiography after myocardial infarction. Radiology 132:155, 1979.

Trobaugh GB, Wackers FJ, Sokole EB, et al: Thallium-201 myocardial imaging: An interinstitutional study of observer variability. J Nucl Med 19:359, 1978.

Zir LM, Miller SW, Dinsmore RE, et al: Interobserver variability in coronary angiography. Circulation·53:627, 1976.

APPLICATIONS

Diagnosis of Chest Pain and Other Cardiac Findings

Ascoop CA, Simoons ML, Egmond WE, et al: Exercise test, history, and serum lipid levels in patients with chest pain and normal electrocardiogrm at rest: comparison to findings at coronary arteriography. Am Heart J 82:609, 1971.

Bartel AG, Behar VS, Peter RH, et al: Graded exercise stress tests in angiographically documented coronary artery disease. Circulation 49:348, 1974.

Campeau L, Bourassa MG, Bois MA, et al: Clinical significance of selective coronary cinearteriography. Can Med Assoc J 99:1063, 1968.

Chaitman BR, Hanson JS: Comparative sensitivity and specificity of exercise electrocardiographic lead systems. Am J Cardiol 47:1335, 1981.

Cutler B, Wheeler H, Paraskos J, et al: Applicability and interpretation of electrocardiographic stress testing in patients with peripheral vascular disease. Am J Surg 141:501, 1981.

Friesinger GC, Smith RF: Correlation of electrocardiographic studies and arteriographic findings with angina pectoris. Circulation 46:1173, 1972.

Gensini GG, Kelly AE: Incidence and progression of coronary artery disease: An angiographic correlation in 1,263 patients. Arch Intern Med 129:814, 1972.

Goldschlager N, Selzer A, Cohn K: Treadmill stress tests as indicators of presence and severity of coronary artery disease. Ann Intern Med 85:277, 1976.

Harris JM: The hazards of bedside Bayes. JAMA 246:2602, 1981.

Helfant RH, Banka V, DeVilla MA, et al: Use of bicycle ergometry and sustained handgrip exercise in the diagnosis of presence and extent of coronary artery disease. Br Heart J 35:1321, 1973.

Kassebaum DG, Sutherland KI, Judkins MP: A comparison of hypoxemia and exercise electrocardiography in coronary artery disease: Diagnostic precision of the methods correlated with coronary angiography. Am Heart J 75:759, 1968.

McConahay DR, McCallister BD, Smith RE: Post-exercise electrocardiography: Correlation with coronary arteriography and left ventricular hemodynamics. Am J Cardiol 28:1, 1972.

McHenry PL, Phillips JF, Knoebel SB: Correlation of computer-quantitated treadmill exercise electrocardiogram with arteriographic location of coronary artery disease. Am J Cardiol 30:747, 1972.

Martin CM, McConahay DR: Maximal treadmill exercise electrocardiograpy: Correlations with coronary arteriography and cardiac hemodynamics. Circulation 46:956, 1972.

Mason RE, Likar I, Biern RO, et al: Multiple-lead exercise electrocardiography: Experience in 107 normal subjects and 67 patients with angina pectoris and comparison with coronary cinearteriography in 84 patients. Circulation 36:517, 1967.

Neill WA, Pantley GA, Nakornchai V: Respiratory alkalemia during exercise reduces angina threshold. Chest 80:149, 1981.

Proudfit WL, Shirey EK, Sones FM: Selective cinecoronary angiography: Correlation with clinical findings in 1,000 patients. Circulation 33:901, 1966.

Roitman D, Jones WB, Sheffield LT: Comparison of submaximal exercise ECG test with coronary cineangiocardiogram. Ann Intern Med 72:641, 1970.

Sheffield LT, Reeves TJ, Blackburn H, et al: The exercise test in perspective (editorial). Circulation 55:681, 1977.

Shephard R: A critique: Coronary disease and exercise stress tests. Can Fam Physician 26:555, 1980.

Sox HC, Margulies I, Sox CH: Psychologically mediated effects of diagnostic tests. Ann Intern Med 95:680, 1981.

Determination of Prognosis and Severity

Bruce RA, DeRouen TA, Hammermeister KE: Noninvasive screening criteria for enhanced 4-year survival after aortocoronary bypass surgery. Circulation 60:638, 1979.

Levites R, Anderson GJ: Detection of critical coronary lesions with treadmill exercise testing: Fact or fiction? Am J Cardiol 42:533, 1978.

McNeer JF, Margolis JR, Lee KL, et al: The role of the exercise test in the evaluation of patients for ischemic heart disease. Circulation 57:64, 1978.

Nixon JV, Lipscomb K, Blomqvist CG, et al: Exercise testing in men with significant left main coronary disease. Br Heart J 42:410, 1979.

Podrid PJ, Graboys T, Lown B: Prognosis of medically treated patients with coronary artery disease with profound ST segment depression during exercise testing. N Engl J Med 305:1111, 1981.

Weiner DA, McCabe CH, Ryan TJ: Identification of patients with left main and three vessel coronary disease with clinical and exercise test variables. Am J Cardiol 46:21, 1980.

Weiner DA, Ryan TJ, McCabe CH, et al: Correlations among history of angina, ST-segment response and prevalence of coronary-artery disease in the coronary artery surgery study (CASS). N Engl J Med 301: 230, 1979.

Evaluation of Treatment

Bartel AG, Behar VS, Peter RH, et al: Exercise stress testing in evaluation of aortocoronary bypass surgery: Report of 123 patients. Circulation 48:141, 1973.

Brown HV, Wasserman K: Exercise performance in chronic obstructive pulmonary diseases. Med Clin North Am 65:525, 1981.

Bruce RA, Eleady-Cole R, Bennett LJ, et al: Divergent effects of antihypertensive therapy on cardiovascular responses and left ventricular function during upright exercise. Am J Cardiol 30:768, 1972.

Detry J, Bruce RA: Effects of nitroglycerin on "maximal" oxygen intake and exercise electrocardiogram in coronary heart disease. Circulation 43:155, 1971.

Franciosa JA, Park M, Levine TB: Lack of correlation between exercise capacity and indexes of resting left ventricular performance in heart failure. Am J Cardiol 47:33, 1981.

Goldman L, Hashimoto B, Cook EF, et al: Comparative reproducibility and validity of systems for assessing cardiovascular functional class: Advantages of a new specific activity scale. Circulation 64:1227, 1981.

McConahay D, Valdes M, McCallister BD, et al: Accuracy of treadmill testing of assessment of direct myocardial revascularization. Circulation 56:548, 1977.

Niederberger M, Bruce RA, Frederick R, et al: Reproduction of maximal exercise performance in patients with angina pectoris despite ouabain treatment. Circulation 49:309, 1974.

Exercise Testing soon after Acute Myocardial Infarction

Atterhog JH, Ekelund LG, Kaijser L: Electrocardiographic abnormalities during exercise 3 weeks to 18 months after anterior myocardial infarction. Br Heart J 33:871, 1971.

Cain HD, Frasher WG, Stivelman R: Graded activity program for safe return to self-care after myocardial infarction. JAMA 177:111, 1961.

Davidson D, DeBusk R: Prognostic value of a single exercise test 3 weeks after uncomplicated myocardial infarction. Circulation 61:236, 1980.

Ericsson M, Granath A, Ohlsen P, et al: Arrhythmia and symptoms during treadmill testing three weeks after myocardial infarction in 100 patients. Br Heart J 35:787, 1973.

Granath A, Sodermark T, Winge T, et al: Early work load tests for evaluation of long-term prognosis of acute myocardial infarction. Br Heart J 39:758, 1977.

Ibsen H, Kjoller E, Styperek J, et al: Routine exercise ECG three weeks after acute myocardial infarction. Acta Med Scand 198:463, 1975.

Koppes GM, Kruyer W, Beckmann CH: Response to exercise early after uncomplicated acute myocardial infarction in patients receiving no medication: Long-term follow-up. Am J Cardiol 46:764, 1980.

Markiewicz W, Houston N, DeBusk RF: Exercise testing soon after myocardial infarction. Circulation 56:26, 1977.

Sami M, Kraemer H, DeBusk RF: The prognostic significance of serial exercise testing after myocardial infarction. Circulation 60:1238, 1979.

Sivarajan ES, Snydsman A, Smith B, et al: Low-level treadmill testing of 41 patients with acute myocardial infarction prior to discharge from the hospital. Arch Phys Med Rehabil 58:241, 1977.

Smith JW, Dennis CA, Gassman A, et al: Exercise testing three weeks after myocardial infarction. Chest 75:12, 1979.

Stang J, Lewis R: Early exercise tests after myocardial infarction (editorial). Ann Intern Med 94:814, 1981.

Theroux P, Waters DD, Halpen C, et al: Prognostic value of exercise testing soon after myocardial infarction. N Engl J Med 301:341, 1979.

Torkelson LO: Rehabilitation of the patient with acute myocardial infarction. J Chronic Dis 17:685, 1964.

Tubau JF, Chaitman BR, Bourassa MG, et al: Detection of multivessel coronary disease after myocardial infarction using exercise stress testing and multiple ECG lead systems. Circulation 61:44, 1980.

Weld FM, Chu K, Bigger JT: Risk stratification with low-level exercise testing 2 weeks after acute myocardial infarction. Circulation 64:306, 1981.

Wohl AJ, Lewis HR, Campbell W, et al: Cardiovascular function during early recovery from acute myocardial infarction. Circulation 56: 931, 1977.

Exercise Testing as a Screening Tool

Allen WH, Aronow WS, DeCristofaro D: Treadmill exercise testing in mass screening for coronary risk factors. Cathet Cardiovasc Diagn 2:39, 1976.

Allen WH, Aronow WS, Goodman P, et al: Five-year follow-up of maximal treadmill stress test in asymptomatic men and women. Circulation 62:522, 1980.

Aronow WS, Cassidy J: Five year follow-up of double Master's test, maximal treadmill stress test, and resting and postexercise apexcardiogram in asymptomatic persons. Circulation 52:616, 1975.

Breslow L, Sommers AR: The lifetime health monitoring program: A practical approach to preventive medicine. N Engl J Med 296:601, 1977.

Bruce RA, McDonough JR: Stress testing in screening for cardiovascular disease. Bull NY Acad Med 45:1288, 1969.

Bruce RA, DeRouen TA, Hossack KF: Value of maximal exercise tests in risk assessment of primary coronary heart disease events in healthy men. Am J Cardiol 46:371, 1980.

Cumming GR, Samm J, Borysyk L, et al: Electrocardiographic changes during exercise in asymptomatic men: 3-year follow-up. Can Med Assoc J 112:578, 1975.

Froelicher VF, Thompson AJ, Yanowitz F, et al: Treadmill exercise testing at the USAF-SAM: Physiological responses in aircrewmen and the detection of latent coronary artery disease. Agardograph No 210. Springfield, Va, NTIS, 1975.

Froelicher VF: The detection of asymptomatic coronary artery disease. Annu Rev Med 28:l, 1977.

Froelicher VF, Thomas M, Pillow C, et al: An epidemiological study of asymptomatic men screened with exercise testing for latent coronry heart disease. Am J Cardiol 34:770, 1975.

Froelicher VF, Thompson AJ, Longo M, et al: The value of exercise testing for screening asymptomatic men for latent CAD. Prog Cardiovasc Dis 18:265, 1976.

Hartley LH, Herd JA, Day WC, et al: An exercise testing program for large populations. JAMA 241:269, 1979.

MacIntyre NR, Kunkler JR, Mitchell RE, et al: Eight-year follow-up of exercise electrocardiograms in healthy, middle-aged aviators. Aviat Space Environ Med 52:256, 1981.

Manca C, Cas LD, Albertini D, et al: Different prognostic value of exercise electrocardiogram in men and women. Cardiology 63:312, 1978.

Maximal or Near-Maximal Exercise Testing with Coronary Angiography

Barnard RJ, Gardner GW, Diaco NV: "Ischemic" heart disease in fire fighters with normal coronary arteries. J Occup Med 18:818, 1976.

Barnard RJ, Gardner GW, Diaco NV, et al: Near-maximal ECG stress testing and coronary artery·disease risk factor analysis in Los Angeles City fire fighters. J Occup Med 17:693, 1975.

Borer JS, Brensike JF, Redwood DR, et al; Limitations of the electrocardiographic response to exercise in predicting coronary artery disease. N Engl J Med 193:367, 1975.

Erikssen J, Enge I, Forfang K, et al: False positive diagnostic tests and coronary angiographic findings in 105 presumably healthy males. Circulation 54:371, 1976.

Froelicher VF, Thompson AJ, Wolthuis R, et al: Angiographic findings in asymptomatic aircrewmen with electrocardiographic abnormalities. Am J Cardiol 39:32, 1977.

New Electrocardiographic Criteria

Chahine RA, Awdeh MR, Mayer M, et al: The evolutionary pattern of exercise-induced ST segment depression. J Electrocardiol 12:235, 1979.

Lozner EC, Morganroth J: New criteria to enhance the predictability of coronary artery disease by exercise testing in asymptomatic subjects. Circulation 56:799, 1977.

Thallium-201 Exercise Testing

Caralis DG, Bailey I, Kennedy HL, et al: Thallium myocardial imaging in evaluation of asymptomatic individuals with ischaemic ST segment depression on exercise electrocardiogram. Br Heart J 42:562, 1979.

Nolewajka AJ, Kostuk WJ, Howard J, et al: Thallium stress myocardial imaging: An evaluation of fifty-eight asymptomatic males. Clin Cardiol 4:134, 1981.

Uhl GS, Kay TN, Hickman JR: Detection of coronary artery disease in asymptomatic aircrewmembers with computer-enhanced thallium-201 scintigraphy. Am J Cardiol 48:1037, 1981.

Radionuclide Left Ventricular Angiography During Exercise

Battler A, Slutsky R, Pfisterer M, et al: Left ventricular ejection fraction changes during recovery from treadmill exercise: A preliminary report of a new method for detecting coronary artery disease. Clin Cardiol 3:14, 1980.

Borer JS, Bacharach SL, Green MV, et al: Real-time radionuclide cineangiography in the noninvasive evaluation of global and regional left ventricular function at rest and during exercise in patients with coronary artery disease. N Engl J Med 296:839, 1977.

Pfisterer ME, Slutsky RA, Schuler G, et al: Profiles of radionuclide left ventricular ejection fraction changes induced by supine bicycle exercise in normals and patients with coronary heart disease. Cathet Cardiovasc Diagn 5:305, 1979.

Pfisterer ME, Williams RJ, Gordon DG, et al: Comparison of rest/exercise ECG, thallium-201 scans and radionuclide angiography in patients with suspected coronary artery disease. Cardiology 66:45, 1980.

Cardiokymography

Silverberg RA, Diamond GA, Vas R, et al: Noninvasive diagnosis of coronary artery disease: The cardiokymographic stress test. Circulation 61:5579, 1980.

Coronary Artery Calcification on Fluoroscopic Examination

Kelley MJ, Juang EK, Langou RA: Correlation of fluoroscopically detected coronary artery calcification with exercise stress testing in asymptomatic men. Radiology 129:1, 1978.

Langou RA, Huang EK, Kelley MJ, et al: Predictive accuracy of coronary artery calcification and abnormal exercise test for coronary artery disease in asymptomatic man. Circulation 62:1196, 1981.

Lipid Screening

Uhl GS, Troxler RG, Hickman JR, et al: Angiographic correlation of coronary artery disease with high density lipoprotein cholesterol in asymptomatic men. Am J Cardiol 48:903, 1981.

Williams P, Robinson D, Bailey A: High density lipoprotein and coronary risk factors in normal men. Lancet 1:72, 1979.

Gated Chest X-Rays

Dinsmore RE, Wernikoff RE, Miller SW, et al: Evaluation of left ventricular free wall asynergy due to coronary artery disease: Use of an interlaced ECG-gated radiography system. AJR 132:909, 1979.

Computerized Probability Estimates

Diamond GA, Forrester JS: Analysis of probability as an aid in the clinical diagnosis of coronary artery disease. N Engl J Med 300:1350, 1979.

Systolic Time Intervals

Boudoules H, Ruff PE, Fulkerson P, et al: Effect of propranolol on post exercise left ventricular time index. Am J Cardiol 48:357, 1981.

Louis RP, Marsh DG, Sherman JA, et al: Enhanced diagnostic power of exercise testing for myocardial ischemia by addition of post exercise left ventricular ejection time. Am J Cardiol 39:767, 1977.

Sugiura T, Doi Y, Haffty B, et al: Noninvasive assessment of left ventricular performance in patients with ischemic heart disease: Ear densitigraphic study during uninterrupted treadmill exercise. Am J Cardiol 48:101, 1981.

Prognosis In Asymptomatic Coronary Disease

Hammermeister KE, DeRouen TA, Dodge HT: Effect of coronary surgery on survival in asymptomatic and minimally symptomatic patients. Circulation 62:98, 1980.

Hickman JR, Uhl GS, Rosa L, et al: Coronary artery disease: Natural history and pathology. Am J Cardiol 45:422, 1980.

Summary

Battler A, Froelicher VF, Gallagher KP, et al: Dissociation between regional myocardial dysfunction and ECG changes during ischemia in the conscious dog. Circulation 62:735, 1980.

Battler A, Gallagher KP, Froelicher VF, et al: Experimental study: Detection of latent coronary stenosis with isoproterenol in conscious dogs using regional functional and electrocardiographic responses. Cardiovasc Res 14:476, 1980.

McHenry PL, Richmond HW, Weisenberger BL, et al: Evaluation of abnormal exercise electrocardiogram in apparently healthy subjects: Labile repolarization (ST-T) abnormalities as a cause of false positive responses. Am J Cardiol 47:1152, 1981.

Theroux P, Franklin D, Ross J Jr, et al: Regional myocardial function during acute coronary artery occlusion and its modifications by pharmacologic agents in the dog. Circ Res 35:896, 1974.

Thompson AJ, Froelicher VF: Kugel's artery as a major collateral channel in severe coronary disease. Aerospace Medicine 45:1276, 1974.

Thompson AJ, Froelicher VF, Longo MR, et al; Normal coronary angiography in an aircrewman with serial exercise test changes. Aviat Space Environ Med 46:69, 1975.

Upton MT, Rerych SK, Newman GE, et al: Detecting abnormalities in left ventricular function during exercise before angina and ST-segment depression. Circulation 62:341, 1980.

CHAPTER

II
Radionuclide Exercise Testing

INTRODUCTION

The addition of radionuclide techniques to exercise testing has opened an exciting new era of investigation. These techniques are leading to a better understanding of cardiovascular physiology and pathophysiology as well as improving cardiac diagnostic capabilities. The two major techniques currently used are (1) imaging after exercise with a radionuclide that behaves metabolically like potassium and (2) left ventricular function analysis during bicycle exercise. Exercise radionuclide left ventricular function analysis is the less expensive of the two techniques, but it has greater technologic variability. It can be performed using either the first-pass procedure or blood-pooling agents that require gating. The first-pass procedure has the best validation by correlation with cardiac catheterization data, but it requires multiple injections for sequential studies, and regional wall motion analysis is best accomplished using a multicrystal camera. Gated blood-pool studies have the advantage of enabling repeated analyses with one injection, but two minutes or longer are required for data gathering in order to obtain sufficient counts. Technetium-99m is used to label red cells or a pooling agent, injected intravenously, and allowed to equilibrate in the bloodstream. Images are collected and indexed by time intervals to gather sufficient counts for viewing during each interval. Before the methodology of these techniques is discussed, it is appropriate to begin with a review of radiation physics.

RADIATION PHYSICS

Each atom possesses at its center a dense, positively charged core, or nucleus. Each nucleus contains two types of particles: positively charged protons and neutral neutrons. Neutrons can change into protons by emitting a beta particle, and this transformation is called beta-ray decay. Outside the nucleus, the atom consists of a swarm of negatively charged electrons arranged in shells. The outer ring contains the valence electrons.

The position of an atom in the periodic table of chemical elements is determined by the number of electrons and protons that an atom contains. The atomic number of an atom is the number of protons in its nucleus. The mass of an atom is the total number of protons and neutrons in the nucleus.

The chemical elements differ from one another by the number of protons in their nuclei. Any individual atom, characterized by a particular atomic number and mass number, is called a nuclide. Atoms differing in atomic weight but not in atomic number (i.e., having the same number of protons) are referred to as isotopes, from Greek words meaning same place, because they occupy the same place in the periodic table. Isotopes of each element differ mainly by the number of neutrons they contain. The word isotope is often colloquially used when nuclide is actually meant. We can certainly speak of one nuclide, but when referring to a single isotope, one might as well speak of one twin.

The neutrons play the role of a glue holding the entire nucleus together in spite of a very strong repulsion exerted by the positive protons. The most complicated nucleus known in nature is the common isotope of uranium (U-238). It contains 92 protons (giving it an atomic number of 92) and 92 electrons. The nucleus also contains 146 neutrons, giving it a mass number of 238. Uranium does not have a stable nuclear configuration. It can become less unstable by splitting off a helium nucleus (an alpha particle). This phenomenon is the basis of the alpha-ray radioactivity of the heavy elements.

Electrons are arranged in shells and in subshells, each of which is characterized by energy level and by number of electrons. The inner-shell electrons are more tightly bound than are the outer-shell electrons. When atoms are bombarded by high-energy particles or radiation, an electron may be knocked out of a neutral atom. The energy expended by electrons moving between shells can be emitted in two ways: either as electromagnetic radiation or as electrons themselves.

Radioactivity is the constant emission of penetrating and ionizing radiation. It is dependent on the spontaneous transformation within the nucleus of neutrons and protons or of their internal arrangement. Knowledge of the properties of the three types of radiation (alpha, beta, and gamma) is based on the effects of collisions of these ionizing radiations with electrons and nuclei. There are five types of transformations that can take place in the nucleus causing radioactivity: alpha decay, beta decay, electron capture, isomeric transition, and spontaneous fission.

Alpha decay is found only in the isotopes of heavy elements. The alpha ray ejected from the nucleus in this type of decay is a fast helium nucleus (i.e, two protons and two neutrons). For a given radionuclide, alpha rays are emitted in one or more monoenergetic groups. Alpha rays are the heaviest particles emitted from nuclei and have the greatest kinetic energy. Radium and radon are typical alpha-ray emitters.

All of the very heavy nuclides (atomic number greater than 83) have a very prolonged radioactive decay in the form of spontaneous nuclear fission. This fission results in the release of alpha rays. All of the nuclides produced by nuclear fission are negatron beta-ray emitters.

Beta rays are high-speed electrons produced in radioactive transformations by one of two types of beta decay. The slightly more common type of beta ray is an ordinary negative electron called a negatron, and the other type consists of a positive electron called a positron. Because many nuclear reactors can only provide a source of neutrons, the most commonly used radionuclides are neutron-rich, negatron beta-ray emitters. The production of positron-emitting radionuclides requires a cyclotron or linear accelerator. These complex devices are particle accelerators and are located only at a few research facilities.

All proton-rich nuclides can accomplish a transformation of a proton into a neutron by capturing an electron. This capture results in a reduction of the atomic number and a change in the isotope's position in the periodic table. If the nuclear transformation leaves the decay-product nucleus at an excited level, then gamma rays will be emitted. All radionuclides that transform by positron beta-ray emission or by electron capture (e.g., thallium), are man-made from particle accelerators. All the naturally occurring radioactive nuclides emit either alpha rays or negatron beta-rays. Man-made radioactive nuclides not found in nature have the advantage for nuclear medicine of having short half-lives since they must be unstable if they do not exist in nature.

Gamma rays are emitted when there are shifts of neutrons or protons within the shells and subshells of the nucleus. Gamma rays originate in nuclei, whereas x-rays originate from the transformation of extranuclear electrons. Every gamma-ray–emitting radionuclide has its own particular gamma-ray energy spectrum that characterizes it. There are a few cases in which an excited state in a nucleus is prolonged, when the gamma-ray transition is delayed by minutes or hours rather than by microseconds. Because the ground level and the excited level have the same number of protons and neutrons, they are called nuclear isomeres, and the transition between them is called isomeric transition. Technetium-99m, which can be produced by commercial nuclear reactors, emits gamma rays in this way.

Alpha or beta rays ionize some of the atoms that lie along their path as they travel through matter. Gamma rays and x-rays interact with matter and produce secondary electrons. Beta rays can travel roughly 100 times farther than alpha particles can. X-rays and gamma rays are electromagnetic radiations. They behave like a stream, called photons, or quanta, rather than as waves. The modes of interaction of x-rays or gamma rays with matter include photoelectric interaction, Compton interaction, and pair-production interaction. The photoelectric interaction is with an atom and produces a single photoelectron. The Compton interaction takes place with an electron and produces both a Compton-recoil electron and a Compton-scatter proton. The pair-production interaction occurs with a nucleus and produces a pair of electrons—one positron and one negatron.

The basic unit of activity for all radionuclides is the curie (Ci). This activity unit is defined as 3.5×10^{10} disintegrating nuclei per second and is not a measure of the number of rays emitted. The energy of nuclear radiations is usually measured in electron volts (eV). The unit of absorbed radiation is the rad, which is equal to 6.25×10^{13} eV per frame of exposed tissue. The rate of decay is a constant for each radionuclide. The so-called decay constant is the probability of disintegration per unit time and per atom. It can be shown that the mean or average, life for a large group of identical atoms is simply the reciprocal of the decay constant. Instead of the mean life, the rate of decay of any radionuclide can be described by its half-life, which is equal to the product of 0.693 and the mean life. Half-life is the time at which one half of any initial amount of radioactive atoms remains undecayed.

The measurement of alpha activity does not play a role in nuclear medicine because the radioisotopes utilized emit only beta and gamma rays. The photoelectrons or Compton electrons originating from gamma-ray absorption or scatter produce ionization and excitation along their paths similar to that produced by beta rays of corresponding energies. Radiation-measuring devices depend on effects mediated through the charged-particle path of ionization or excitation. There are three principal classes of such devices—a gas, a liquid, or a solid. Gas devices such as ion chambers and Geiger tubes are now only used for dosing applications. They have been largely replaced by liquid and crystal scintillation cameras or scintigraphs. An Anger camera uses one crystal, whereas various other cameras use multiple crystals.

MYOCARDIAL IMAGING WITH POTASSIUM-LIKE RADIONUCLIDES (COLD-SPOT IMAGING)

The radionuclides that metabolically behave like potassium (including potassium-43, cesium-129, rubidium-81, and thallium-201) are either cyclotron or accelerator produced, making them expensive. The optimal gamma-emitting potassium-like radionuclide would have its major energy peak in the range of technetium-99m (i.e., 140 kev) and, like technetium, be produced by commercial nuclear reactors. With the exception of thallium-201, all of the potassium-like radionuclides have a relatively high-energy spectrum of gamma-ray emission, which requires special shielding and collimation of the scintillation camera for efficient imaging. Potassium-43 and rubidium-81 provide relatively poor myocardial-to-background ratios and have limited availability. Also, potassium-43 has a relatively high beta emission, which leads to a high radiation dose for a patient. Cesium-129 is not extracted rapidly enough to detect transient ischemia. The lowest energy can be obtained from thallium-201 for which imaging is centered around 80 kev (actually, x-ray emissions from a mercury breakdown product of thallium). Thallium-201 clearly is the best analog available since it produces diagnostic quality images on currently available scintillation cameras using standard collimation. It is produced by bombarding stable thallium-203 in a cyclotron.

Myocardial imaging with radioactive cations (cold-spot imaging) has been used to identify (1) previous infarction, (2) acute infarction, and (3) areas of transient ischemia. When patients are studied at rest a reduction in regional activity corresponds to areas of scar, most likely secondary to myocardial infarction. When radioactive cations are injected intravenously after the onset of angina pectoris or fatigue during exercise, a new region of decreased activity identifies an ischemic area secondary to an obstructed coronary artery. The radionuclide materials used for analysis of regional myocardial perfusion have been termed cold-spot agents because the areas of decreased myocardial perfusion are identified by a decrease in regional radioactivity, or a cold spot.

An intravenous line is inserted prior to exercise, and the patient is allowed to exercise maximally to the point of angina or severe fatigue. At this point, thallium is injected into the infusion line. Exercise is continued for an additional minute to allow adequate distribution of the radionuclide even if the work load must be decreased. Imaging is begun thereafter as quickly as possible so that ischemia is not missed. Patients must exercise to a maximal effort for the test to have maximum sensitivity. Patients should be studied in multiple views: anterior and 45° and 70° left anterior obliques. The 45° oblique view is of value in separating inferolateral from anteroseptal defects. The 45° left anterior oblique view is especially valuable for quantitative techniques, and sometimes inferior wall defects are best seen in this view. We have replaced the 60° left anterior oblique and the lateral views with a single 70° left anterior oblique. This maneuver helps to visualize transient ischemia by decreasing imaging time. Ischemia can be missed if imaging is delayed after exercise. Care should also be taken so that the diaphragm does not cause a pseudodefect. The resting view is usually obtained when redistribution occurs four hours after the exercise study without requiring a second injection of thallium on another day. A defect at the time, however, can be due to severe ischemia instead of scar. We have added immediate-delay films to follow the rate of redistribution.

The regional myocardial potassium-sodium ratio was studied during acute coronary occlusion in animals. A fall from the normal ratio of 5 to less than 3 in the central ischemic zone occurs 15 minutes after occlusion. At 60 minutes, this ratio falls to less than 2, and at 24 hours it is less than 0.5. Parallel changes or ones of lesser magnitude occur in border zones. Abnormalities in transmyocardial potassium flux have also been noted in humans during ischemia. The regional myocardial uptake of potassium-like radionuclides is based on regional myocardial blood flow and the myocardial extraction of these cations. Potassium is extracted efficiently by cardiac muscle. Following intracoronary injection, approximately 70% of the potassium is extracted. Rubidium has a similar extraction, whereas thallium extraction is higher. Peak myocardial concentration of these radionuclides is generally reached in five minutes after intravenous injection. Cesium is cleared much more slowly and peak myocardial uptake takes much longer. The myocardial biologic half-life of potassium is approximately one hour, and for cesium seven hours. Therefore, cesium cannot be used for exercise scintigraphy. Thallium also has a lesser hepatic and gastric uptake than either rubidium or potassium. The two major unfavorable physical properties of thallium are its half-life of 73 hours, which is much longer than required for clinical measurements, and its emissions are less energetic than gamma photons, which results in a higher likelihood of absorption and scatter within the body. These properties result in unnecessary radiation exposure and poor imaging characteristics.

Uptake of potassium-like radionuclides tends to underestimate the flow in conditions of hyperemia. Extraction will vary with the degree of flow and will increase as flow decreases. This phenomenon is not reflected by increased uptake in low-flow regions, since the amount of cation presented to the low-flow zone is decreased. Extraction or uptake patterns cannot be altered without changes in flow. For instance, the infusion of glucose and insulin leads to significant increases in the uptake of potassium and its analogues. Hypercapnea and respiratory acidosis are said to result in increased myocardial potassium accumulation. In a recent animal study, extraction of thallium by the myocardium was evaluated as a function of heart rate, coronary blood flow, hypoxia, changes in pH, and after administration of propranolol, insulin, and strophanthin. Under basal conditions, the extraction fraction measured 88% and was unchanged by pacing, alterations in pH, and administration of propranolol, insulin, and digitalis. Hypoxia caused a significant decrease in extraction fraction, to 78%. When coronary blood flow was increased in excess of the demand due to drugs, extraction fraction fell logarithmically. Thus, for clinical purposes, if an image were obtained immediately after thallium administration, the regional concentration in the myocardium would be representative of blood flow. In another study comparing thallium-201 and radiolabeled microspheres, variable areas of ischemia were assessed in 16 closed-chest dogs. An excellent correlation between thallium and the microspheres with ischemic segments was found. The major limitation of thallium was the inconsistent detection of small profusion defects. Figure 1 shows the relationship of the heart and coronary arteries to the thallium images.

Forty-four normal subjects were studied at both rest and exercise by Zaret. In all, homogeneous myocardial images were noted under both conditions. Decreased uptake in the apical region was found to be a normal variant. This result occurred in approximately 20% of normal subjects and is probably due to thinning of the apex of the heart. Thirteen healthy adults were studied by Cook and colleagues after administration of thallium-201, both at rest and at maximal exercise. On the rest scan, the left ventricular myocardium, liver, and spleen were seen. In two subjects with a resting tachycardia, the right ventricle was slightly visualized. When the nuclide was administered during exercise, the left ventricular activity was more homogeneous, and the left ventricle was better defined on the scan. The left ventricle-to-lung background activity ratio increased from 2.4 at rest to 3.4 during exercise. The right ventricle myocardium was seen on the exercise scan. Phantom studies showed that small lesions are best defined when viewed either straight on or at a tangent. The usual dose of thallium given for cardiac scanning is 2 mCi. When studying healthy persons who can easily

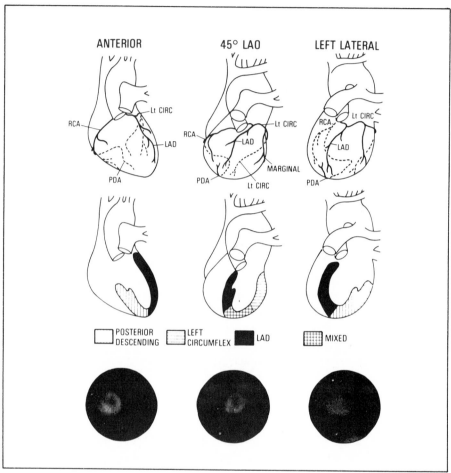

Figure 1.   Relation of regions of the heart and coronary arteries to the thallium images. LAD = left anterior descending artery; RCA = right coronary artery; PDA = posterior descending artery; LT CIRC = left circumflex artery.

tolerate a prolonged scanning period, the dose administered can be reduced to 1 mCi per scan. Although the total body dose is low, the renal and gonadal doses should be a major consideration when studying normal volunteers.

Zaret and associates studied nine patients with exercise-induced ST-segment depression who had normal coronary angiography. Potassium-43 was administered intravenously during treadmill exercise at the time when abnormal electrocardiographic changes were present. Myocardial images in nine patients showed a normal homogeneous pattern of radioisotope distribution. Bulkley and co-workers used exercise thallium scans in six normal volunteers and in five patients with systemic sarcoidosis and cardiac dysfunction. The scans were normal in the volunteers; segmental defects were found in the left ventricle compatible with infiltrative disease of the myocardium in three of the patients with sarcoidosis. Segmental myocardial infiltration by sarcoid was confirmed by autopsy in one of these patients and by an operation in another. They concluded that thallium myocardial perfusion defects can be secondary to myocardial sarcoidosis.

Cold-Spot Exercise Imaging with Angiographic Correlation. Clinical studies (summarized in Table I) have evaluated the sensitivity and specificity of rest and exercise cold-spot imaging, with coronary angiography as the diagnostic reference. Most of these studies also included the results of rest and exercise electrocardiography. Significant coronary artery disease was considered equal to or greater than 50% or 75% reduction of the luminal diameter of one or more of the three major coronary arteries; some of the investigators mentioned that similar results were obtained using either criterion. Most of the exercise tests were performed with only one electrocardiographic lead recorded, which lowered the sensitivity of exercise electrocardiography. Also, other diagnostic end points of exercise testing, including ST elevation, usually were not considered.

Berman and associates reported their results in 40 patients studied with rest and exercise rubidium-81 scans, exercise electrocardiography, and coronary angiography. During the exercise tests, leads I, II, aVF, and V_5 were recorded. In 33 patients with significant coronary disease, the rubidium-81 scan was abnormal in 88%, whereas 58% showed abnormal ST-segment depression. In seven patients with less than 50% narrowing, the scans showed no defects, but two of the seven had abnormal ST-segment depression.

Rosenblatt and co-workers performed rest and exercise thallium-201 scans, single-lead exercise electrocardiography, and coronary angiography on 15 patients with severe coronary disease, 12 patients with mild coronary disease, and 3 patients with normal coronary arteries. Forty percent of the patients with severe coronary artery disease had abnormal treadmill tests, whereas 93% had positive exercise myocardial scans. Correlation between scan defects and sites of coronary lesions was poor in patients with two- and three-vessel disease as compared with those with single-vessel disease. The one patient with a false-negative scan had three-vessel disease. The scans of patients with diffuse disease were characterized by generalized poor uptake. The scans after exercise, however, exhibited greater uptake. Of the four

TABLE I
EXERCISE COLD-SPOT STUDIES WITH ANGIOGRAPHIC CORRELATION
DEMONSTRATING SENSITIVITY AND SPECIFICITY

Principal Investigator	N	Sensitivity	Specificity	Comments
Berman	40	88%	100%	Rubidium
Rosenblatt	30	93%	71%	Unprocessed analog images
Bailey	83	75%	100%	Manual quantification of analog images
McGowan	160	83%	82%	Potassium or rubidium
Ritchie	101	76%	92%	Unprocessed analog images
Collaborative Study	190	78%	88%	Some images interpreted after 20%–25% background subtraction
Turner	64	68%	97%	Unprocessed Polaroid film; no myocardial infarction patients
Verani	82	78%	97%	Unprocessed analog images; no delayed images obtained
Botvinick	65	85%	92%	Unprocessed analog images using rubidium
McCarthy	128	85%	79%	Five-point smooth, 30% background subtraction on Polaroid film
Zeppo	30	70%	—	Unprocessed Polaroid film; patients with triple-vessel disease only
Caldwell	52	85%	100	Unprocessed Polaroid film
Jengo	58	93%	94%	Unprocessed Polaroid film
Uhl	100	75%	89%	Processed images; large sample of asymptomatic patients
Total	1,183	79%	92%	

patients without lesions exceeding 50% narrowing, one had both an abnormal ST-segment response to exercise and an abnormal myocardial scan. Another patient had an abnormal scan in spite of normal left ventricular contraction and minimal coronary disease. Three patients with chest pain but with normal coronaries and left ventriculograms had normal myocardial scans.

Bailey and colleagues studied 20 healthy subjects and 63 coronary artery disease patients using treadmill testing with thallium-201 scans and simultaneously recorded 12-lead electrocardiograms. The studies in the healthy subjects were all normal. Small inhomogeneities of thallium-201 uptake were frequent, but they were not equal to 15% of the left ventricular circumference in any projection. None of these subjects developed a new perfusion defect on the exercise image. When the electrocardiograms (Q waves at rest or ST-segment depression during exercise or both) and abnormal myocardial scans (perfusion defect at rest or a new defect with exercise or both) in patients with coronary artery disease were compared, the sensitivity for the electrocardiographic studies was 65% versus 75% for the thallium scans. In those with single-vessel disease, the sensitivities were 46% versus 71%, in those with two-vessel disease 70% versus 65%, and in those with three-vessel disease 93% versus 93%. If the development of precordial chest pain with the exercise test was also considered an abnormal response, the sensitivity of the routine exercise test was similar to that of the exercise myocardial imaging. Two patients with left bundle branch block and coronary disease had abnormal scans. Eleven percent of the patients with significant coronary artery disease failed to develop chest pain, a scan defect, or ST-segment depression during exercise.

McGowan and co-workers reported 160 patients studied with rest and exercise myocardial imaging using potassium-43 or rubidium-81 single-lead exercise electrocardiography and coronary angiography. Fifty-one of 62 patients with insignificant coronary disease had normal imaging studies, 81 of 98 patients with significant coronary disease had normal imaging studies, and 81 of 98 patients with significant coronary disease had abnormal imaging studies.

Ritchie and colleagues reported 101 patients studied with rest and exercise myocardial imaging using thallium-201, single-lead exercise electrocardiography, and coronary angiography. Of 25 patients with insignificant coronary disease, one had a resting defect and one had an exercise defect. Four of these had exercise-induced ST-segment depression. Among the 76 patients with significant coronary disease, 76% had a defect on either the rest or exercise thallium image. Forty-five percent of them had exercise-induced ST-segment depression. Of the patients with coronary disease, 91% had either an abnormal thallium study, an abnormal resting electrocardiogram, or an abnormal electrocardiographic response to exercise testing. Image defects corresponded to a coronary lesion in all patients with single-vessel disease. In patients with two- or three-vessel disease, the image defect was always associated with a lesion; however, other high-grade lesions were often present, but image defects did not develop in these regions.

Botvinick and associates reported results in 65 patients studied with rest and exercise myocardial imaging using rubidium-81 single-lead exercise electrocardiography and coronary angiography. Thirty-four patients had significant coronary artery disease. Myocardial imaging had a sensitivity of 85% and a specificity of 92%, whereas exercise electrocardiography had a sensitivity of 79% and a specificity of 64%. Myocardial imaging was more sensitive than exercise electrocardiography in the patients with one- and two-vessel disease; the converse was true in those with three-vessel disease. There were two patients with false-positive myocardial scans who had documented anterior infarctions without significant coronary disease. The three false-negative images occurred in one patient with one-vessel disease and well-established coronary collaterals, one patient with severe three-vessel disease, and one patient with a prior infarct.

In a collaborative study involving six institutions, Ritchie and colleagues used myocardial imaging with thallium-201 in patients with angina pectoris or acute myocardial infarction. Ninety of 111 patients (81%) with acute myocardial infarction had image defects, compared with 71 (64%) who had new electrocardiographic Q waves. Patients with enzymatically large infarctions and anterior infarcts were more commonly detected than were those with smaller or inferior infarcts. In patients presenting with angina pectoris, 42 patients had no coronary lesion with greater than 50% luminal narrowing, and five of them had an abnormal rest or exercise defect, a specificity of 88%. Among the 148 patients with significant coronary lesions, image defects occurred at rest or with exercise in 115. New exercise image defects were more common than were exercise ST-segment depression. The false-positive responses occurred in one patient with catheter-induced spasm, one with an isolated distal 40% narrowing left anterior descending lesion, and one with normal coronary arteries but with both angina and exercise-induced ST-segment depression. Exercise imaging was particularly useful in the patients with digitalis effect or left bundle branch block. Thirteen of 16 such patients had exercise thallium-201 defects. Imaging also localized the site of ischemia.

McLaughlin reported 76 thallium-201 myocardial perfusion studies performed on 25 patients to assess reproducibility and the effects of varying levels of exercise on the results of imaging. Of 70 segments among the 14 patients assessed by two maximal exercise tests, 64 (91%) were reproducible. Only 51% of the ischemic defects present at maximal exercise were seen in the submaximal exercise study in 12 patients studied at two exercise levels.

Dunn and colleagues studied 76 consecutive patients with documented normal coronary arteries who had thallium exercise studies. The thallium scintigrams had been judged to be normal in 79% and abnormal in 21%. Analysis of the locations of thallium defects in the 16 normal subjects with abnormal scintigrams revealed a pattern consistent with coronary disease in five (including four with an abnormal left ventricle) and a pattern that suggested soft tissue attenuation in nine (diaphragm, breast, or adipose tissue), whereas the other two had apical defects. Consistent defects were defined as: anterior, if seen in more than one projection and extending into the apical segment; inferior, if seen in more than one projection; and lateral, if associated with inferior defects. This mannner of interpretation appears to improve the specificity of the thallium test.

Thallium scanning and exercise electrocardiography have been said to complement each other by being strong in the situation of the other's weakness. Thallium was thought to be more sensitive in single-vessel disease because of the greater chance of contrast between poorly and well-perfused areas than in triple-vessel disease. The opposite situation would apply in exercise electrocardiography, which is clearly more sensitive in multivessel disease. Also, thallium studies were thought to be helpful in patients with chronotropic incompetence or with poor exercise tolerance. Recent studies have shown that false-negative thallium scans usually occur in patients with inadequate heart rates and in those with single-vessel disease. Thus, it appears that both procedures have some similar limitations. Iskandrian and Segal evaluated the impact of exercise thallium studies in 71 patients who had inconclusive, or equivocal, exercise electrocardiograms. The thallium exercise test had a sensitivity of 79% and a specificity of 95% in these patients and thus was comparable to the results in patients who had exercise electrocardiographic studies that were unequivocal.

Previous studies evaluating the sensitivity and specificity of exercise electrocardiography, using coronary angiography or follow-up coronary events, have established its sensitivity to be 60% to 70% and its specificity to be 90%. This level of specificity was obtained by avoiding the conditions that can cause false-positive responses. The low specificity of exercise electrocardiography in the studies reviewed here was due to the inclusion of patients likely to have false-positive exercise electrocardiographic responses. The greater sensitivity of exercise thallium imaging compared with ST-segment depression can be partially explained by the inclusion of patients with myocardial damage. The thallium exercise test is of particular value in patients with chronotopic incompetence, poor exercise tolerance, or abnormal resting electrocardiograms. Another situation in which cold-spot imaging has particular value is in patients who develop ventricular dysrhythmias during exercise without significant ST-segment depression. Since ventricular dysrhythmias have a poor predictive value for the diagnosis of coronary disease, a radionuclide study can help make a diagnostic decision in such patients. Patients with left bundle branch block can have septal fibrosis not due to coronary disease and thus have septal cold spots.

Rigo and colleagues evaluated the diagnostic value of thallium exercise testing in 141 patients with and without a previous myocardial infarction but all with angiographically proved coronary disease. One hundred one had a previous myocardial infarction, and 40 did not. In the patients without infarction, the sensitivity for detecting left anterior descending and right circumflex and left circumflex coronary artery occlusions was 66%, 53%, and 24%, respectively. In those without a previous infarction, the sensitivity for demonstrating disease in the artery corresponding to the site of infarction was 100% for the left anterior descending, 79% for the right circumflex, and 63% for the left circumflex coronary artery. In patients with a prior anterior infarction, concomitant right or left circumflex coronary artery lesions were detected in only one of 12 cases, whereas in those with a prior inferior infarct, the sensitivity for left anterior disease was 69%. Thallium exercise testing was useful for identifying multivessel disease in patients with previous inferior infarction but had relatively no value in detecting right or left circumflex disease in patients with a prior anterior infarction and in patients without previous myocardial infarction. Overall, in the group without previous infarction, 76% had an abnormal exercise scintigram, and in the group with a previous myocardial infarction, 96% had abnormal scintigrams at rest or during exercise.

Rehn and colleagues assessed thallium exercise testing for identifying left main coronary artery disease by studying 24 patients with left main disease and 80 patients with narrowing of other vessels. Ninety-two percent of those with left main disease had abnormal exercise scintigrams, but the patterns of perfusion defects were not specific. This finding was compounded by the fact that lesions in other vessels were found in all patients with left main disease, so it is unlikely that improvement in technique would have been of further help.

Exercise thallium scanning has been shown to be a valuable diagnostic technique, and it is to be hoped that the technique will become less expensive. In the future the use of positron emitters will result in the ability to obtain cross-sectional tomographic images. Also, gating to avoid motion artifact, availability of new radionuclides, computerized image enhancement, and computerized quantification of ischemic areas should all lead to improvement of cold-spot imaging. Gating makes possible the visualization of wall motion abnormalities using thallium, but currently this requires long periods of data-gathering to obtain sufficient counts in both systole and diastole. Recent studies have evaluated the lung uptake of thallium in patients with exercise-induced subclinical congestive heart failure. Such observations may be helpful in identifying left ventricular failure as the cause of dyspnea on exertion.

RADIONUCLIDE VENTRICULAR ANGIOGRAPHY DURING BICYCLE EXERCISE

Evaluation of cardiac contraction by qualitative and quantitative techniques has been of particular interest to physicians involved in the care of patients with heart disease. Until the advent of echocardiography and radionuclide angiography, these types of analyses were performed with direct injection of radiopaque contrast material into the left ventricle. Now, however, these two noninvasive methods can supply much of the data generated from contrast ventriculograms and can be repeated without harm to the patient.

Wall motion, ventricular function (ejection fraction), and ventricular volume can be derived from radionuclide angiograms by geometric or count-based techniques. Much of the original work in radionuclide imaging involved application of the traditional area-length formula to left ventricular images to derive left ventricular volumes and ejection fraction. Area-length calculations are difficult and dependent on geometric assumptions. Thus, count-based methods for evaluation of left ventricular size and function have been developed. These techniques involve external imaging of the cardiac blood pool with an external imaging device, such as a probe or gamma scintillation camera.

Two methods of radionuclide analysis of left ventricular function have been utilized. In the first method, the transit of a bolus of a radionuclide material as it passes through the central circulation is observed. In the second method, the left ventricle is visualized using radioactive substances that

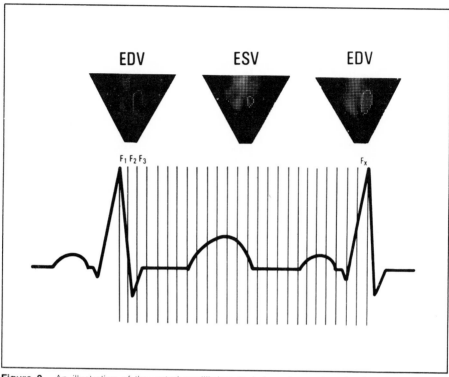

Figure 2. An illustration of the gated equilibrium technique for noninvasive imaging of the left ventricle using technetium tagged to red blood cells or a pooling agent. EDV = end-diastolic volume; ESV = end-systolic volume.

circulate in the blood in a steady state. This equilibrium technique requires gating of multiple RR intervals to produce a summed, composite cardiac cycle (Figure 2).

A variety of ^{99m}Tc-labeled radiopharmaceuticals may be used for these procedures. First-transit, or first-pass, studies can be done with any agent that is not filtered out by the lungs. Any pharmaceutical that can be injected in a bolus is suitable. If repeated studies are needed, two agents should be used: one is excreted by the kidneys and one extracted by the liver. For equilibrium studies, any blood-pool–imaging agent is suitable, including human serum albumin and in vitro or in vivo labeled red blood cells.

First-transit studies can be performed with standard single-crystal Anger cameras. The use of multicrystal cameras increases the count rate with loss of resolution. A dedicated nuclear computer system is needed to perform the analyses. Gated or equilibrium studies are usually performed with single-crystal cameras and dedicated computer systems.

The first-pass approach requires the evaluation of the radioactive bolus as it passes through the right and left ventricle. A variety of camera projections can be used, the requirements being that the left ventricle can be clearly seen and that the aorta and mitral valve plane can be located. Data are acquired in list, or serial, mode at a sampling frequency equal to or greater than 20 frames per second. Usually the right and left ventricular time-activity curves are separated. The computer operator then assigns a fixed left ventricular and background region of interest, from which a time-activity (volume) curve is generated. Ejection fraction can thus be calculated by averaging the end-diastolic and end-systolic data points. This technique has been shown to correlate well with contrast ventriculography. Gating must be used for imaging with a first-pass agent when using a single-crystal camera if wall motion and volume estimates are to be made.

The equilibrium techniques can be used after the blood-pool–imaging radionuclide passes through the heart numerous times and reaches a stable concentration in the circulation. An electrocardiographic gate is utilized to initialize time blocks in the cardiac cycle. The electrocardiographic gate is used to accumulate two frames, either end diastole or end systole—now more commonly, multiple frames throughout the entire cycle—based on short acquisition intervals phased from a fiducial point on the electrocardiogram. When multiple RR intervals are summed and the resulting frames viewed in sequence, a cine format produces the illusion of ventricular contraction. The left ventricle can be assigned manually or with a variety of edge-detection algorithms. Ejection fraction and ventricular volume can be quantitated from the time-activity curves.

Using a single-crystal camera, the first-pass angiogram can reliably estimate both right and left ventricular ejection fractions. However, because the end-diastolic and end-systolic regions of interest have less than 200 counts per 0.04 second frame, visualization of the ventricular silhouette and wall motion analyses are difficult. Analysis of ventricular volume is even more difficult, although area-length methods have been successfully applied to first-pass angiograms derived from multicrystal cameras. First-pass ejection fractions can be obtained in the right anterior oblique position so that single-plane wall motion analyses can be performed. Intervention studies require multiple injections, and wall motion analyses require higher doses of radionuclides.

Gated radionuclide studies, unlike first-pass techniques, cannot be performed in the right anterior oblique projection for the purpose of evaluating left ventricular function because the right ventricle overlies the left ventricle in this projection. Studies of ventricular function and wall motion must therefore be performed in the left anterior oblique projection, in which the right and left ventricle are clearly separated. Visual interpretation of the ventricular silhouette in this view is not as informative as the right anterior oblique view because the anterolateral and inferior walls are not well seen. Still, one dose of a radionuclide can produce multiple studies for up to four hours after injection. It has been thought that the right ventricle could best be evaluated by first-pass techniques, but equilibrium angiograms can also produce estimates of right ventricular ejection fraction and volume. The advantages and disadvantages of these two techniques are summarized in Table II.

While attempts have been made to utilize the posttreadmill exercise period to evaluate left ventricular performance, most investigators have utilized either supine or erect bicycle exercise. The investigations that evaluated the hemodynamic response to supine exercise using invasive techniques have shown that there is a marked difference between the body's response to acute exercise in the supine and erect positions. In normal subjects, stroke volume and end-diastolic volume do not change significantly during supine bicycle exercise from rest, whereas in the erect position, both increase during mild work and then plateau. When angina patients perform identical submaximal bicycle work loads, supine and erect, heart rate is higher in the supine position. Maximal work load is lower in the supine position and angina develops at a lower double product. In angina patients, left ventricular filling pressure is more likely to increase during exercise in the supine position than in the erect. Also, ST-segment depression is greater in the supine position. The linear relationship of cardiac output to oxygen consumption during supine bicycle exercise has been used to separate patients with ventricular dysfunction from normal subjects. Exercise factor (the increase of cardiac output for an increase in oxygen consumption) is based on studies of healthy individuals. For every 100 ml increase in oxygen consumption, cardiac output should increase by 500 ml. This measurement has been replaced by the measurement of ejection factor in most clinical practice except in Germany, where the response of the exercise fraction and end-diastolic pressure are used to quantitate disability. Left ventricular filling pressure does not increase in proportion to work in normal subjects, but it very often increases during supine work in abnormal subjects.

In general, supine protocols for radionuclide imaging have consisted of two to four exercise levels, three or four minutes in duration, to fatigue or

---

TABLE II
COMPARISON OF TWO NONINVASIVE TECHNIQUES OF
RADIONUCLIDE LEFT VENTRICULAR ANGIOGRAPHY

The First-Pass (Transit) Technique

Disadvantages
1. Multiple injections are required for intervention studies, with time allowed between injections for clearance of the previously injected material.
2. In general, a multicrystal scintillation camera is needed for regional wall motion studies. However, some investigators have gated and used a standard camera. This camera is immobile, expensive, delicate, and less commonly available.
3. Imaging cannot be done during exercise because of motion artifact. The radionuclide is injected during exercise immediately before stopping, and imaging is begun after stopping. The ejection fraction can normalize quickly after exercise.
4. Volume measurements are less reproducible.

Advantages
1. Can be done in the right anterior oblique or anterior projections, enabling evaluation of wall motion of the anterior left ventricular wall.
2. Easier to account for interference from the right ventricle and left atrium.
3. Short data acquisition time (about 10 sec).
4. Can be performed with a scintillation probe ("nuclear stethoscope").

Gated Blood-Pool Studies

Disadvantages
1. The optimal pooling agent has not been demonstrated.
2. Requires left anterior oblique imaging to avoid the right ventricle, so regional wall motion abnormalities of the anterior left ventricular wall cannot be assessed while ejection fraction is measured.
3. The left atrium is difficult to account for during imaging.
4. Relatively long acquisition time (2 min or more) required for sufficient counts.
5. Correlation studies have suggested that ejection fraction is lower using this technique because of interference from the left atrium.

Advantages
1. After one injection, serial studies can be performed for 4 hours or longer.
2. Wall motion can be assessed using a conventional Anger scintillation camera.
3. Ejection fraction and volume can be followed through exercise and recovery after one injection of a radionuclide.
4. Ejection fraction and volume can be determined serially after treadmill testing.

---

angina. They have been continuous and progressive. Usually scintigraphic data are obtained during the last few minutes of each stage to minimize heart rate variation while collecting the gated images. Erect exercise has been used in similar fashion, though mostly by investigations with multicrystal cameras. Arguments over which method is more suitable for diagnostic testing at present remain unresolved, though one study found no difference in diagnostic value between the two positions. Although supine exercise is not as physiologic as erect exercise, it is technically easier to perform and is associated with increased venous return, cardiac dilatation, and greater resting left ventricular wall stress. Positioning of the camera is extremely critical, and four-chamber separation should be achieved for optimal calculations; such separation is much easier to accomplish in supine patients.

The response of the left ventricle to acute exercise depends on the functional reserve of the left ventricle, myocardial perfusion, as well as the exercise performed. The following is a review of studies that have investigated the role of exercise in the evaluation of heart function using radionuclide left ventricular angiography.

Ejection Fraction Response to Exercise in Normal Subjects and in Patients with Coronary Heart Disease. Borer and colleagues studied ten men and one woman with angiographic coronary artery disease and normal resting left ventricular function confirmed by angiography. Fourteen normal subjects were also studied. Gated radionuclide angiography was performed in the supine position at rest and during exercise. Human serum albumin labeled with 10 mCi of radioactive technetium was administered intravenously. A conventional Anger camera was oriented in a modified left anterior oblique position to isolate the left ventricle. Ejection fractions by this technique were consistently lower than those determined by contrast angiography, but there was a correlation coefficient of .86. Imaging was performed during exercise for at least two minutes near-maximum effort. Ejection fraction increased from rest during exercise in all normal subjects, with the increase ranging from 7% to 30%. In patients with coronary disease, ejection fraction during exercise diminished in all but one patient, and in that patient it remained unchanged. At least one new region of left ventricular dysfunction developed during exercise in each of the patients with coronary artery disease.

Rerych and colleagues studied 30 normal volunteers (mean age 34 years) using the first-pass technique and maximal upright bicycle exercise. An increase of the ejection fraction from a resting value of 66% to 80% obtained at peak exercise was reported for mean values. Similar values were obtained by these same investigators when evaluating college swimmers before and after training. They found a rest to peak exercise ejection fraction increase from 73% to 87% before training and a similar increase (67% to 86%) following training. Port and colleagues studied 12 subjects in the upright position during maximal exercise and found all subjects to increase exercise ejection fraction above the resting value. Bodendeimer and co-workers employed isometric handgrip exercise to evaluate 19 subjects without coronary artery disease. Although global function was found to be of limited value (only 3 of 19 subjects increased exercise ejection fraction by more than 5%), the authors found assessment of relative changes in regional ejection fraction to be useful.

Conflicting results were reported by Foster and colleagues who studied the response of nine healthy male volunteers to maximal upright bicycle ergometry. Using the first-pass technique and progressive exercise, they found a mean ejection fraction increase from rest to peak exercise (67% to 73%) and decrease in one from 85 to 83%. In addition, all of these normal subjects decreased their peak ejection fraction when subjected to sudden strenuous exercise. The fact that the subjects were stressed to their true maximal effort, that the ejection fraction was obtained during the last minute of exercise (as opposed to immediately after), and that they started with high ejection fraction may possibly explain these results.

Few studies have examined the ejection fraction response in coronary heart disease patients with respect to the nature or severity of their disease (angina, infarct, or vessels involved). However, Battler and co-workers reported that 20 patients with typical angina decreased their ejection fraction from a resting value of 57% to 47% at peak supine exercise. Only three patients failed to decrease their ejection fractions by more than three ejection fraction units. Similar results were obtained by Borer and co-workers in 44 patients who experienced chest pain during supine exercise. The resting mean left ventricular ejection fraction of 48% decreased to 39% during chest pain. Five of the 44 patients did show an increase in the exercise ejection fraction, whereas one remained unchanged. The remaining 38 patients decreased their exercise ejection fraction response.

Puluido and colleagues reported that patients several months after inferior wall myocardial infarctions had normal ejection fraction responses to exercise, whereas those with anterior wall myocardial infarctions showed a decrease in ejection fraction response to exercise. There is a large individual difference in the ejection fraction response in patients who have sustained a myocardial infarction due to differences in the size of the myocardial infarction, number and severity of vessel involvement, and the presence of collateral circulation. In a group of 21 patients with documented myocardial infarctions, Jengo and co-workers reported that 14 decreased their ejection fraction response to upright bicycle exercise, 5 remained unchanged, and 2 increased. In agreement with these findings, Rerych and associates found that 9 of 13 patients decreased their exercise ejection fraction, 2 remained unchanged, and 2 increased. Borer also noted that among the coronary patients who had Q waves, all had regional dysfunction. Most patients with angina pectoris decrease left ventricular ejection fraction response from rest to peak exercise. However, patients with myocardial infarction either decrease their ejection fraction during exercise or show no change, depending on the location and extent of their infarction. Patients with angiographic evidence of coronary heart disease but without angina or infarction usually do not significantly increase peak exercise ejection fraction value from the resting value. Figure 3 is an illustration of this finding from a study by our group. Table III summarizes the studies that have investigated the sensitivity and specificity of exercise ventriculography for coronary heart disease using coronary angiography as the gold standard. One of the problems with comparing results is that the criteria for abnormal differ among these studies.

Detection of Wall Motion Abnormalities. Left ventricular contraction is a series of sequential contractions of muscle bundles; abnormal contraction, which can be regional or global, is due to disorganization of the contraction sequence. Regional contraction or wall motion abnormalities are characteristically seen in CAD patients and are due to disorganized contraction in a localized area. Asynergy is usually classified as hypokinesia (decreased motion), akinesia (no motion), or dyskinesia (bulging during systole). The exact relationship of these findings to pathologic aneurysms is uncertain. Regional contraction abnormalities can be found in more than one half of all patients with coronary disease and in more patients when midsystole or early systole are considered. In general, regional wall motion disturbances induced by exercise are due to inadequate coronary perfusion and those present at rest are due to scar. However, some abnormalities present at rest can be reversed with nitroglycerin and thus are due to resting ischemia. There is a progressively higher prevalence of asynergy with occlusion of more coronary vessels. However, asynergy is a dynamic event and may be induced by a variety of pharmacologic and physiologic interventions. The ability to analyze resting and stress-induced wall motion abnormalities enhances the ability to discern the severity and location of coronary lesions.

Ventricular asynergy can be seen in any location, although the apex is the most common site. The prevalence of asynergy has not been altered by

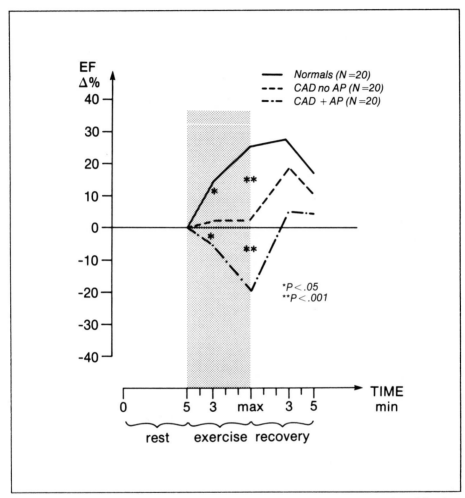

Figure 3. Profiles of ejection fraction response to supine bicycle exercise. Illustration of the ejection fraction response to exercise of normal subjects, coronary disease (CAD) patients with angina pectoris (AP), and those without angina. It must be remembered that patients with other types of heart disease can behave similarly to coronary patients. However, coronary disease is characterized by regional dysfunction, which theoretically should be unusual in other diseases. Δ %EF = percent change in ejection fraction from the resting value.

the addition of the left anterior oblique view, and biplane ventriculography is found to add only a few additional abnormally contracting zones to the right anterior oblique single-plane view. However, visual interpretation of single-plane left anterior oblique equilibrium radionuclide angiograms provides less

TABLE III
RESULTS OF 5 STUDIES USING EXERCISE RADIONUCLIDE VENTRICULOGRAPHY WITH
CORONARY ANGIOGRAPHIC CORRELATION

Principal Investigator	N	Sensitivity	Specificity	Method (1) and Criteria (2) for Normal
Borer	25	100%	100%	(1) Gated (2) Exercise EF $\geq$ 7% above rest
Berger	73	87%	100%	(1) First pass (2) Wall motion, rest EF $\geq$ 55%, exercise EF $>$ 5% above rest
Brady	89	93%	100%	(1) Gated (2) Exercise EF $>$ rest
Pfisterer	40	95%	55%	(1) Gated (2) Rest EF $>$ 50%, exercise EF $\geq$ 10% above rest
Caldwell	52	93%	54%	(1) Gated (2) Rest EF $\geq$ 50%, exercise EF $>$ 5% above rest
Jengo	58	98%	94%	(1) First pass (2) Wall motion, exercise EF $>$ 10% above rest
Jones	387	90%	58%	(1) First pass (2) Rest EF $>$ 50%; predicted exercise EF, end-systolic volume, wall motion
Total	724	92%	70%	

EF = ejection fraction.

information than do first-pass right anterior oblique radionuclide angiograms. But to be practical, there is an excellent relation between wall motion disturbances seen by first-pass and gated blood-pool studies. Assessment of wall motion abnormalities has relied on visual interpretation of radionuclide images, although computer programs for regional ejection fraction and phase analysis are currently being validated. These techniques rely on area or time analysis of pie-shaped wedges of the left ventriculogram. Regional ejection fractions correlate well with regional wall motion abnormalities detected by contrast ventriculography, as do phase analysis abnormalities. However, it appears that regional wall motion abnormalities are not specific for coronary disease, i.e., they can occur in other forms of heart disease. In some views the normal septum appears akinetic. These techniques have not yet been applied during exercise and would be difficult to validate since no other technique exists for analyzing wall motion during exercise. Digital imaging with small amounts of contrast injected into a peripheral vein or using two-dimensional echocardiography may make validation possible.

Right Ventricular Ejection Fraction Response to Exercise. Recently, there has been interest in assessing right ventricular ejection fraction in patients with coronary heart disease. Slutsky and co-workers studied 20 normal subjects and 50 patients with coronary heart disease using equilibrium radionuclide angiography. The resting right ventricular ejection fraction did not differ between these two groups (49% versus 46%). Both groups were then maximally exercised in the supine position. The normal subjects increased their ejection fraction from 49% at rest to 64% at peak exercise, whereas those patients with right coronary occlusion either alone or with other vessel involvement showed no increase in right ventricular ejection fraction (46% to 45%). Those patients with coronary artery disease but with no evidence of right coronary artery occlusion increased the right ventricular ejection fraction from a resting value of 46% to 53% at peak exercise. Right ventricular dysfunction was probably related to both local ischemia and an increased load due to left ventricular dysfunction.

Slutsky and co-workers studied 10 normal subjects and 37 patients with mild to severe chronic obstructive lung disease, some with and some without coronary disease, using first-pass radionuclide angiography. Despite a mean left ventricular ejection fraction above 51% in all three groups, the patients with severe chronic obstructive pulmonary disease without coronary heart disease and those with coronary disease had mean resting right ventricular ejection fractions of 46% and 43%, respectively. Berger and colleagues studied 36 patients with chronic obstructive pulmonary disease also using the first-pass technique and reported a wide variation in the resting right ventricular ejection fraction. More than half had normal values. All ten chronic obstructive pulmonary disease patients with cor pulmonale had an abnormal resting right ventricular ejection fraction.

Matthay and colleagues evaluated the right and left ventricular ejection fraction responses to exercise in 24 chronic obstructive pulmonary disease patients. Twenty failed to increase their right ventricular ejection fraction more than five ejection fraction units above the resting value with exercise. Only 7 of these 24 patients demonstrated an abnormal exercise left ventricular ejection fraction. Slutsky and co-workers found a similar decrease in the exercise right ventricular ejection fraction in 11 patients with severe chronic obstructive lung disease (43% to 36% with exercise). Volume and pulmonary pressures were also assessed, and patients with severe chronic obstructive pulmonary disease often dilated the right ventricle and therefore decreased the ejection fraction with exercise. These changes correlated with pulmonary pressure. Olvey and co-workers studied the effects of oxygen administration on exercise function in 18 patients with chronic hypoxic lung disease. These investigators concluded that while oxygen does not alter right ventricular performance at rest, it can improve the function during exercise.

Ejection Fraction Response in Valvular Heart Disease. Radionuclide angiography is helpful in evaluating patients with valvular heart disease. Employing the first-pass technique, it is useful to identify flow patterns and transit times. Regurgitant fraction can be calculated from right and left ventricular stroke volume and counts. Using gated equilibrium, Borer and co-workers studied 34 patients with severe aortic regurgitation. Although 14 of the 21 symptomatic patients had a normal resting left ventricular ejection fraction, only one patient had a normal response to exercise. In the 22 asymptomatic patients, 21 had a normal resting left ventricular ejection fraction and only 13 responded normally to supine exercise. This technique could be useful for following ventricular function in patients with aortic regurgitation.

DETERMINATION OF LEFT VENTRICULAR VOLUME

The determination of left ventricular volume provides a better understanding of the pathophysiology of heart disease than does ejection fraction alone. In clinical practice, left ventricular volume is of proven value as a prognostic index in patients with heart disease. The ability to assess left ventricular volume changes in response to exercise, drug administration, or other interventions is exciting because it impacts on wall tension, one of the major determinants of myocardial oxygen. Both noninvasive radionuclide approaches to visualizing the left ventricle can be used for volume assessment.

Ventricular Volume Using the First-Pass Method. The study of heart function using the first pass of a radionuclide bolus through the central circulation has been described. In brief, radioactivity in the left or right ventricle during the first circulation of a radionuclide tracer is proportional to the amount of blood in the chamber at any time. By sampling left ventricular radioactivity over time using a standard gamma camera and a dedicated computer, it is possible to obtain a time-activity curve for each heartbeat during several cardiac cycles. The time-activity curve is the radioactivity (counts over time) and usually contains three to eight heartbeats with peaks and valleys of counts until equilibrium occurs. After subtraction of the background activity, a time-activity curve with a high sampling rate (25 points per second) is obtained. It consists of a succession of peaks and valleys in which the peaks correspond to end diastole and the valleys to end systole. Images obtained at 25 to 50 msec intervals from several cardiac cycles of similar duration and characteristics are superimposed to obtain high-fidelity images that can be displayed in cine format for qualitative analysis of wall motion. Left ventricular volumes can then be obtained by planimetry of the end-diastolic frame images using a similar technique for contrast ventriculography. This method postulates that the left ventricular cavity can be represented by an ellipsoid. The same methodology can be applied to the radionuclide angiogram in the anteroposterior or right anterior oblique projection.

Rezych and co-workers used this method to derive cardiac output from the ejection fraction, left ventricular end-diastolic volume, and heart rate (cardiac output = EF × LVEDV × HR). The correlation coefficient between simultaneous dye cardiac output and calculated radionuclide cardiac output was .95. Resting and exercise values for the same patient were included in the correlation coefficient analysis, making this technique appear better than it really is.

A second method for calculating ventricular volume using the first-pass approach is to consider only the first transit of the radionuclide through the central circulation. A simple calculation of cardiac output using this method is based on the indicator-dilution principle. A curve similar to the one obtained using dye and a densitometer is generated by using a gamma camera to sample a radionuclide passing through the heart. The integration of the area under the curve is proportional to cardiac output and correlates well with the dye technique. It is possible to use the cardiac output and ejection fraction to derive left ventricular volume: LVEDV = cardiac output/(EF × HR).

Ventricular Volume Using the Equilibrium Gated Technique. This technique is based on the administration of technetium linked to human serum albumin or red cells that remains relatively stable in the circulation for a period of four to six hours. Stannous salt helps technetium bind to red cells. Using a standard gamma camera and a computer, the radioactivity in the left ventricle can be assessed throughout the cardiac cycle. Because the amount of radioactivity in one cycle is insufficient for imaging, the study requires the accumulation of counts through 300 or more heartbeats.

Once the radioactive substance has reached equilibrium in the blood pool, the study is performed in the following way. Using a fiducial point on the electrocardiogram, the RR interval is divided into equal portions (12, 36, or more portions have been used) and the information from each corresponding portion of each cycle are added, forming composite images based on all 300 cycles. The movie format display of the images is used for the assessment of wall motion, and the count-rate changes through the cycle are used for constructing a time-activity curve. Ejection fraction is then obtained by the formula EF equals end-diastolic counts minus end-systolic counts (all background-corrected values) divided by end-diastolic counts. End diastole and end systole are considered the highest and lowest values of the curve. A point-by-point comparison of the left ventricular volume curve obtained by contrast ventriculography and the time-activity curve correlate well ($r = .93$). If it is possible to convert counts to milliliters, the volume calculated by this method would be of great value because, in addition to being noninvasive, it is less influenced by the inherent errors of geometric assumptions. The following will be a review of several methods already being used for research purposes using this technique.

If the distribution of the radioactive tracer in the blood is homogeneous, the radioactivity per milliliter of a sample of peripheral blood may be used to calculate the counts in the left ventricle at any time during the cardiac cycle with the actual volume. Left ventricular volume equals total counts in the left ventricle (at a particular time of the heart cycle) divided by activity per milliliter of the blood sample. To make an appropriate conversion several factors are important: (1) the time during which the reference blood sample and the left ventricle counts are obtained should be normalized, (2) the radioactive decay should be considered when there is a significant time difference between the sampling of peripheral blood and the performance of the radioactivity assay of the sample, and (3) attenuation factors must be considered.

The first two factors are relatively easy to account for in calculating volume. In brief, the radioactivity (counts at end diastole) is theoretically the same for all cycles processed; so if the time per frame (RR interval in seconds divided by number of frames) and the number of heartbeats proc-

TABLE IV
STATISTICAL ANALYSIS OF METHODS USING RADIONUCLIDE VENTRICULOGRAPHY TO ESTIMATE LEFT VENTRICULAR VOLUME

Center	N	*r* Value		SEE (ml)	
		EDV	ESV	EDV	ESV
University of California, San Diego	17	.97	.98	12	7
Dallas	22	.98	.98	16	15
Boston	13	.86	.91	36	22
Johns Hopkins	22	.94	.95	—	—
Johns Hopkins*	22*	.96	.96	33	33

*Accounting for attenuation.   *r* = correlation with contrast ventriculography

SEE = standard error of estimation; EDV = end-diastolic volume; ESV = end-systolic volume.

essed are known, the counts at end diastole per single beat per unit of time can be easily calculated. The second factor involves a very simple calculation using a decay constant, assuming a half-life of six hours and knowing the time between the blood sampling and counting.

The most controversial factor is attenuation. In an intuitive way, it is obvious that the reference blood sample should be counted at a similar distance from the camera as the left ventricle. In addition, there is lung and soft tissue between the heart and the camera that may equally influence the amount of radioactivity arriving at the camera. The main factors influencing the amount of radioactivity seen by the camera include (1) the distance and (2) the kind of tissue interposed between the heart and the camera. If we assume a source at a distance d, separated from the camera by a tissue with attenuation characteristics defined by a coefficient r, the counts arriving at the camera (Cc) will be equal to the real counts (Cr) times e^{-rd}. When considering a ellipsoid source like the left ventricle, it is obvious that the distance will be shorter for the anterior portion of the ventricle compared with the most posterior portion. The radioactivity from the posterior regions of the left ventricle will have to cross the whole thickness of blood inside the left ventricle in addition to the soft tissue, so the left ventricular geometry may play a significant role in the calculation of ventricular volumes. The complexity of the issue has resulted in two approaches to the problem: one that does not account for attenuation and a second that does. The methods that do not involve attenuation factors are summarized in Table IV. These methods are very similar to one another, and they consider all other factors except attenuation. They have been published by groups in San Diego, Dallas, and Boston.

In brief, the background-corrected counts in the left ventricle are obtained from the time-activity curve using a semiautomated computer program or by manually assigning a region of interest around the left ventricle at end diastole and end systole. A blood sample (3 to 5 ml) is drawn in the middle of the study and counted in front of the camera. The background-corrected counts per milliliter are used to calculate volume units from counts in the left ventricle: LV unit = LV counts divided by counts per milliliter of blood sample. The reports have shown a good correlation between the radioactive volume units and the left ventricular volumes calculated from contrast ventriculography performed within 24 to 48 hours. The equation obtained from the regression line can be used to convert volume units into milliliters. Using this methodology, the calculation of volumes was possible, but the difference between radionuclide and angiographic volumes was significant, as assessed by the standard error of the estimate values (SEE).

Two methods have been proposed that consider attenuation. The theoretic advantage is avoiding the utilization of a regression equation that has the potential error of disparities between the reference population used to calculate the equation and subsequent patients. One of the methods developed at Johns Hopkins University utilizes an attenuation factor obtained through the calculation of the distance between the camera and the theoretic center of the left ventricle, based on the linear attenuation coefficient of water. The volume is then calculated from the formula:

$$\mathrm{LVEDV} = \frac{\text{count rate from LV in end diastole}/e^{-md}}{\text{count rate per milliliter of blood sample}}$$

Calculation of the distance d is relatively simple (Figure 4). A radioactive point source is positioned over the left ventricle in the 40° left anterior oblique projection and fixed on the chest. The left ventricle and the source are imaged in the posterior-anterior view. Calculation of d = x divided by sin 40°, where x is the frontal plane length. Using this method, very good correlation was obtained with contrast angiography ($r = .96$). The standard error of the estimate was not different from that obtained by other investigators who did not consider attenuation. In fact, in this particular study the correlation was similar whether considering attenuation factors or not. When estimating the distance from the camera to the left ventricle, a difference of 1 cm represented a 14% change in the calculated LV volume. No correlation was found between the distance and the calculated volume, the body surface area, or body morphology that could improve the calculation.

The Seattle group has proposed correcting for attenuation by calculating the thickness of soft tissue between the left ventricle and the skin using

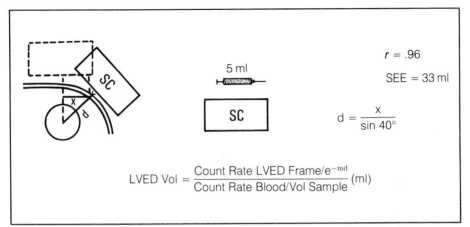

Figure 4. Illustration shows the method to correct for attenuation in estimating left ventricular end-diastolic volume (LVED Vol) using angulation of the scintillation image. The measurement of the projection of d on the frontal plane x is measured over the computer's television screen in pixels and converted to centimeters by a conversion factor. SEE = standard error of estimation.

an x-ray along the camera axis (Figure 5). The correction factor would be incorporated when imaging the blood sample at the same distance that the camera was from the chest and with the interposition of the same thickness of material with an attenuation similar to soft tissue.

The response of left ventricular volume to exercise remains controversial. At the University of California, San Diego, we have made volume measurements during supine and erect exercise in the same individuals, but our results have been complicated by a wide scatter of the volume data. Part of this was due to the fact that our patients were first studied supine and then erect one hour later. Patients do not become basal within this time frame both because of sympathetic stimulation and because of fluid shifts out of the vascular tree. However, much of the scatter is due to methodologic difficulties with the technique. From our studies and a review of the literature, the following analysis seems reasonable. In the supine position, end-diastolic volume is close to maximal, particularly if the feet are elevated (i.e, up on bicycle pedals)—meaning that there will be little change in volume in response to exercise. In the erect position, end-diastolic volume begins at its lowest possible value but increases with exercise as venous return increases. At near-maximal levels, end-diastolic volume plateaus and possibly can even drop. There are some coronary patients and normal subjects who increase end-diastolic volume at maximal exercise in either position, but we have yet to explain this observation. It is hard to imagine that the ventricle becomes

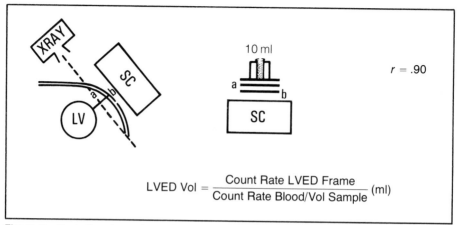

Figure 5.   Illustration shows the method for correcting for attenuation in estimating left ventricular end-diastolic volume (LVED VOL) by calculating the thickness of soft tissue between the left ventricle and the skin using an x-ray image taken along the axis of the scintillation camera (SC). The distance from the skin to the left ventricle is assessed by an orthogonal six-foot x-ray film. The source is imaged through air (b) and "soft tissue" of thickness a. (With permission of the Western J Med.)

so dyskinetic that it bulges in such a manner that total left ventricular end-diastolic volume is markedly increased. It appears that there is a variable response of end-diastolic volume during submaximal exercise in both positions, probably due to sympathetic tone and venous return. It is doubtful that changes in end-diastolic volume during exercise have much diagnostic impact because of their great variability.

Okada and colleagues used multigated blood-pool images at rest and during supine bicycle exercise to determine the pulmonary blood volume ratio in patients being evaluated with angiography for chest pain. The mean exercise-to-rest pulmonary blood volume ratio was lower for persons without coronary artery disease and for those with only right coronary artery disease, as compared with all others with coronary artery disease. A pulmonary blood volume rest-exercise ratio equal to or greater than 1.06, that is, an increase in pulmonary volume with exercise, had a sensitivity of 79% for coronary disease in their population.

CONCLUSION

Left ventricular volume measurements in addition to ejection fraction are very important for the assessment of left ventricular performance. The use of percentage changes in volume has already been very reliable and helpful, but in certain circumstances it is important to obtain an accurate absolute value, particularly for estimates of prognosis. First-pass methods using area-length analysis are less reproducible than are equilibrium methods because of the difficulty in planimetry of a small image. In addition, this method encounters more problems when used to assess several interventions in the same patient because it requires several injections of radionuclide tracer. Equilibrium methods have problems as well. Radionuclide measurements underestimate angiographic volumes when the region of interest around the left ventricle is defined semiautomatically with a computer algorithm, in contrast to one defined manually. Although the methods described here seem to be very promising, they are time consuming and their reproducibility, interobserver variability, and accuracy in larger patient populations need to be assessed before they become routine clinical tools. Calibration of volume changes during exercise is tenuous because of the lack of reliable correlative techniques.

Dynamic radionuclide angiography provides an approach for evaluating left ventricular function, volume, and wall motion at rest and during exercise. It can be performed with the standard single-crystal camera available in most hospitals using the first-pass or gated blood-pool techniques or using the more expensive and delicate multicrystal cameras. Use of these techniques in the evaluation of the response to exercise is augmenting our knowledge of physiology and pathophysiology. Noninvasive assessment of pharmacologic intervention and cardiac surgery and rehabilitation are all good reasons for using these techniques, in addition to their diagnostic potential.

The use of dynamic radionuclide angiography for the evaluation of patients with chest pain syndromes remains controversial. It must be remembered that left ventricular dysfunction without ischemia during exercise can be caused by other cardiac diseases. Regional wall motion is more sensitive and specific for ischemic disease, but it is more difficult to analyze and less reproducible than is ejection fraction. Criteria for an abnormal ejection fraction response to exercise vary from institution to institution. Understanding these problems makes it apparent that, whereas the sensitivity of this technique for diagnosing coronary heart disease may be high, its specificity may be unacceptably low. When used in conjunction with thallium scintigraphy, specificity may be improved, but at a high cost. Thallium exercise testing appears to have a sensitivity of 80% and a specificity of 90%, and exercise radionuclide ventriculography has a sensitivity of about 90% and a specificity of 50%. These values were obtained in academic centers that have the time and personnel for exceptional standards. It is apparent that these two noninvasive radionuclide procedures certainly increase the data base available for patient management beyond that available from standard clinical and exercise test assessment.

Radionuclide left ventricular angiography during bicycle exercise and thallium treadmill imaging are exciting new techniques that need further research to optimize their methodology and interpretation and to establish their limitations. However, the ability to assess noninvasively left ventricular function, scarring, and perfusion and to obtain the same prognostic information previously available only from invasive left ventricular angiography is an exciting diagnostic advance.

The radiation dose for the gated cardiac blood-pool scan using 20 mCi of technetium, calculated by the absorbed fraction method is approximately 300 mrad to the whole body, 170 mrad for the gonads, and 520 mrad for bone marrow. Using 2 mCi of thallium gives 70 mrad to the whole body and 250 mrad to the kidneys and gonads. In comparison, cardiac catheterization with left ventricular angiography delivers 200 mrad to the gonads and up to 4,000 mrad to the bone marrow. The fact that even a small radiation exposure is involved limits the subjects examined and the number of serial examinations. In this increasingly environmentally alert society, radiopharmaceuticals are viewed suspiciously. Perhaps probes and solid-state imaging devices will reduce the radionuclide dosage needed.

Problems with methodology center around interference from other structures, the delay imposed by sequential single-plane imaging, selection of areas of interest and background, and the development of computer programs to analyze optimally the data gathered. These imaging techniques require technical expertise. Reproducibility and reliability require experience with computers, with reading the images themselves, and with angiographic interpretation. Institutional quality control is of great importance and requires rigorous laboratory standards. It is uncertain if these requirements can be met in standard nuclear medicine departments that do not have the time for or interest in research. These problems may possibly be solved before too much money is spent going down blind alleys and utilizing expensive but ill-suited equipment. A technique will probably evolve that will provide measurements of ejection fraction and perfusion every 30 seconds and enable the reliable analysis of localized wall motion abnormalities and volume at maximal exercise and during recovery, but such a technique is not available today.

At the present time, it would appear that radionuclide ventriculography can best be used for evaluating patient prognosis because the resting ejection fraction has considerable data gathered from cardiac catheterization in this regard. At this point, the exact value of exercise-induced ejection fraction changes or of wall motion abnormalities that have prognostic value is uncertain. Most likely those with ejection fractions that drop will have a worse prognosis than those with an ejection fraction that rises. However, the methodology and the exercise-testing protocol used can greatly effect this response, and this procedure does not have standardized methodology or techniques. In contrast, thallium treadmill testing has been more widely used and has a fairly standard methodology. Many studies have shown it to have both a sensitivity and a specificity approaching 90%. This exceeds the sensitivity of standard exercise electrocardiography, while retaining a high specificity. The major studies with exercise ventriculography suggest a greater sensitivity for it, but a much lower specificity, possibly approaching 50%. Thus, currently using exercise ventriculography for identifying normal subjects is equivalent to flipping a coin.

REFERENCES
CHAPTER II

INTRODUCTION

Beller GA: Radionuclide techniques in the evaluation of the patient with chest pain. Mod Concepts Cardiovasc Dis 50:43, 1981.

Berger HJ, Zaret BL: Nuclear cardiology. N Engl J Med 305:799, 1981.

Strauss H, McKusick K, Bingham J: Cardiac nuclear imaging: Principles, instrumentation and pitfalls. Am J Cardiol 46:1109, 1981.

Radiation Physics

Asimov I: Understanding Physics. New York, New American Library, 1969.

Rhodes B: Radiopharmaceuticals, in Strauss HB, Pitt B (eds): Cardiovascular Nuclear Medicine. St. Louis, C. V. Mosby, 1979, p 57.

Myocardial Imaging with Potassium-like Radionuclides (Cold-Spot Imaging)

Abenavoli T, Rubler S, Fisher V, et al: Exercise testing with myocardial scintigraphy in asymptomatic diabetic males. Circulation 63:54, 1981.

Aizawa Y, Kamei K, Shibata A: Quantitative analysis of thallium-201 uptake and the effect of heart rate. Jpn Circ J 44:863, 1980.

Ashburn W, Tubau J: Myocardial perfusion imaging in ischemic heart disease. Radiol Clin North Am 18:467, 1980.

Berger BC, Watson DD, Taylor GJ, et al: Quantitative thallium-201 exercise scintigraphy for detection of coronary artery disease. J Nucl Med 22:585, 1981.

Blood DK, McCarthy DM, Sciacca RR, et al: Comparison of single-dose and double-dose thallium-201 myocardial perfusion scintigraphy for the detection of coronary artery disease and prior myocardial infarction. Circulation 58:777, 1978.

Boucher CA, Zir LM, Beller GA, et al: Increased lung uptake of thallium-201 during exercise myocardial imaging: Clinical, hemodynamic and angiographic implications in patients with coronary artery disease. Am J Cardiol 46:189, 1980.

Bulkley BH, Hutchins GM, Bailey I, et al: Thallium-201 imaging and gated cardiac blood pool scans in patients with ischemic and idiopathic congestive cardiomyopathy: A clinical and pathologic study. Circulation 55:753, 1977.

Bulkley BH, Rouleau JR, Whitaker JQ, et al: The use of thallium for myocardial perfusion imaging in sarcoid heart disease. Chest 72:27, 1977.

Dunn R, Freedman B, Bailey I, et al: Exercise thallium imaging: Location of perfusion abnormalities in single-vessel coronary disease. J Nucl Med 21:717, 1980.

Gordon DG, Pfisterer M, Williams R, et al: The effect of diaphragmatic attenuation on thallium images. Clin Nucl Med 4:150, 1979.

Hecht H, Hopkins J, Rose J, et al: Reverse redistribution: Worsening of thallium-201 myocardial images from exercise to redistribution. Radiology 140:177, 1981.

Kirshenbaum HD, Okada RD, Boucher CA, et al: Relationship of thallium-201 myocardial perfusion pattern to regional and global left ventricular function with exercise. Am Heart J 101:734, 1981.

Lenaers A: Thallium-201 myocardial perfusion scintigraphy during rest and exercise. Cardiovasc Radiol 2:195, 1979.

Lenaers A, Block P, vanThiel E, et al: Segmental analysis of Tl-201 stress myocardial scintigraphy. J Nucl Med 18:509, 1977.

Mueller TM, Marcus ML, Ehrhardt JC, et al: Limitations of thallium-201 myocardial perfusion scintigrams. Circulation 54:640, 1976.

Pohost GM, Alpert NM, Ingwall JS, et al: Thallium redistribution: Mechanisms and clinical utility. Prog Cardiovasc Dis 22:70, 1980.

Stolzenberg J, Kaminsky J: Overlying breast as cause of false-positive thallium scans. Clin Nucl Med 3:229, 1978.

Strauss HW, Harrison K, Langan JK, et al: Thallium-201 myocardial imaging: Relation of thallium-201 to regional myocardial perfusion. Circulation 51:641, 1975.

Turner JD, Schwartz KM, Logic JR, et al: Detection of residual jeopardized myocardium 3 weeks after myocardial infarction by exercise testing with thallium-201 myocardial scintigraphy. Circulation 61:729, 1980.

Verani MS, Marcus ML, Spoto G, et al: Thallium-201 myocardial perfusion scintigrams in the evaluation of aorto-coronary saphenous bypass surgery. J Nucl Med 19:765, 1978.

Wackers FJ, Sokole EB, Samson G, et al: Anatomy of the normal myocardial image, in Ritchie JL, Hamilton GW, Wackers FJT (eds): Thallium-201 Myocardial Imaging. New York, Raven Press, 1978, p 50.

Cold-Spot Exercise Imaging with Angiographic Correlation

Bailey IK, Griffith LS, Rouleau J, et al: Thallium-201 myocardial perfusion imaging at rest and during exercise: Comparative sensitivity to electrocardiography in coronary artery disease. Circulation 55:79, 1977.

Berman DS, Salel AF, Denardo GL, et al: Noninvasive detection of regional myocardial ischemia using rubidium-81 and the scintillation camera: Comparison with stress electrocardiography in patients with arteriographically documented coronary stenosis. Circulation 52:619, 1975.

Bodenheimer MM, Banka VS, Fooshee CM, et al: Comparative sensitivity of the exercise electrocardiogram, thallium imaging and stress radionuclide angiography to detect the presence and severity of coronary artery disease. Circulation 60:1270, 1979.

Botvinick EH, Taradash MR, Shames DM, et al: Thallium-201 myocardial perfusion scintigraphy for the clinical clarification of normal, abnormal and equivocal electrocardiographic stress tests. Am J Cardiol 41:43, 1978.

Botvinick EH, Shames DM, Gershengorn KM, et al: Myocardial stress perfusion scintigraphy with rubidium-81 versus stress electrocardiography. Am J Cardiol 39:364, 1977.

Bulkley BH, Rouleau JR, Whitaker JQ, et al: The use of thallium-201 for myocardial perfusion imaging in sarcoid heart disease. Chest 72:27, 1977.

Caldwell JH, Hamilton GW, Sorensen SG, et al: The detection of coronary artery disease with radionuclide techniques: A comparison of rest-exercise thallium imaging and ejection fraction response. Circulation 61:610, 1980.

Dunn R, Wolff L, Wagner S, et al: The inconsistent pattern of thallium defects: A clue to the false positive perfusion scintigram. Am J Cardiol 48:224, 1981.

Iskandrian A, Segal B: Value of exercise thallium-201 imaging in patients with diagnostic and non-diagnostic exercise electrocardiograms. Am J Cardiol 48:233, 1981.

Jengo JA, Freeman R, Brizendine M, et al: Detection of coronary artery disease: Comparison of exercise stress radionuclide angiocardiography and thallium stress perfusion scanning. Am J Cardiol 45:535, 1980.

McGowan RL, Martin ND, Zaret BL, et al: Diagnostic accuracy of noninvasive myocardial imaging for coronary artery disease: An electrocardiographic and angiographic correlation. Am J Cardiol 40:6, 1977.

McLaughlin P, et al: Reproducibility of thallium myocardial imaging. Circulation 55:497, 1977.

Pfisterer M, Muller-Brand J, Cueni T: Prevalence and significance of reversible radionuclide ischemic perfusion defects in asymptomatic aortic valve disease patients with or without concomitant coronary disease. Am Heart J 103:92, 1982.

Pfisterer ME, Williams RJ, Gordon DG, et al: Comparison of rest/exercise ECG, thallium-201 scans and radionuclide angiography in patients with suspected coronary artery disease. Cardiology 66:43, 1980.

Rehn T, Griffith L, Achuff S, et al: Exercise thallium-201 myocardial imaging in left main coronary artery disease: Sensitive but not specific. Am J Cardiol 48:217, 1981.

Rigo P, Bailey I, Griffith L, et al: Stress thallium-201 myocardial scintigraphy for the detection of individual coronary arterial lesions in patients with and without previous myocardial infarction. Am J Cardiol 48:209, 1981.

Ritchie JL, Trobaugh GB, Hamilton GW, et al: Myocardial imaging with thallium-201 at rest and during exercise: Comparison with coronary arteriography and resting and stress electrocardiography. Circulation 56:66, 1977.

Ritchie JL, Zaret BL, Strauss HW, et al: Myocardial imaging with thallium-201: A multicenter study in patients with angina pectoris or acute myocardial infarction. Am J Cardiol 42:345, 1978.

Rosenblatt A, Lowenstein JM, Kerth W, et al: Post-exercise thallium-201 myocardial scanning: A clinical appraisal. Am Heart J 94:463, 1977.

Shimokawa H, Matsuguchi T, Koiwaya Y, et al: Variable exercise capacity in variant angina and greater exertional thallium-201 myocardial defect during vasospastic ischemic ST segment elevation than with ST depression. Am Heart J 103:142, 1982.

Zaret BL, Stenson RE, Martin ND, et al: Potassium-43 myocardial perfusion scanning for the noninvasive evaluation of patients with false-positive exercise tests. Circulation 48:1234, 1973.

Radionuclide Ventricular Angiography During Bicycle Exercise

Battler A, Ross J Jr, Slutsky R, et al: Improvement of exercise-induced left ventricular dysfunction with oral propranolol in patients with coronary heart disease. Am J Cardiol 44:318, 1979.

Battler A, Slutsky R, Karliner J, et al: Left ventricular ejection fraction changes during recovery from treadmill exercise: A new method for detecting coronary artery disease. Clin Cardiol 3:14, 1980.

Berger H, Reduto L, Johnstone D, et al: Global and regional left ventricular response to bicycle exercise in coronary artery disease: Assessment by quantitative radionuclide angiography. Am J Med 66:13, 1979.

Berger H, Sand M, Davies R, et al: Exercise left ventricular performance in patients with chest pain, ischemic-appearing exercise electrocardiograms, and angiographically normal coronary arteries. Ann Intern Med 94:186, 1981.

Borer JS, Kent KM, Bacharach SL, et al: Sensitivity, specificity and predictive accuracy of radionuclide cineangiography during exercise in patients with coronary artery disease. Circulation 60:572, 1979.

Jengo J, Oren V, Conant R, et al: Effects of maximal exercise stress on left ventricular function in patients with coronary artery disease using first-pass radionuclide angiography: A rapid, non-invasive technique for determining ejection fraction and segmental wall motion. Circulation 59:60, 1979.

Pulido JI, Doss J, Twieg D, et al: Submaximal exercise testing after acute myocardial infarction: Myocardial scintigraphic and electrocardiographic observations. Am J Cardiol 42:19, 1978.

Rerych S, Scholz P, Newman G, et al: Cardiac function at rest and during exercise in normals and patients with coronary heart disease. Ann Surg 187:449, 1978.

Rerych SK, Scholz PM, Sabiston DC, et al: Effects of exercise training on left ventricular function in normal subjects: A longitudinal study by radionuclide angiography. Am J Cardiol 45:244, 1980.

Slutsky R, Ackerman W, Karliner J, et al: Right and left ventricular dysfunction in patients with chronic obstructive lung disease. Am J Med 68:205, 1980.

Slutsky R, Karliner J, Battler A, et al: The reproducibility of ejection fraction and ventricular volume by gated radionuclide angiography after acute myocardial infarction. Radiology 132:153, 1979.

Sorensen S, Caldwell J, Ritchie J, et al: "Abnormal" reponses of ejection fraction to exercise, in healthy subjects, caused by region-of-interest selection. J Nucl Med 22:1, 1981.

Upton M, Rerych S, Roeback J, et al: Effect of brief and prolonged exercise on left ventricular function. Am J Cardiol 45:1154, 1980.

Ejection Fraction Response to Exercise in Normal Subjects and in Patients with Coronary Heart Disease

Caldwell J, Hamilton G, Sorensen S, et al: The detection of coronary artery disease with radionuclide techniques: A comparison of rest-exercise thallium imaging and ejection fraction response. Circulation 61:610, 1980.

Diamond GA, Forrester JS: Improved interpretation of a continuous variable in diagnostic testing: Probabilistic analysis of scintigraphic rest and exercise left ventricular ejection fractions for coronary disease detection. Am Heart J 102:189, 1981.

Foster C, Anholm J, Hellman C, et al: Left ventricular function during sudden strenuous exercise. Circulation 63:592, 1981.

Freeman MR, Berman DS, Staniloff H, et al: Comparison of upright and supine bicycle exercise in the detection and evaluation of extent of coronary artery disease by equilibrium radionuclide ventriculography. Am Heart J 102:182, 1981.

Gibbons RJ, Lee KL, Cobb F, et al: Ejection fraction response to exercise in patients with chest pain and normal coronary arteriograms. Circulation 64:952, 1981.

Newman G, Rerych S, Upton M, et al: Comparison of electrocardiograpic and left ventricular functional changes during exercise. Circulation 62:1204, 1980.

Pfisterer ME, Battler A, Swanson S, et al: Reproducibility of ejection-fraction determinations by equilibrium radionuclide angiography in response to supine bicycle exercise: Concise communication. J Nucl Med 20:491, 1979.

Pfisterer ME, Slutsky RA, Schuler G, et al: Profiles of radionuclide left ventricular ejection fraction changes induced by supine bicycle exercise in normals and patients with coronary heart disease. Cathet Cardiovasc Diagn 5:305, 1979.

Port S, Cobb F, Coleman R, et al: Effect of age on the response of the left ventricular ejection fraction to exercise. N Engl J Med 303:1133, 1980.

Port S, Cobb FR, Jones RH: Effects of propranolol on left ventricular function in normal men. Circulation 61:358, 1980.

Rerych S, Scholz P, Newman G, et al: Cardiac function at rest and during exercise in normals and in patients with coronary heart disease. Ann Surg 187:449, 1978.

Slutsky R, Battler A, Gerber K, et al: The effect of nitrates on left ventricular size and function during exercise: Comparison of sublingual nitroglycerin and nitroglycerin paste. Am J Cardiol 45:831, 1980.

Slutsky R, Curtis G, Froelicher V, et al: The effect of sublingual nitroglycerin on left ventricular function at rest and during spontaneous angina pectoris: Assessment with a radionuclide approach. Am J Cardiol 44:1365, 1979.

Detection of Wall Motion Abnormalities

Bodenheimer M, Banka V, Fooshee C, et al: Comparison of wall motion and regional ejection fraction at rest and during isometric exercise. J Nucl Med 20:724, 1979.

Bodenheimer M, Banka V, Fooshee C, et al: Detection of coronary heart disease using radionuclide determining regional ejection fraction at rest and during exercise: Correlation with coronary arteriography. Circulation 58:640, 1978.

Bodenheimer M, Banka V, Fooshee C, et al: Quantitative radionuclide angiography in the right anterior oblique view: Comparison with contrast ventriculography. Am J Cardiol 41:718, 1978.

Bodenheimer M, Banka V, Helfant R, et al: Radionuclide angiographic assessment of left ventricular contraction: Uses, limitations, and future directions. Am J Cardiol 45:661, 1980.

Hecht HS, Hopkins JM: Exercise induced regional wall motion abnormalities on radionuclide angiography are not specific for coronary artery disease (abstract). Circulation 62:147, 1980.

Johnson L, Ellis K, Schmidt D, et al: Volume ejected in early systole. Circulation 52:378, 1975.

Leighton R, Pollack M, Welch T: Abnormal left ventricular wall motion at mid-ejection in patients with coronary heart disease. Circulation 52:238, 1979.

Maddox D, Holman B, Wynne J, et al: The ejection fraction image: A non-invasive index of regional left ventricular wall motion. Am J Cardiol 41:1230, 1978.

Maddox D, Wynne J, Uren R, et al: Regional ejection fraction: A quantitative radionuclide index of regional left ventricular performance. Circulation 59:1001, 1979.

Okada R, Kirschenbaum H, Kushner F, et al: Observer variance in the qualitative evaluation of left ventricular wall motion and the quantitation of left ventricular ejection fraction using rest and exercise multigated blood pool imaging. Circulation 61:128, 1980.

Slutsky R, Karliner J, Battler A, et al: Comparison of early systolic and holosystolic ejection phase indices by contrast ventriculography in patients with coronary heart disease. Circulation 61:1083, 1980.

Right Ventricular Ejection Fraction Response to Exercise

Berger H, Matthay R, Loke J, et al: Assessment of cardiac performance with quantitative radionuclide angiography with right ventricular ejection fraction with reference to findings in chronic obstructive pulmonary disease. Am J Cardiol 41:897, 1980.

Berger HJ, Matthay RA, Pytlik LM, et al: First-pass radionuclide assessment of right and left ventricular performance in patients with cardiac and pulmonary disease. Semin Nucl Med 9:275, 1979.

Maddahi J, Berman D, Matsomoko D, et al: A new technique for assessing right ventricular ejection fraction using multiple-gated equilibrium cardiac blood pool scintigraphy: Description, validation, and findings in coronary artery disease. Circulation 60:581, 1979.

Maddahi J, Berman DS, Matsuoka DT, et al: Right ventricular ejection fraction during exercise in normal subjects and in coronary artery disease patients: Assessment by multiple-gated equilibrium scintigraphy. Circulation 62:133, 1980.

Matthay R, Berger H, Davies R, et al: Effect of steady state exercise on right and left ventricular performance in chronic obstructive pulmonary disease. Chest 77:303, 1980.

Olvey S, Reduto L, Stevens P, et al: First pass radionuclide assessment of right and left ventricular performance in chronic pulmonary disease. Effect of oxygen upon exercise reserve (abstract). Chest 76:362, 1979.

Slutsky R, Ashburn W, Karliner J: Right ventricular volume: Analysis by equilibrium radionuclide angiography in normal subjects and patients with coronary disease (abstract). Am J Cardiol 45:412, 1980.

Slutsky R, Hooper W, Gerber K, et al: Assessment of right ventricular function at rest and during exercise in patients with coronary artery disease: A new approach using equilibrium radionuclide angiography. Am J Cardiol 45:63, 1980.

Tobrinick E, Schelbert H, Henning H, et al: Right ventricular ejection fraction in patients with acute anterior and inferior myocardial infarction. Circulation 57:1078, 1978.

Ejection Fraction Response in Valvular Heart Disease

Bough EW, Gandsman EJ, North DL, et al: Gated radionuclide angiographic evaluation of valvular regurgitation. Am J Cardiol 46:423, 1980.

Iskandrian S, Hakki A, Kane S, et al: Quantitative radionuclide angiography in assessment of hemodynamic changes during upright exercise: Observations in normal subjects, patients with coronary artery disease and patients with aortic regurgitation. Am J Cardiol 48:239, 1981.

Johnson LL, McCarthy DM, Sciacca RR, et al: Right ventricular ejection fraction during exercise in patients with coronary artery disease. Circulation 60:1284, 1979.

Sorensen SG, O'Rourke RA, Chaudhuri TK: Non-invasive quantitation of valvular regurgitation by gated equilibrium radionuclide angiography. Circulation 62:1089, 1980.

Determination of Left Ventricular Volume

Ashburn WL, Schelbert H, Verba J: Left ventricular ejection fraction—A review of several radionuclide angiographic approaches using the scintillation camera, in Holman BL, Sonnenblick EH, Leach M (eds): Principles Of Cardiovascular Nuclear Medicine. New York, Grune & Stratton, 1978, p 171.

Caldwell J, Stewart D, Dodge H, et al: Left ventricular volume during maximal supine exercise: A study using metallic epicardial markers. Circulation 58:732, 1978.

Dehmer G, Lewis J, Hillis LD, et al: Nongeometrical determinations of left ventricular volumes from equilibrium blood pool scans. Am J Cardiol 45:293, 1980.

Froelicher VF, Goldberger A, Tubau JF, et al: New non-invasive approaches to evaluating coronary heart disease. Specialty Conference, University of California, San Diego. West J Med 135:104, 1981.

Konstam M, Wynne J, Holman L, et al: Quantitation of left ventricular output in patients with and without left sided valvular regurgitation using equilibrium (gated) radionuclide ventriculography (abstract). J Nucl Med 22:620, 1981.

Links J, Becker L, Shindledlecker G, et al: Left ventricular volume determined from gated blood pool studies using an attenuation corrected count rate method. Circulation 65:82, 1982.

Okada R, Pohost G, Kirshenbaum H, et al: Radionuclide-determined change in pulmonary blood volume with exercise improved sensitivity of multigated blood pool scanning in detecting coronary artery disease. N Engl J Med 301:569, 1979.

Rerych J, Schulz P, Newman G, et al: Cardiac function at rest and during exercise in normals and in patients with coronary heart disease. Ann Surg 187:449, 1978.

Sandler H, Dodge HT: The use of single plane angiocardiograms for the calculation of left ventricular volume in man. Am Heart J 75:325, 1968.

Slutsky R, Karliner J, Ricci D, et al: Left ventricular volumes by gated equilibrium radionuclide angiography: A new method. Circulation 60:556, 1979.

Slutsky R, Karliner J, Ricci D, et al: Response of left ventricular volume to exercise in man assessed by radionuclide equilibrium angiography. Circulation 60:565, 1979.

Sorensen S, Ritchie J, Caldwell J, et al: Serial exercise radionuclide angiography—Validation of count-derived changes in cardiac output and quantitation of maximal exercise ventricular volume change after nitroglycerin and propranolol in normal men. Circulation 61:600, 1980.

III

The Cardiovascular Effects of Chronic Exercise

INTRODUCTION

Chronic exercise or an exercise program has also been called training or physical conditioning. This can be defined as maintaining a regular habit of exercise at levels greater than those usually performed. Exercise can be designed for increasing muscular strength, muscular endurance, or dynamic performance. The type of exercise that results in an increase in muscular strength is isometric exercise or developing muscular tension against resistance. Though this results in an increase in muscular mass along with strength, such exercises do not benefit the cardiovascular system. They result in a pressure load on the heart rather than a flow load because mean pressure is elevated, but not cardiac output. Dynamic exercise, also called isotonic, involves the rhythmic movement of large groups of muscles and requires an increase in cardiac output, ventilation, and oxygen consumption. Such exercise is also called aerobic because it must be performed with sufficient oxygen present. This is the type of exercise that results in the cardiovascular changes that will be described.

The features of an aerobic exercise program that must be considered include the mode, the duration, the intensity, and the frequency of the exercise. In general, the mode of exercise must involve movement of large muscle groups, such as with bicycling, walking, running, skating, cross-country skiing, and swimming. The exercise should be carried out in at least three sessions a week and should be spread out through the week. Duration should be 30 minutes to 60 minutes. Intensity should be at least 50% of the maximal oxygen consumption and involve at least 300 kcal of energy expenditure per session. The percentage of maximal oxygen consumption being performed can be approximated by heart rate and perceived exertion.

The results of such an aerobic exercise program include hemodynamic, morphologic, and metabolic changes. The hemodynamic consequences of an exercise program include a decrease in resting heart rate, a decrease in the heart rate and systolic blood pressure at any matched submaximal work load, an increase in work capacity and maximal oxygen consumption, and a faster recovery from a bout of exercise. It is argued whether these changes are due to peripheral or to central adaptations, but probably they are due to both. Peripheral adaptations are more important in older individuals and in patients with heart or lung disease, whereas central adaptations are more of a factor in younger individuals. Central hemodynamic changes that have been observed in some instances include enhanced cardiac function and cardiac output.

The morphologic changes that occur with an exercise program are clearly age-related. These changes occur most definitely in younger individuals and may not occur in older individuals. The exact age at which the response to chronic exercise is altered is uncertain, but it would seem to be in the early 30s. Morphologic changes include an increase in myocardial mass and left ventricular end-diastolic volume. Paralleling these changes are increases in coronary artery size and the myocardial capillary to fiber ratio. These changes are clearly beneficial, making it possible for the heart to function more efficiently and to have greater perfusion during any stress. In older individuals there can be a decrease in myocardial mass resulting in an improvement in capillary to muscle fiber ratio, but no change in coronary artery size. No studies have shown an exercise program to decrease atherosclerotic plaques once they are present. However, a recent monkey study has shown that exercise can offset the impact of an atherogenic diet.

The metabolic alterations secondary to an aerobic exercise program are summarized below. Total serum cholesterol level is not affected, but high-density lipoproteins (which remove cholesterol from the body) are increased. Serum triglyceride and fasting glucose levels are decreased. In addition, it appears that there are favorable alterations in insulin and glucagon responses. Diabetics need less insulin if they maintain a regular exercise program. Also, after an exercise program, blood catecholamine levels are lower in response to any stress. The fibrinolytic system seems to be enhanced and, since coronary thrombosis is no longer a misnomer, this would seem to be beneficial in preventing myocardial infarction.

TABLE I
RESULTS OF ANIMAL STUDIES INVESTIGATING THE EFFECTS OF CHRONIC EXERCISE

Age-dependent myocardial hypertrophy
Myocardial microcirculatory changes
Proportional increase in coronary artery size
Mixed results when studying changes in coronary collateral circulation
Improved cardiac mechanical and metabolic performance
Favorable changes in skeletal muscle mitochondria and respiratory enzymes
Mixed results with myocardial mitochondria and enzyme changes
Little effect on established atherosclerotic lesions or risk factors
Improved peripheral blood flow during exercise

Note: These results are strong support for the exercise hypothesis. Perhaps if people were as "compliant" as animals, the benefits of exercise to humans would be more apparent.

Although it is said that exercise enhances psychologic well-being and can even produce the "runner's high," few scientific studies have been performed in this area. It would seem, however, that exercise does have a tranquilizing effect and increases pain tolerance, which may be beneficial in some individuals. This chapter presents the studies that have investigated the effects of chronic exercise on the heart in animals and humans. The hemodynamic, echocardiographic, and exercise electrocardiographic testing results are described.

ANIMAL STUDIES OF THE EFFECTS OF CHRONIC EXERCISE

Animal studies provide some of the strongest evidence for the health benefits of regular exercise. The many effects listed in Table I have been demonstrated in various studies, and a review of some of these follows.

Myocardial Hypertrophy. Numerous studies have demonstrated that vigorous exercise can produce cardiac hypertrophy in animals. Heart-body ratios are invariably larger in wild animals as compared with the domestic form of an animal species. Heart hypertrophy is due to exercise in young rats, whereas in older rats, exercise causes a decline in heart weight due to a loss of myocardial fibers or a decrease in fiber mass.

The cellular morphologic mechanism of exercise cardiac hypertrophy has not been determined. There is even controversy regarding pathologic cardiac hypertrophy, which has been investigated more extensively in animal experiments. In exercise hypertrophy, the increased cardiac weight could be due to myocardial fiber hyperplasia, fiber hypertrophy, or both. The classic belief has been that myocardial fiber hyperplasia does not occur beyond the immediate postnatal period. There are several studies involving rat and human myocardial tissue, however, that support the concept that myocardial fiber hyperplasia occurs beyond this time. Also, an increase in fiber length has been demonstrated in biventricular hypertrophy secondary to pulmonary artery banding.

Hyperplasia and fiber lengthening, which could result in increased cardiac mass without fiber thickening, are advantageous as compared with fiber thickening, which occurs with pathologic cardiac hypertrophy. Maintenance of normal fiber diameter is important, since the diffusion distance from surrounding capillaries to central myofibrils is not increased. Exercise studies have shown a constant myocardial fiber diameter, favoring hyperplasia or fiber lengthening as the cellular morphologic mechanism of exercise-induced hypertrophy.

Myocardial Microcirculatory Changes. In comparing tame with wild animals (i.e., tame rabbit to hare, domesticated rat to wild rat), the density of muscle cells and capillaries was found to be much greater in the more active wild animals. In an experiment utilizing surgical constriction of the aorta, there was a 35% increase in heart weight in one-month-old rabbits and in adult rabbits. In the young rabbits, the hypertrophied hearts showed a normal capillary density; in the adult rabbits it was decreased. From these observations, Poupa hypothesized that in young animals, cardiac hypertrophy is secondary to fiber hyperplasia, whereas in older animals it is secondary to cellular hypertrophy. Also, he hypothesized that the capillary bed responds to growth stimuli most markedly if applied at an early age.

Tomanek studied the age-related response of the ventricular capillary bed and myocardial fiber width in male albino rats to chronic exercise. Eighty male rats, aged 40 days (young), 130 days (adult), or 575 days (old), were assigned to experimental or to control groups. The exercised rats ran on a treadmill six days a week for approximately 40 minutes for 12 weeks. The rats developed a resting bradycardia with this exercise program. At autopsy, the myocardial fiber width was constant at about 12 μ, whereas the capillary-fiber ratio increased in the exercised rats over the control rats in all age groups. The capillary density decreased with age and was increased over the controls only in the young exercised rats.

Leon and Bloor also performed rat experiments to study the effects of chronic exercise on the heart at different ages. Male rats aged 1 to 12 months were divided into three age groups equivalent to teen years, the 20s to 40s, and the 50s to 70s in humans. Each of these age groups was subdivided into a control group, a group that swam for one hour daily and a group that swam for an hour two days a week. After ten weeks, the animals were killed. They concluded that, although the response of the rat heart to chronic exercise varies with age, the capillary-fiber ratio increases at all ages. Their data regarding capillary changes are in agreement with the findings of Tomanek.

The only studies of the effects of an experimental program of exercise on myocardial capillary density using a species other than the rat have been those of Petren and associates and of Hakkila. Both used guinea pigs, but Petren's study showed an increase in capillary density, whereas Hakkila found a decrease.

After injecting radioactive thymidine in rats exercised by swimming, Ljungqvist and Unge studied capillary proliferation in the heart and skeletal muscle by radioautography. Swimming led to hypertrophy of the myocardium and limb muscle fibers. They found a significant new formation of myocardial capillaries in swimming-induced cardiac hypertrophy, whereas capillary neoformation in hypertrophied skeletal muscles was insignificant.

McElroy and colleagues reported an exercise-induced reduction in myocardial infarction size after coronary artery occlusion in the rat. Rats, forced to swim one hour a day five days a week for five weeks, were sacrificed and the myocardial capillary bed was perfused with carbon black. When compared with sedentary controls, the capillary to muscle fiber ratio was increased by 30% in exercised rats. This training effect occurred in the absence of hypertrophy or increased fiber diameter. An additional 27 exercised rats and 25 control rats underwent left coronary artery occlusion and were sacrificed 48 hours later. Myocardial infarct size was measured by planimetry of the left ventricle. In exercised rats, 22% of the left ventricle was infarcted compared with 31% in the control rats. Exercise training resulted in a 30% reduction of myocardial infarct size after coronary artery occlusion, which suggests an increased myocardial vascularity.

Wexler and Greenberg reported the effects of exercise on myocardial infarction in young versus old rats. Subcutaneous injections of isoproterenol were given to induce acute myocardial ischemia and infarction in both groups. Exercise improved the survival rates of the old rats. In addition, the exercised old rats manifested cardiac hypertrophy, reduced infarction enzyme levels, and less evidence of arrhythmias or extensive myocardial infarction on their electrocardiographic tracings.

Coronary Artery Size Changes. Tepperman and Pearlman studied the effects of exercise on the coronary tree of rats by the corrosion-cast technique. One group of rats ran approximately one mile a day for 36 days, and another group swam for 30 minutes a day for 10 weeks. When the animals were killed, their hearts were weighed, then the coronary arteries were injected with vinyl acetate. The hearts were digested with potassium hydroxide, and the casts of the coronary arteries were weighed alone. Compared with the controls, both groups had an increased heart–body weight ratio and an increased coronary tree cast weight–heart weight ratio.

Stevenson and co-workers used the same corrosion-cast technique to ascertain the effects of exercise of different types, frequency, and duration. Their conclusion was that in the rat, forced exercise caused an increase in the coronary tree size as compared with the cardiac weight, provided the exercise was not too strenuous or frequent.

Leon and Bloor demonstrated that swimming exercise in rats resulted in an increased luminal cross-sectional area of the main coronary arteries in the animals that experienced an increase in ventricular weight, that is, only the young and strenuously exercised adult rats. These results are supported by the studies of Kerr and colleagues that demonstrated coronary artery enlargement in rats with cardiac hypertrophy induced by hypoxia, aortic constriction, and thyroxin. In addition, it has been demonstrated that the relationship between the total heart weight and the diameter of the coronary arteries and ostia is linear in humans up to the upper weight limit of physiologic hypertrophy.

Coronary Collateral Circulation. Eckstein performed the classic study of the effect of exercise and coronary artery narrowing on coronary collateral circulation. He surgically induced a constriction in the circumflex artery of approximately 100 dogs. Various degrees of narrowing were induced, but only dogs that developed electrocardiographic changes were included in the study. After one week of rest, the dogs were divided into two groups. One group was exercised on a treadmill one hour a day, five days a week for six to eight weeks. The other group remained at rest in cages. The extent of arterial anastomoses to the circumflex artery was then determined as follows. The animals were anesthetized, a second thoracotomy was performed, and their blood pressure was stabilized mechanically. The circumflex artery was isolated and divided beyond the surgical constriction. The flow rate through the constriction and the flow rate from the distal end of the artery were measured. The flow rate through the constriction was inversely related to the degree of constriction.

When these values were plotted against one another, it was shown that the less the antegrade flow (or the greater the constriction), the greater the retrograde or collateral flow. Also, the exercised dogs had a greater value for retrograde flow than did the rested dogs for any degree of constriction. Eckstein concluded that moderate and severe arterial narrowing results in collateral development proportional to the degree of narrowing and that exercise leads to even greater coronary anastomosis.

Burt and Jackson used similar methods to study the effects of exercise on the collateral vessels of normal dogs. Twenty dogs were used, 13 rested and 7 exercised. Prior constriction of a coronary artery was not performed, as was in Eckstein's experiment. After one month of treadmill exercise, surgery was performed and retrograde flow measured from the distal portion of the circumflex artery with its proximal end ligated. There was no difference found in retrograde flow between the two groups. The authors concluded that exercise alone in the absence of an ischemic lesion is not sufficient to stimulate coronary collateral growth.

Kaplinsky and co-workers studied the effects of physical training in dogs after coronary artery ligation. Forty dogs were surgically subjected to complete occlusion of the left anterior descending coronary artery. Twenty-six dogs survived and after one week of rest were divided into exercise and control groups. The exercised dogs were run on a treadmill for one hour, six days a week for five weeks, and then both groups were put to death. A training effect was demonstrated in the exercise group. Selective cineangiography and postmortem coronary injections demonstrated extensive collateral formation, but there was no difference between the two groups. The authors concluded that exercise may not enhance collateralization when a large vessel is totally occluded.

Cobb and associates studied the effects of exercise on acute coronary occlusion in dogs with a prior partial occlusion. The anterior descending coronary artery was partially occluded (35% to 70%) in 50 dogs, and then they were divided into a control and an exercise group. The exercise consisted of treadmill running for 40 minutes a day for three months. Subsequently, a complete occlusion of the anterior descending artery was surgically produced. The animals were monitored for arrhythmias for six days, then sacrificed, and their hearts removed. The coronary vessels were injected and the collateral vessels were quantitated radiographically. The two groups did not differ as to the extent of the infarct relative to the partial occlusion, the frequency of arrhythmias, or the extent of radiographically quantitated collaterals.

Malik reported the effects of exercise training on coronary blood flow and cardiac output in rats at rest and during stress induced by breathing a mixture of 5% oxygen and 95% nitrogen for five to seven minutes. Training decreased the resting heart rate and coronary blood flow and increased resting cardiac output and coronary vascular resistance. During hypoxic stress, arterial pressure, heart rate, and cardiac output fell in both the trained and sedentary rats; coronary blood flow also fell in sedentary rats but did not change in trained rats. Decreases in perfusion during hypoxia in both endocardium and epicardium were found solely in sedentary rats. The unchanged coronary blood flow during hypoxia in trained rats was associated with a greater decrease in coronary vascular resistance. Malik concluded that exercise training leads to greater coronary dilatation during hemodynamic stresses and thereby maintains coronary flow.

Spear and colleagues studied coronary blood flow in exercised and sedentary rats using labeled microspheres during hypoxemic conditions designed to develop coronary dilatation. Rats trained for 12 to 18 weeks had a significantly greater blood flow than did sedentary rats. Even though cardiac hypertrophy was found in the trained rats, this increase in perfused mass accounted for only one third the increase in total coronary blood flow. Thus, there was a greater coronary blood flow per unit mass of the myocardium in the trained rats.

Sanders and colleagues reported the effects of endurance exercise on coronary collateral blood flow in miniature swine. Coronary collateral blood flow was measured in ten sedentary control pigs and in seven exercised pigs trained for ten months by running approximately 35 km a week. Using acute, open chest preparations, radiolabeled microspheres were injected into the left atrium during each of three conditions: control, total occlusion of the left circumflex artery, and total occlusion plus mechanically elevated aortic pressure. Ten months of endurance exercise training did not have an effect on the development of coronary collaterals, as assessed by microsphere blood flow measurements in the left ventricle of the pigs.

Heaton and colleagues studied the effect of physical training on collateral blood flow in 14 dogs with chronic coronary occlusions. Regional blood flow was measured using injected radionuclide microspheres at rest and during exercise. One half of the dogs subsequently trained for six weeks while the other half remained inactive in kennels. After six weeks, myocardial blood flow was not significantly changed in control animals. After training, however, myocardial blood flow to the underperfused endocardium of collateral-dependent zones was 39% greater than it was before training.

Scheel and colleagues studied ten control beagles, ten exercised beagles, eight beagles with occluded circumflex arteries for five months, and seven beagles similar to the last group but exercised. Using an isolated heart preparation, they found no increase in collaterals in the normal dogs, but doubled collateral conductance in the exercised ischemic dogs.

There is some question whether middle-aged patients with coronary artery disease can accomplish enough physical exertion to stimulate collateral development greater than the ischemia secondary to their disease. Neill and Oxedine studied the effects of exercise training on coronary collaterals developing in response to gradual coronary occlusion in dogs. Ameroid constrictors were used, which initially were nonobstructive but slowly absorbed body fluids and gradually expanded over two to three weeks. After placement of a constrictor on the proximal left circumflex coronary artery, 33 dogs were randomly assigned to exercise or to sedentary groups. After two months, the exercised dogs developed greater epicardial collateral connections to the occluded left circumflex as judged by higher blood flow and less distal pressure drop. However, no difference in collaterals was found angiographically. Injected microspheres demonstrated that exercised dogs were not better protected against subendocardial ischemia induced by increased heart rate in the myocardium supplied by the collaterals. These investigators concluded that exercise can promote coronary collateral development without improving perfusion of ischemic myocardium. These results raise an additional question: Even if collateral development does occur, does it significantly influence myocardial perfusion?

Cardiac Mechanical and Metabolic Performance. Penpargkul and Scheuer reported the effect of physical training on the mechanical and metabolic performance of the isolated rat heart. Rats were exercised by swimming for $2\frac{1}{2}$ hours a day, five days a week for two months. The exercised rats and controls were killed and their hearts isolated in a perfusion apparatus with cannulas inserted for life support, pressure and flow measurement, and metabolic analysis. When compared with sedentary controls, the hearts from conditioned rats had higher levels of cardiac work and output. Atrial pacing at increased rates caused greater differences in those parameters, and left ventricular pressures and dp/dt became higher in conditioned hearts. Atrial pacing also resulted in greater oxygen consumption in conditioned hearts, whereas higher lactate and pyruvate concentrations occurred in sedentary hearts. Raising atrial filling pressures resulted in ventricular function curves that were superior in the conditioned hearts. Also, there were greater increments in oxygen consumption, a higher aerobic to anaerobic energy production ratio, and increased coronary artery flow. The authors concluded that in physically trained rats, the function of the heart as a pump is improved and that this effect is at least partially due to improved oxygen delivery.

Crews and Aldinger also presented data to support the concept that the exercise-hypertrophied heart is functionally superior to the normal heart. They randomly divided 30 female rats into control and exercise groups of 15 each. The exercised rats swam for six hours a day for approximately one month. Then a thoracotomy was performed and isometric systolic tension was measured while the animals were physiologically supported. This measurement was felt by the authors to reflect potential contractility and cardiac work. Measurements were also made of left ventricular pressure before and during aortic constriction. The animals were sacrificed and body weight, ventricular thickness, cardiac weight, and cardiac volume determined. All of these parameters were significantly increased in the exercise group as compared with the control rats. Aldinger has reported a similar study involving a control and exercised group of rats receiving digitoxin. This study demonstrated that unlike the pathologic hypertrophy of disease, exercise hypertrophy and the increment in myocardial function concomitant with hypertrophy are not altered by digitoxin.

Tomoike and colleagues reported regional myocardial dynamics during brief strenuous bouts of running in 12 conscious dogs using telemetry before and after partial circumflex coronary artery obstruction. Regional myocardial dimensions were measured using surgically embedded ultrasonic crystals in a control segment and in a segment that would be made ischemic. In control exercise runs, heart rate, left ventricular systolic pressure, and dp/dt increased markedly. Also, segment length at end diastole increased along with augmentation of regional myocardial performance. During circumflex constriction, exercise resulted in a similar heart rate, but left ventricular systolic pressure and dp/dt changes were significantly reduced. Shortening of the nonischemic segment did not change significantly, but ischemic segment power and stroke work were depressed. In two dogs, ventricular fibrillation occurred during and immediately after running. Abnormal regional wall motion during and following exercise appeared to be a specific indicator of limited coronary reserve. This animal model has potential for evaluating changes secondary to training.

Carew and Covell reported indices of left ventricular function and diastolic compliance in ten conscious, exercise-trained greyhounds with left ventricular hypertrophy. High-fidelity micromanometers and ultrasonic crystals were implanted, and left ventricular contractility was measured and found to be similar to that measured previously in normal dogs. During volume loading, changes in contractility approximated those in normal dogs. Left ventricular diastolic stiffness did not differ from that of normal dogs. Left ventricular function in exercise-induced left ventricular hypertrophy was substantially normal.

Bershon and Scheuer reported the effects of chronic exercise on the response of the rat heart to ischemia. Sedentary and swimming-trained rats were sacrificed, and their hearts were perfused in an isolated working-heart apparatus under aerobic and ischemic perfusion conditions. During ischemia, coronary blood flow diminished by approximately 40%, and oxygen consumption was similar in the two groups. During oxygenated conditions, end-diastolic pressures and volumes were similar in exercised and sedentary rats. The hearts of the exercised rats had better responses of stroke volume and left ventricular systolic pressure to increases in atrial filling pressure. During ischemia, stroke volume was 30% greater in hearts of exercised rats than in sedentary controls, and left ventricular systolic pressure was also significantly higher. Relaxation was faster during aerobic and ischemic perfusion in hearts of exercised rats. The duration of diastole was increased in hearts of exercised rats under ischemic and aerobic conditions. Under these highly controlled loading conditions, hearts of chronically exercised rats continued to perform better during ischemia than did hearts of sedentary controls. This result did not seem to be due to altered diastolic pressure–volume relationships and may be related to an intrinsic improvement in myocardial function.

Wyatt and colleagues studied the influence of physical training on myocardial contractility in six cats. After training, right ventricular papillary muscles were studied in vitro, and adenylate cyclase activity was determined from ventricular muscle. Physical training did not alter the intrinsic contractile function or the contractile response to paired or frequency stimulation. However, training might have improved the catecholamine-induced enhancement of myocardial contractility and adenylate cyclase activity.

Stone reported the effects of exercise training on cardiac function in conscious dogs that were instrumented so that ascending aortic flow, left ventricular pressure, and left atrial pressure could be measured. A standardized submaximal test was performed before and after training. The heart rate in the trained animals was reduced by an average of 20 beats/min. The maximum derivative of left ventricular pressure increased in the trained animals. Ventricular function curves were lower in trained animals because of a reduction in heart rate response. These results indicate a reflex adaptation of the nervous system with training to improve cardiac function. The earliest changes found were in stroke volume and cardiac output. Later, changes occurred in the heart rate response to volume loading and the contractility of the left ventricle associated with the test. The early changes in stroke volume could be associated with change in ventricular end-diastolic volume, whereas changes in contractility and heart rate could be consistent with a change in the balance of autonomic innervation of the heart. Reflex changes in heart rate with volume loading indicate that there may have been some integrative changes in the central nervous system pathways associated with this reflex. In conscious dogs, the cardiac effect of exercise training tended to lower the submaximal energy requirements of the heart and to increase maximal pumping capacity of the heart.

Dowell and colleagues, using chronically instrumented dogs, studied myocardial contractility and adenosine triphosphatase (ATPase) activity of cardiac contractile proteins before and after exercise training. Before training, heart rate and the maximal rate of left ventricular pressure development were measured at rest and during submaximal exercise. Animals were then subjected to an eight- to ten-week treadmill running program. After training, maximal dp/dt was within normal limits at rest but significantly elevated by submaximal exercise. When maximal dp/dt was plotted as a function of heart rate, either at rest or during submaximal exercise, a marked elevation of maximal dp/dt at any given heart rate was observed following training. Myofibrillar protein content and ATPase activity of left ventricular myocardium were nearly identical before and after training. Although exercise training by treadmill running improved myocardial contractility in the unanesthetized dog, this response does not involve alterations in myofibrillar ATPase activity.

Bershon and Scheuer studied hemodynamics and ventricular performance in hearts from sedentary and swimming-trained rats. They used an isolated working-heart apparatus modified to measure end-diastolic volume by dye dilution. In addition, instantaneous aortic flow, left ventricular pressure, and oxygen consumption were measured. Heart rate and mean aortic pressure were kept constant, and atrial filling pressure was varied. Heart weights were equal and end-diastolic pressures and volumes were similar to all atrial pressures. However, ejection fraction and circumferential fiber work were both greater in hearts of conditioned rats. Maximal negative dp/dt was also greater at all three loads. Maximal oxygen consumption of trained rats increased in proportion to the increase in work. These results indicated that the improved pumping performance of trained hearts is due to a change in ventricular function. Faster cardiac relaxation is a prominent effect of physical training and may foster more complete filling at high heart rates.

Dowell and colleagues studied the functional responses of the rat heart to pressure overload in exercised and sedentary rats. The rats were trained with a moderate treadmill running program. Left ventricular RNA, DNA, and cyctochrome C levels were unchanged. After training, when subjected to a pressure overload by sustained aortic constriction, exercised animals maintained or increased myocardial contractility. Exercised animals fully regained a normal cardiac output after the acute overload was relieved, but the cardiac output remained approximately 10% below control in sedentary animals. The improved ability of previously exercised animals to withstand pressure overload appears to be due to alterations in adaptation rather than augmentation of metabolism or function.

Ritzer and colleagues studied the effects of ten weeks of treadmill exercise on left ventricular performance in nine dogs chronically instrumented with left ventricular pressure transducers. At similar exercise heart rates, the trained dogs had greater left contractility indices than the sedentary dogs.

Skeletal Muscle Mitochondria and Respiratory Enzyme Changes. The changes that occur in chronically exercised skeletal muscles have been confirmed by numerous investigators, whose work has been reviewed by Holloszy. Mitochondria are increased in number, size, and the number of cristae. Amounts of mitochondrial protein and respiratory enzymes are also increased per gram of fresh muscle. There is an increased capacity for ATPase production and aerobic metabolism of many substrates. Myoglobin concentration is increased. This adaptation must partially account for the increased aerobic work capacity and for the decreased muscle blood flow at any level of submaximal exercise that occurs secondary to chronic exercise.

Tibbits and colleagues reported the results of 11 weeks of progressive treadmill exercise in rats. In the trained rats, gastrocnemius cytochrome C oxidase activity was 38% higher in the controls. They found that endurance training of this type did not necessarily increase myofibrillar ATPase activity or the time course of the isometric twitch of the rat papillary muscle. However, tension per unit area did increase and appeared to be due to a greater amount of calcium being made available to the contractile apparatus.

Myocardial Mitochondria and Respiratory Enzyme Changes. Arcos and his colleagues studied female rats, using a protocol similar to that used by Aldinger. The rats were separated into a control group and three swimming groups, with total swimming time ranging from 60 to 500 hours. The rats who exceeded 300 hours of total swimming could not continue swimming 6 hours a day, so their daily time had to be decreased. The rats were sacrificed and their hearts analyzed by various methods. Mitochondrial mass was increased only in the rats that swam for approximately 160 hours. Electron microscopy showed increased size and number of mitochondria in this group, whereas mitochondrial degeneration was noted in rats exercised for a longer time. No change in the respiratory rate of myocardial homogenates was found between the groups. The microscopic and histochemical sections showed evidence of myocardial degeneration in the exercised rat hearts. The authors suggested that the increase in mitochondrial mass is a compensatory response to exercise and that this increase brings about focal regions of hypoxia during overexercise causing degenerative changes.

Aldinger and Sohal repeated the previous experiment but with the total swimming time increased to between 400 and 1,500 hours. Also, a control and an exercise group treated with digitoxin were included again, and mitochondrial degenerative changes were seen in the myocardium of the nontreated swimmers; however, the swimmers receiving digitoxin showed no degenerative changes. In fact, they had an increase in the size of the mitochondria and in the number of mitochondrial cristae. In addition, the following subcellular changes occurred in the myocardium of both swimming groups: (1) increased mitochondrial-myofibril ratio, (2) occasional areas of myocardial hemorrhage, (3) increased distance between nuclei, and (4) dilatation and vesicle formation within intercalated discs. The authors suggested that some of these changes did not appear beneficial but concluded that the morphologic integrity of the myocardial mitochondria is better preserved in the swimming rat receiving digitoxin than in the untreated swimming rat.

Banister, Tomanek, and Cvorkov reported a study of the effects of chronic exercise on rat heart mitochondrial morphology using the electron microscope. Male rats were run to exhaustion on a motor-driven treadmill for one hour a day over a 65-day period. Throughout the training period four animals were sacrificed on certain days. The four consisted of one control, one trained animal killed immediately after exercise, one killed 30 minutes after exercise, and one killed 24 hours after exercise. On the first training day, exhaustive running resulted in mitochondrial degeneration in the animal killed immediately and in the one killed 30 minutes after exercise. The rat killed 24 hours after exercise showed mitochondrial morphology similar to the unexercised control rat. The effects of training began to appear after ten days of training. Fewer altered mitochondria were seen in the trained rats sacrificed at any period after exercise. This study demonstrates that with physical training, exhaustive exercise has a less damaging effect on myocardial mitochondria, suggesting that this organelle adapts to exercise.

Oscai, Mole, and Holloszy studied rats using various exercise protocols including the same swimming protocol used by Arcos and Aldinger. They could not confirm an increase in mitochondrial protein or respiratory enzymes in the myocardium of exercised rats. They suggested that the capacity for aerobic metabolism of normal, untrained rat myocardium is adequate to meet the increased demands for ATPase imposed by an exercise program without augmenting mitochondrial mass or respiratory capacity. They found that respiratory enzyme levels are approximately five times higher in the heart than in the gastrocnemius muscle of the sedentary rat. They also confirmed the interesting finding that exercise depresses the appetite of male rats and does not affect the appetite of female rats. Because of problems with growth differences secondary to this phenomenon between control and exercised rats, some investigators have used only female rats.

Tibbits and colleagues found tension per unit area increased in the papillary muscle of exercised rats, but this effect appeared to be due to a greater amount of calcium being made available to the contractile apparatus. Scheuer and co-workers have measured increased cardiac glycogen stores in conditioned rat hearts but found no increase in the concentration of high-energy phosphate compounds.

Effects on Atherosclerosis and Risk Factors. McAllister and colleagues reported an experiment that demonstrated an accelerating effect of muscular exercise on experimental atherosclerosis. Ten mongrel dogs were placed on identical high-cholesterol diets of equal caloric value and 150 mg of thiouracil daily. The diet and the thyroid antagonist were used to shorten the time period of the study. The dogs were treated identically, except that five were trained to run five miles a day at five miles per hour on a treadmill. At the end of one year, angiograms were performed, the dogs were sacrificed, and their arteries were analyzed for the extent of atherosclerosis. During the course of the study period, the serum cholesterol levels progressively rose with the runners having higher values. The runners also showed more atherosclerosis than did the sedentary dogs in all vessels, including the coronaries.

Myasnikov reported the results of studies performed by himself and his colleagues in Russia. Ten rabbits were given a high-cholesterol diet, 25 rabbits received the same diet but were run to exhaustion daily on an electric treadmill, and 8 rabbits received no cholesterol but were exercised. The exercised rabbits on a high-cholesterol diet had lower serum cholesterol levels than did those not exercised. At the end of six months, the animals were sacrificed and visual estimation showed that the physical exercise reduced to some extent the development of atherosclerosis in the aorta and coronary arteries. However, for unknown reasons, there were more marked pathologic changes in the myocardium of the exercised rabbits receiving cholesterol than in either of the other groups.

Kobernick and his co-workers reported the results of a similar study. Eighteen rabbits were fed high-cholesterol diets and exercised ten minutes a day, while a nonexercised matched group received the same diet. Serial serum cholesterol values did not differ between the groups. After 13 weeks, the rabbits were sacrificed and their aortas inspected visually for atherosclerosis and chemically analyzed for cholesterol. The exercised rabbits had greater muscle mass, less body fat deposits, and less aortic atherosclerotic involvement than did the nonexercised rabbits.

Warnock and colleagues reported an exercise study using young male roosters. All of the birds were caged and fed an atherogenic diet. Ten remained caged while 14 were taken from the cage and forced to walk briskly for one hour a day (approximately four miles a week). Weekly serum cholesterol values were determined and found to be lower in the exercised birds. The food consumption was equal in both groups, but the exercised birds were heavier. After 14 weeks, the birds were sacrificed and the aorta, its main branches, and samples of brain and liver were assayed for cholesterol. Cholesterol content was lower in the assayed vessels and liver of the exercised than of the nonexercised birds. Coronary arteries were not studied.

Carlson reported the results of strenuous exercise on the serum cholesterol levels of old rats. The trained group ran three hours daily for one month. At the end of this period, the serum cholesterol level averaged 186 mg/100 ml in the trained group and 250 mg/100 ml in controls. The extent of atherosclerotic involvement was not studied. Faris and his co-workers performed a similar study in young rats. Both the control and the exercised animals had serum cholesterol readings of about 45 mg/100 ml, and there was no statistical difference between the groups. Neither investigator discussed the diet fed their rats, but Carlson stated that lipid levels in rats increased with age, as they do in humans.

The influence of training on resting blood pressure in rats who were normotensive, borderline hypertensive, genetically hypertensive, or hypertensive but receiving drugs was investigated. Training resulted in lower blood pressure in normal rats. In the borderline hypertensive and genetically hypertensive rats, exercise training appeared to delay the onset of hypertension as well as the magnitude of systolic pressure, but exercise was unable to normalize the resting pressure.

Rasmussen and Hostmark studied cholesterol and triglycerides in two groups of rats with widely different levels of physical activity. Cholesterol and triglycerides were measured from the age of three to eight months in females and from three months to one year in males. A pronounced increase in lipids with age was observed in the active male rats. In the inactive male rats and in all females there was no major change in lipid levels. The data for male rats showed an association between the inherited tendency to perform spontaneous high levels of physical activity and an age-related increase in plasma lipids. However, running did not have any influence on the level of cholesterol or triglycerides.

Pedersoli reported the effects of physical exercise and of an atherogenic diet of serum lipids in swine. Twenty-two pigs were exercised daily, and 22 pigs served as controls. All were fed an atherogenic diet. Exercise training alone did not produce any change in serum lipids.

Kramsch and colleagues randomly allocated 27 young adult male monkeys into three groups. Two groups were studied for 36 months, and one group was studied for 42 months. Of the groups studied for 36 months, one was fed a vegetarian diet for the entire study, whereas the other was fed the vegetarian diet for 12 months and then an isocaloric atherogenic diet for 24 months. Both were designated as sedentary because their physical activity was limited to a single cage. The third group was fed the vegetarian diet for 18 months and then the atherogenic diet for 24 months. This group exercised regularly on a treadmill for the entire 42 months. Because two of the monkeys on the atherogenic diet, one sedentary and one exercising, did not develop elevated serum cholesterol levels, they were excluded from the study. For three years the animals were observed for objective evidence to support the protective value of periodic and regular exercise. Total serum cholesterol levels remained the same, but HDL cholesterol levels were higher in the exercise group. Ischemic electrocardiographic changes, angiographic size of coronary artery narrowing, and sudden death were observed only in the sedentary monkeys fed the atherogenic diet. In addition, postmortem examination revealed marked coronary atherosclerosis and stenosis in this group. Exercise was associated with substantially reduced overall atherogenic involvement, lesion size, and collagen accumulation. These results demonstrate that exercise in young adult monkeys produces increases in heart size, left ventricular mass, and the diameter of coronary arteries. Additionally, the subsequent experimental atherosclerosis, induced by the atherogenic diet administered for two years, was substantially reduced. Exercise before exposure to the atherogenic diet delayed the development of the manifestation of coronary heart disease. The important question this study raises is: At what point comparable to the human life span were these studies initiated, and what percentage of that life span was represented by the three years of observation?

Goodrick studied 140 rats that were maintained in either wheel-cage units or cage units for their entire life span. Body weight increment or growth rate was negatively related to longevity, whereas growth duration was positively related to longevity. Rats who performed wheel exercise had a significantly increased mean longevity compared with controls.

Changes in Peripheral Blood Flow in Response to Acute Exercise. Fixler and colleagues studied the distribution of cardiac output in six dogs at rest and during mild and moderate exercise. Organ blood flows were measured using radioactive microspheres. The greatest change was in diaphragmatic flow, which increased by 275% with mild exercise and increased by 500% with moderate exercise. Flow to intercostal muscles increased by 160% and 269%, to the exercising gastrocnemius muscle by 153% and 224%, and to the cardiac muscle by 57% and 109%, all during mild and moderate exercise, respectively. Renal and cerebral flows did not change. Significant decreases in flow occurred in the small and large intestines during moderate exercise. These results demonstrate that the increase in cardiac output during submaximal exercise was redistributed in a manner that limited blood flow to brain, intestines, and kidneys and increased the flow to the diaphragm, to the heart, and to the limb muscles. This organ blood flow measurement technique should prove to be useful in studying the peripheral adaptations to exercise brought about by training.

Summary. Animal studies add considerable data to our knowledge of the effects of chronic exercise on the heart. They demonstrate that there are morphologic and metabolic changes that make the cardiovascular system better able to withstand stress, possibly even that imposed by atherosclerosis. These favorable adaptations are more marked in young animals than in older animals. The data regarding beneficial effects of chronic exercise on the atherosclerotic process or on serum cholesterol levels are only suggestive, however, and better studies are required to confirm this effect. A recent study by Kramsch and colleagues provides the strongest evidence for a favorable impact of exercise on the primary prevention of coronary disease. In this study, exercise lessened ischemic manifestations, but only diet stopped progression of coronary atherosclerosis. Nevertheless, the therapeutic and preventive use of exercise is supported by animal studies, but such efforts should be adjunctive to modification of the risk factors that have a well-demonstrated influence on the atherosclerotic process.

HEMODYNAMIC STUDIES OF THE EFFECTS OF AN EXERCISE PROGRAM

The effects of an exercise program can be studied by the cross-sectional approach, comparing athletes to normal people, and by the longitudinal approach, comparing individuals before and after a training program. Both of these approaches have limitations and difficulties. The cross-sectional approach is the easier of the two because the trouble and expense of organizing a training program can be avoided. However, athletes are endowed with biologic attributes and motivation that make them capable of superior performance. Also, they undergo long periods of physical training that usually begin at a young age when dimensional and morphologic changes are more apt to occur. This fact makes comparison with normal people rather questionable since most trained normal individuals cannot reach an athlete's level of cardiovascular function or performance. For these reasons, only longitudinal studies are reviewed here.

Besides the expense and difficulty in organizing and maintaining an exercise program, there are other problems encountered in longitudinal studies. Volunteers often are athletic and differ from randomly selected normal people. An exercise program can modify significant variables, such as body weight and smoking habits, and results can be biased by dropouts. In persons with coronary heart disease, a placebo effect on hemodynamics has been documented and a training program may select a healthier group.

In any training program, the end result depends on a number of factors. These factors include the level of fitness, physical endowment, previous physical training, age, sex, and health of the individual entering the program. The changes are greater in sedentary individuals, as compared with those somewhat physically fit, and greater in younger individuals than in older individuals. It has been hypothesized that diseased hearts are not modified by chronic exercise and that peripheral circulatory changes associated with exercise training are more important in persons with coronary heart disease. The most important of these variables will be evaluated in this review by including discussions of normal trainees of different ages and of persons with coronary heart disease.

The structure of an exercise program is important. Intensity and duration of the work periods must be considered, as well as the overall time of exercise. Individuals with coronary heart disease must be carefully selected for an exercise program. During training they must be closely monitored and should follow a less demanding exercise protocol because of the danger of exercise-induced sudden death. An exercise program can be aimed at improving or increasing muscle strength and anaerobic or aerobic performance. Only the latter effect is dependent on the improvement of the oxygen-transporting system (i.e., blood, lungs, heart, and blood vessels) and comes about mainly because of an improvement in the overall capacity of the cardiovascular system.

Muscle strength can be improved by repetitious isotonic or isometric muscle contractions of a few seconds duration and against resistance. This type of exercise does not produce an improvement in cardiovascular function, as shown by relatively normal-size hearts, normal resting and exercise heart rates, and unexceptional maximal oxygen intakes of those athletes who only train in this manner.

Anaerobic capacity is necessary for short activities of high intensity or for activities that require more energy than is available from the oxygen transport system. This energy is derived from high-energy phosphate compounds that result from breakdown of glycogen to lactic acid without oxygen utilization. Athletes, such as sprinters, who require relatively infrequent short bursts of high-intensity activity acquire this capacity and often do not improve their overall cardiovascular function. Training aimed at developing anaerobic capacity should consist of maximal work periods of short duration (10 to 60 sec). This type of training requires much motivation because it is difficult and painful. As mentioned, cardiovascular performance is not significantly improved.

Aerobic performance depends on an increase in the oxygen transport system, which is developed principally through adaptations in the cardiovascular system and the skeletal muscles. Large muscle masses are usually called into play, so the greatest demand for oxygen is made. Physical activity ranging from work periods of a few seconds repeated quickly to hours of continuous work may induce an improvement in aerobic performance. The following patterns have been reported to be effective in this regard:

1. Dash training—maximal effort (i.e., running full speed, preferably uphill) for 30 to 60 sec and repeated 5 to 10 times with several minutes of low-level activity between each dash. This pattern also improves anaerobic performance.

2. Interval training—slightly less effort than maximal (80% of dash effort), lasting 3 to 7 minutes repeated 3 to 7 times with low-level activity periods of 6 to 8 minutes between each interval.

3. Continuous training—submaximal effort for 45 to 75 minutes. Heart rates should range from 130 to 170 beats/min with maximal rates achieved at certain times.

These training patterns are applicable to walking, running, bicycling, swimming, or isotonic arm exercises. Isometric exercises such as weight lifting are not aerobic, and they can be dangerous for coronary heart disease patients because of the excessive level of myocardial pressure work associated with them.

The exercise prescription for cardiovascular changes and fitness must consider the frequency, duration, and intensity of aerobic exercise. Three times a week for at least 30 minutes is recommended. Less exercise may be suitable for maintenance, and more exercise is associated with an increased incidence of injuries. For cardiac patients, a warmup and a cool-down are important. Starting slowly can usually be substituted for the stretching ritual in normal subjects. Intensity should be at 60% to 80% of maximal oxygen uptake. This level is most easily monitored by heart rate, which is linearly related to oxygen consumption. The Karvonen technique for determining training heart rate most closely approximates the appropriate exercise intensity. It is calculated by subtracting basal heart rate from maximal, multiplying by 75%, and adding the product to the basal value. Perceived exertion levels of 13 to 14 seem to approximate an exercise intensity for achieving a training effect (Table II). For cardiac patients on beta blockers or with symptoms or signs that are maximal end points, an exercise effect can be achieved by backing off five to ten beats from the heart rate at the end point (i.e., at angina).

There are only a few reported studies that have evaluated the hemodynamic consequences of exercise training using arterial and venous catheterization during exercise testing, the Douglas bag technique for collection of expired air, accurate oxygen measurement, and the Fick or dye dilution technique for estimation of cardiac output. Cardiac catheterization is necessary for accurate pressure measurement and determination of cardiac output. Central aortic pressure is necessary for obtaining hemodynamic measurements to estimate myocardial oxygen consumption, but most studies have been performed with brachial artery catheters. The Fick technique is the standard of reference for determining cardiac output, but it requires right heart catheterization for sampling of mixed venous blood. The dye dilution technique is not as accurate as the Fick method, but it does not require blood gas analysis or right heart catheterization. Radionuclide techniques do not appear to be as accurate as either of these techniques. Currently, paramag-

---

TABLE II
BORG RATING OF PERCEIVED EXERTION SCALE

6	
7	Very, very light
8	
9	Very light
10	
11	Fairly light
12	
13	Somewhat hard
14	
15	Hard
16	
17	Very hard
18	
19	Very, very hard
20	

Adding a zero to each number will give the heart rate during exercise in young men, in association with a perceived level of exertion; it then becomes readily apparent how the scale was derived.

---

netic oxygen measurement techniques are very accurate, though the older chemical methods (Haldane, Scholander) are still the standards of reference. Direct gas flowmeter measurement of air flow during exercise is not accurate enough to replace the Douglas bag technique. The validity of hemodynamic measurements during exercise with catheters has been established. Even if the cardiac output, maximal oxygen intake, and heart rate are reduced in the catheterized exercising subject, the effect is consistent and influences results similarly after as well as before the exercise program.

Studies of Normal Subjects. The Dallas study included five male subjects aged 19 to 21. Three were classified by their activity habits as sedentary and two as active. The former had maximal oxygen uptakes of 33 to 45 ml/kg/min prior to training, and the latter 61 and 47 ml/kg/min. The training program lasted for 55 days with workouts held twice each weekday and once on Saturday. The workouts consisted principally of running and were either interval patterned, with periods of maximal effort for two to five minutes repeated four to ten times with two-minute periods of rest, or continuous training, with running at a constant pace until exhaustion for longer than ten minutes. Before and after training, hemodynamic measurements were determined at rest and during exercise with catheters in a peripheral arm vein and in the brachial artery. Both treadmill and supine bicycle ergometer testing were performed with maximal oxygen uptake measured. The previously sedentary trainees had the greatest measured changes.

The Stockholm study included eight sedentary male subjects aged 19 to 27. Maximal oxygen uptakes prior to training ranged from 36 to 50 ml/kg/min. The training program lasted for 120 days and consisted of cross-country running three times a week in dash, interval, and continuous patterning. Before and after training, hemodynamics were measured. Testing was done with the subject sitting on a bicycle ergometer and exerting maximal effort at work loads calculated to 25%, 50%, and 75% of the maximal oxygen uptake measured prior to training.

Tabkin and colleagues at the University of Vermont studied nine members of the university cross-country team before and after three months of daily training in preparation for competition. Training consisted of daily warmup exercises, sprints, and five miles of running. The radial artery and a peripheral vein were catheterized. Measurements were made at rest and while walking on a treadmill at three miles per hour on the level and at 4%, 8%, 12%, and 14% elevation. No changes were noted other than a lowering of the cardiac output at the two lowest levels of exercise. The fact that the subjects were athletes explained this lack of significant change.

Frick and colleagues studied 14 men aged 19 to 26 before and after "hard" basic military training. The exact nature of this training was not described. Oxygen consumption was not measured, and cardiac output was estimated with Evans blue by a dye dilution technique using earlobe density changes. Physical work capacity was significantly increased after training. Hemodynamic measurements were made via a brachial artery catheter during supine bicycle exercise at 400 kpm/min for six minutes.

The Stockholm-Gothenburg Study was designed to evaluate the effects of an exercise program on middle-age men. Sixty-eight employees of an insurance company who considered themselves to be healthy but who were judged to be inactive by their response to a questionnaire were asked to participate in a ten-week physical training program. The program consisted of two miles of intermittent or continuous running two to three times a week for a total time of about 18 hours and 55 miles of running. Twenty percent of the subjects dropped out for medical or other reasons. Of those who completed the program, half had significant orthopedic problems. Forty-two of the group had noninvasive studies performed, and 15 had venous and arterial catheterization. Maximal effort and multiple predetermined levels of sub-maximal exercise were performed sitting on a bicycle ergometer.

Hanson and colleagues studied the hemodynamic response of 25 normal men aged 40 to 49. Ten of these men could not perform a three-minute walk at three miles per hour and 14% elevation and had a similar response to the treadmill test. They exhibited high resting oxygen consumption and stroke volume, then raised cardiac output excessively with level walking and maintained it throughout higher work loads. They demonstrated an initial overshoot and subsequent poor adaptation to exercise. These investigators assumed this response was due to prolonged physical inactivity. Seven of the ten men completed a physical training program consisting of three hourly sessions a week of competitive paddleball for 29 weeks. Catheterization was repeated and hemodynamic measurements made while walking on a treadmill at three miles per hour level and at elevations of 4%, 8%, 12%, and 14%. Maximal work capacity and maximal oxygen consumption were increased following training.

Rerych and colleagues studied 18 athletes before and after six months of training for competitive swimming. They were studied during erect bicycle exercise using the first-pass technique and a multicrystal camera. Total blood volume increased after training, as did end-diastolic volume. Cardiac output at maximal exercise increased because of an increased diastolic volume with the same heart rate and ejection fraction. The reliability of this technique is questionable, particularly since one athlete reached a maximal cardiac output of 56.6 L/min. It appears, however, that exercise training in this group of healthy young college athletes resulted in no change in cardiac function but did induce an increase in left ventricular end-diastolic volume.

Studies of Coronary Heart Disease Patients. Varnauskas and colleagues at the University of Gothenburg studied the hemodynamics of five patients with coronary heart disease before physical conditioning, after one month, and then after six months of physical conditioning. Coronary heart disease was diagnosed by clinical evaluation and coronary angiograms. The patients were exercised on a bicycle ergometer for one-half hour three times a week, with the work load gradually increased according to individual tolerance and heart rate response. Measurements were made via catheters in the brachial artery and subclavian vein with the trainees sitting on a bicycle ergometer at rest and at 5 and 25 minutes while pedaling against an individualized work load. The dye dilution technique was used to estimate cardiac ouput and AV O_2 difference was calculated from the oxygen consumption and cardiac output. Plasma volume measured with ^{131}I-tagged albumin, total blood volume, and red cell mass calculated from the hematocrit, all increased with training. The hemodynamic changes were more significant after six months of training than after one month. Cardiac output decreased at the submaximal level, and the AV O_2 difference increased. The investigators suggested that this favored a peripheral circulatory mechanism rather than a direct cardiac mechanism as the explanation for the increased work capacity in persons with coronary heart disease after training. However, Hanson and others have demonstrated this overshoot phenomenon in deconditioned persons. The exaggerated cardiac output and narrowed AV O_2 difference are returned to normal by an exercise program, just as they are in persons with vasoregulatory asthenia.

Frick and Katila studied six men aged 37 to 55 before and after an exercise program that began two to four months after a documented myocardial infarction. The exercise program consisted of pedaling a bicycle ergometer three times a week at progressive work loads. Each session consisted of 15 minutes of exercise at a heart rate of 100 beats/min and then for 15 minutes at a heart rate of 150 beats/min or until chest pain. Hemodynamic measurements were made while pedaling a bicyle ergometer in the supine position for six minutes at one or two individualized submaximal work loads. The resting mean heart volume did not change for the group, but two trainees with enlarged hearts had significant decreases in heart volume. Most of the subjects had abnormal hemodynamic measurements in response to acute exercise before and after the training program. This finding is in accord with the criteria of Donald and Reeves for cardiac output and pulmonary wedge pressure response to supine exercise. All subjects increased their exercise capacity, however, and those with angina increased their angina-free work capacity.

Clausen and Trap-Jensen reported the effects of physical conditioning on hemodynamic measurements including hepatic and muscle blood flow during exercise in nine men with coronary heart disease. The men were aged 36 to 57 and had either a myocardial infarction or angina. The aim of the study was to determine the role of peripheral circulatory changes. The authors had demonstrated that in normal subjects, abdominal viscera perfusion was less reduced during exercise in trained subjects, as compared with untrained subjects, and that muscle blood flow was reduced during exercise after training. The exercise program consisted of pedaling a bicycle ergometer in an intermittent pattern for 30 minutes, five days a week for four to ten weeks. The work load was individualized but progressively increased. For testing, catheters were placed in the brachial artery, superior vena cava, and right hepatic vein. Testing was performed sitting on a bicycle ergometer pedaling at work loads initially at 60% of and then equal to the pretraining maximal work load. Hepatic blood flow was estimated using indocyanine green and blood gas analysis, cardiac output was estimated using ^{131}I-tagged iodohippuric acid, and the blood flow in the vastus lateralis muscle was measured using the ^{133}Xe local clearance technique. The cardiac output at the lowest exercise level clearly demonstrated the overshoot phenomenon and this hyperkinetic response was normalized after training. At the higher submaximal exercise level, there was no change in cardiac output. Muscle blood flow was reduced at submaximal loads, and hepatic blood flow was less reduced during submaximal exercise after the training program.

Detry and colleagues collaborated on a study of patients from the University of Washington, Seattle, and the University of Louvain, Belgium. Six men with angina pectoris and six men with documented healed myocardial infarction underwent right heart catheterization and brachial artery cannulation before and after three months of exercise. Their ages ranged from 34 to 68 years, with a mean of 48 years. The exercise program consisted of 45-minute sessions three times a week utilizing various submaximal exercises including walking and running. Maximal exercise was done on a bicycle ergometer or treadmill prior to the hemodynamic studies. Hemodynamic measurements were made while sitting on a bicycle ergometer at rest and during seven-minute exercise periods with work loads equal to 45% and then 75% of the pretraining maximal oxygen consumption. Surprisingly, arterial oxygen content was higher after training, indicating the possibility that improved oxygenation rather than improvements in the peripheral circulation made possible the increased AV O_2 difference. All of the trainees subjectively improved, and two previously limited by symptoms of angina pectoris were no longer symptomatic at any exercise level. These results favor the hypothesis of a peripheral mechanism for improved work tolerance of persons with coronary heart disease.

Bruce and colleagues performed invasive hemodynamic studies in coronary patients who had been in a long-term exercise program. Although all patients had improvement in exercise capacity and were able to perform at an exercise level satisfactory to themselves, some of the patients exhibited deterioration of cardiac function. This study points out the inability to detect worsening of cardiac function by using the treadmill test to evaluate functional changes.

Ferguson and colleagues studied the effects of six months of bicycle ergometry training on coronary sinus blood flow and left ventricular oxygen consumption in ten patients with exertional angina pectoris. After training, the patients increased physical work capacity by 18% at the same submaximal heart rate of approximately 114 beats/min. Coronary blood flow, myocardial oxygen consumption, and the rate-pressure product were not significantly different despite this increase in work load. Symptom-limited maximal exercise capacity increased by 43% with training. The posttraining increase in exercise tolerance in patients with angina pectoris did not depend on an augmented myocardial oxygen delivery but was related to a reduction in coronary flow requirement for a work load.

Sim and Neill studied eight patients with exertional angina pectoris due to coronary disease before and after a three- to four-month exercise program. The double product for angina was determined for upright bicycle exercise and for atrial pacing. This rate-pressure product at the exercise angina threshold was higher after conditioning, suggesting that conditioning increased the maximal myocardial oxygen supply during exercise. However, when the angina was induced by atrial pacing, heart rate, arterial blood pressure, coronary blood flow, myocardial oxygen consumption, and the angina threshold were the same before and after conditioning. Myocardial lactate extraction was still abnormal during pacing, and there were no changes in coronary obstruction or collaterals as judged by coronary angiograms. The increase in anginal threshold during exercise appears to be due to functional adaptation either in myocardial oxygen supply or in the relation between hemodynamic work and myocardial oxygen consumption. The adaptation was limited to exercise and did not occur during atrial pacing, a different stress to myocardial oxygen supply. The effects of conditioning appear to be due to functional adaptation in either delivery or utilization of oxygen in the myocardium rather than to a static alteration in the coronary circulation. This classic study demonstrated an increase in the maximal rate-pressure product at the anginal threshold during exercise after training, but there was no change after atrial pacing. Hemodynamics at rest, left ventricular volumes, and ejection fractions remained unchanged as did the coronary angiogram. These findings constitute a strong argument against a training effect on maximal coronary flow, but it is possible that coronary flow during exercise did increase. An alternate explanation is that changes affecting determinants of myocardial oxygen demand occurred that are not accounted for by the rate-pressure product (e.g., catecholamine levels, less prominent increase in contractile state during exercise) and can explain the increased capacity after the exercise program.

Lee and colleagues studied the hemodynamic effects of physical training on coronary heart disease patients with impaired ventricular function. Eighteen coronary heart disease patients with an ejection fraction of 40% or less were entered into an exercise training program. Maximal symptom-limited exercise testing and cardiac catheterization were performed initially and at 12 to 14 months after exercise training. Functional capacity improved, and resting and submaximal heart rates were significantly lowered; however, there was no significant change in pulmonary artery or left ventricular end-diastolic pressure, cardiac index, stroke index, left ventricular end-diastolic volume, or ejection fraction. An increase in work capacity was not correlated with improvement in ventricular function, and exercise training did not cause deterioration of ventricular function. They concluded that exercise training can be beneficial even for patients with impaired ventricular function.

Carter and Amundsen compared infarct size estimated from serum creatine kinase elevations with the functional exercise capacity for 22 myocardial infarction patients. The patients were studied 2.5 to 4.5 months after acute myocardial infarction. Eleven of the 22 entered an exercise program for three to four months and were subsequently retested on a bicycle ergometer. Prior to this exercise training, a significant correlation was demonstrated between aerobic capacity and estimated infarct size ($r = -.68$), but the correlation was higher ($r = -.84$) after training. Infarct size was not a predictor of the capacity of a patient to obtain a training effect. These results suggest that more accurate comparisons of training responses may be made when both infarct size and the time after infarction are considered.

DeBusk and colleagues studied the cardiovascular effects of exercise training very early after a clinically uncomplicated myocardial infarction. At 3 to 11 weeks after infarction, 28 men underwent gymnasium training, 12 trained at home, and 30 were followed as controls. Patients with ventricular gallops and other evidence of heart failure were avoided, and they were highly selected. Patients were "randomized" to the training programs only after stratification. If they had ST-segment depression or angina pectoris they were only assigned to gymnasium training or to no training. By the 11th week, functional capacity increased significantly in all three groups: gymnasium training 66%, home training 41%, and controls 34%. Aerobic capacity at 11 weeks was 11 METs, 10.3 METs, and 9.4 METs, respectively in the three groups. Functional capacity increased more in the gymnasium-trained group than in the no-training group, but this difference was significant only in patients without exercise-induced ST-segment depression or angina. All three groups lowered their heart rate response to submaximal work. These authors concluded that (1) symptom-limited treadmill testing is safe and provides useful guidelines for cardiac rehabilitation, (2) patients who demonstrate nonischemic responses to treadmill testing soon after infarction may safely undergo unsupervised exercise training at home, and (3) supervised training may not be required to restore functional capacity to near-normal values soon after a myocardial infarction in selected patients. This report is rather exciting because exercise has traditionally commenced no sooner than six to eight weeks after a myocardial infarction. Sample size and careful patient selection, however, make it difficult to form convincing conclusions. Also, the control subjects did a considerable amount of walking on their own.

Nolewajka and colleagues studied 20 male patients three to six months postmyocardial infarction. One half of the patients were randomly assigned to an exercise program. The exercise program was maintained five days a week at a heart rate of 60% to 70% of maximal heart rate obtained during a bicycle ergometer test. They were considered to have a training effect if their heart rate dropped at least 10 beats/min at an oxygen consumption of 1.2 L/min. Both groups underwent coronary angiography, invasive resting left ventricular function studies, and intracoronary artery injection of radionuclide microspheres before and after a seven-month period. No differences were found to suggest an improvement in disease progression, resting myocardial perfusion or function, or myocardial collateralization.

Paterson and colleagues studied 79 patients under 54 years of age 3 to 12 months postmyocardial infarction, with CO_2 rebreathing during submaximal bicycle exercise both before and after 6 and 12 months of exercise training. Thirty-seven were randomized to a low-intensity activity as controls. Over the year of training, only predicted maximal oxygen consumption of the high-intensity training group increased. At six months, their heart rates were significantly reduced at each work load, with a widened AV O_2 difference, but there was no change in stroke volume. By the end of the year, their stroke volume had increased by 10%. These observations were interpreted to mean that only peripheral changes occur in such patients after six months of high-intensity training, whereas longer periods can result in an increase in myocardial contractility.

Discussion. Consistent hemodynamic results of a regular exercise program include a resting bradycardia, a decrease in heart rate and systolic blood pressure at any matched submaximal work load, an increase in maximal oxygen consumption and maximal cardiac output, and a more rapid return toward normal in recovery. It is somewhat controversial whether exercise can lower maximal heart rate. It appears that some athletes who develop cardiomegaly with an increase in left ventricular end-diastolic volume and in mass may well lower their maximal heart rate, but this is not a consistent finding.

From the submaximal testing results, it is apparent that peripheral adaptations during acute exercise secondary to an exercise program are important. Lactic acid concentration during submaximal exercise was decreased in spite of an unchanged or decreased cardiac output. Adaptations in the peripheral circulation were demonstrated by a decrease in active skeletal muscle blood flow and by a smaller decrease in liver blood flow. These changes in perfusion and aerobic metabolism are partially explained by morphologic and enzymatic adaptations in skeletal muscle.

The peripheral response to training is important for another reason. Clausen and Trap-Jensen have demonstrated that the training bradycardia is operative only when using trained skeletal muscles. They trained two groups of men using similar bicycle ergometer protocols, except that one group used their arms while the other used their legs. When tested with alternating arm and leg exercises after training, the trainees demonstrated a lower heart rate during exercise only when using the trained limbs. These investigators also trained individuals with fixed-rate ventricular pacemakers. These subjects responded to training with an increased work capacity in spite of a fixed ventricular rate. Interestingly, the atrial rate decreased after training in response to a similar submaximal work load. Frick has demonstrated that individuals with congenital bradycardia respond to training by increasing stroke volume. These findings suggest that an exercise program induces a neural signal or a vascular response in the periphery that modifies the chronotropic and inotropic control of the heart during acute exercise.

The AV O_2 difference was either increased or unchanged in normal subjects during submaximal exercise after training. In coronary heart disease patients, Detry and Varnauskas demonstrated an increase in the AV O_2 difference, whereas Frick found no change. Clausen did not measure AV O_2, but his data suggest that there was no change. Some investigators have suggested that the increase in AV O_2 difference supports the concept that peripheral changes rather than changes in cardiac function are of primary importance for the increased work capacity of trained coronary heart disease patients. It is conceivable that some hearts are so badly damaged that they cannot be modified by training. In which case, peripheral circulatory changes and enzymatic and morphologic changes in skeletal muscle would be of primary importance. However, Frick and Paterson demonstrated improvement in cardiac function in coronary heart disease patients after an exercise program. Frick's data include changes in left ventricular stroke work versus pulmonary capillary wedge pressure during submaximal exercise (Sarnoff function curves), as well as increases in cardiac output for a given oxygen consumption in response to supine exercise. Thus, there appears to be evidence that an exercise program can improve ventricular function in selected patients with coronary heart disease.

In normal subjects, Braunwald and Ross have shown that the cardiovascular response to acute exercise involves the integrated effects on the myocardium of tachycardia, sympathetic stimulation, and the Frank-Starling mechanism. The effects of an exercise program on these responses, as well as on the morphology of the heart, require delineation in humans. Along with exercise-induced ventricular hypertrophy, an increase in sympathetic tone could also explain an increase in contractility with training. Evidence for an increase in contractility secondary to an exercise program in humans is limited; however, the mean rate of systolic ejection increases, as does the dp/dt in the brachial artery and, in some cases, also the ejection fraction. Another point to be considered is that venous return could be facilitated by an exercise program, the end-diastolic volume for a given work load increased, and thus ventricular function increased.

Cardiac output was unchanged at identical submaximal work loads by an exercise program in normal subjects, except in the study by Hanson. However, this group of older normal individuals demonstrated a cardiac output overshoot phenomenon that was hypothesized to be secondary to prolonged physical inactivity. Approximately half the coronary heart disease trainees had a similar overshoot phenomenon and lowered their cardiac output response to submaximal exercise, while the others did not. The correction of the exaggerated cardiac output and narrowed AV O_2 difference by an exercise program was similar to its effects on the abnormal hemodynamics of vasoregulatory asthenia. The lowering of cardiac output and widening of the AV O_2 difference in response to submaximal exercise are not the major effects of an exercise program, since this does not occur in all individuals who experience an increase in work capacity.

Measurement of myocardial oxygen consumption is technically difficult at rest, and there are many problems with its measurement during exercise. However, estimations can be made by blood pressure, heart rate, and ejection time. Blood pressure and ejection time can be lessened to some extent by an exercise program, but the major change is a lowering of heart rate. Because of lowered heart rate, hemodynamic values approximating changes in myocardial oxygen consumption will decrease after training. However, there is evidence that cardiac function improves with training, even in coronary heart disease patients. An increase in the contractile state of the myocardium or an increase in end-diastolic volume (Frank-Starling mechanism) would increase myocardial oxygen consumption and invalidate approximations using hemodynamic calculations. Myocardial work is a determinant of myocardial oxygen consumption; however, it is not sufficient to estimate this value alone. For instance, although calculated work might increase or not change if stroke volume increased and blood pressure decreased, myocardial oxygen consumption would decrease. This effect is due to myocardial flow work requiring less oxygen than does pressure work. However, even if myocardial oxygen consumption is not decreased by an exercise program, the training bradycardia is an important physiologic benefit. The concomitant increase in diastolic time increases the time available for myocardial perfusion. Myocardial changes brought about by an exercise program most likely are subtle and will only be apparent during stress, such as exercise testing.

ECHOCARDIOGRAPHIC STUDIES OF THE EFFECTS OF AN EXERCISE PROGRAM

The echocardiogram is a diagnostic tool that can be used to evaluate the effects of an exercise program on the heart since it allows for the noninvasive measurement of chamber size, wall thickness, and function. Echocardiographic studies have demonstrated morphologic and functional cardiac changes secondary to aerobic exercise training. These changes appear beneficial, and so most of the studies appear to support the exercise hypothesis. Some of the cross-sectional and longitudinal studies of exercise training using echocardiography are summarized here.

Cross-Sectional Studies Comparing Echocardiographic Measurements of Normals and of Athletes (Table III). Gilbert and colleagues at Emory University compared M-mode echocardiographic measurements of 20 endurance runners with 26 young sedentary subjects. A modest degree of right and left ventricular chamber enlargement and left ventricular hypertrophy was observed in endurance runners. There were no significant differences, unless differences in body size were accounted for with the use of indices based on body surface area. There was no significant difference in resting measurements of ventricular performance. This study suggests that isotonic leg training results in adaptive changes in ventricular volume and mass, slower heart rates that may be associated with more efficient function (increased stroke volume) and insignificant alterations in resting ejection phase indices of left ventricular function.

Parker and colleagues at the University of Missouri compared 12 long-distance runners with 12 normal control subjects using multiple noninvasive techniques. The athletes showed a higher prevalence of third and fourth heart sounds and electrocardiographic and vectorcardiographic abnormali-

TABLE III

CROSS-SECTIONAL ECHOCARDIOGRAPHIC STUDIES COMPARING ATHLETES TO CONTROLS

Emory University Echocardiographic Study

	Controls	Athletes
LVPWT	9.8	10.9
LVVIED	62	72
VO_2	43	71
EF	72%	68%
Resting HR	62	51

University of Missouri Echocardiographic Study

	Controls	Athletes
LVPWT	9	11
LVEDD	52	57
LVESD	37	34
$\dot{V}O_2$	47	74
EF	64%	78%
Resting HR	61	50
MVCFS	0.9	1.2

National Institutes of Health Echocardiographic Study

	Aerobic athletes	Isometric athletes	Normals
LVPWT	11	13.7	10
Septum	10.8	13	10.3
LVEDD	55	48	46

University of California, San Diego, Echocardiographic Study

	Controls	Athletes
RVEDD	13	21
Septum	13	14
LVPWT	10	11
LVEDD	50	54
LVESD	31	32
EF	76%	79%
MVCFS	1.13	1.18

LVPWT = left ventricular posterior wall thickness; LVVIED = left ventricular volume index at end diastole in ml; $\dot{V}O_2$ = maximal oxygen consumption; EF = ejection fraction; HR = heart rate; LVESD = left ventricular end-systolic dimension; MVCFS = mean ventricular circumferential fiber shortening; LV or RVEDD = ventricular end-diastolic dimension. All dimensions are in millimeters, HR in beats/minute, oxygen consumption in ml O_2/kg-min, and MVCFS in circ/sec.

ties consistent with right and left ventricular hypertrophy. Echocardiographic examination of the athletes revealed an increase in wall thickness, left ventricular muscle mass, diastolic volume, and ventricular function.

Morganroth and colleagues at the NIH studied 56 athletes 18 to 24 years of age with M-mode echocardiography. Mean left ventricular end-diastolic volume and mass increased in aerobic athletes (runners, swimmers), whereas isometric athletes (wrestlers) had increased wall thickness and mass. The former had changes suggestive of chronic volume overload, and the latter had changes similar to those of chronic pressure overload.

Roeske and colleagues at the University of California, San Diego, studied ten professional basketball players and ten matched subjects. Right and left ventricular enlargement were often present in aerobically trained athletes, but left ventricular performance was normal at rest.

Echocardiography Before and After an Exercise Program (Table IV). Ehsani and co-workers at Washington University reported rapid changes in left ventricular dimensions and mass in response to physical conditioning and deconditioning. Two groups of healthy young subjects were studied. The training group consisted of eight competitive swimmers who were studied serially for nine weeks. Mean left ventricular end-diastolic dimension increased by 4.3 mm in the first week. A total of 3.3-mm increase from the pretraining value was demonstrated by the ninth week of training. Mean left ventricular posterior wall thickness increased 0.7 mm by the end of the training period. There was no change in ejection fraction. The deconditioned group consisted of six competitive runners who stopped training for three weeks. Left ventricular end-diastolic dimension decreased 4.7 mm and posterior wall thickness decreased 2.7 mm by the end of the three-week period. Deconditioning did not influence ejection fraction. The authors concluded that exercise training–induced adaptive changes in left ventricular dimensions occur rapidly and mimic the pattern of chronic volume overload and that modest degrees of exercise-induced left ventricular enlargement are reversible after cessation of training. Surprisingly, changes in left ventricular dimension occurred early during endurance training, but there was no significant increase in measured left ventricular posterior wall thickness until the fifth week of training. Estimated left ventricular mass significantly increased after the first week of training. The rapidity of this change make one doubt its validity.

DeMaria and colleagues at the University of California, Davis, reported the results of M-mode echocardiography in 24 young normal subjects before

TABLE IV
SERIAL ECHOCARDIOGRAPHIC STUDIES (LONGITUDINAL OR PROSPECTIVE)
EVALUATING THE CARDIAC EFFECTS OF EXERCISE TRAINING

Washington University Study (college athletes)	8 swimmers trained for 9 wks		3 runners detrained for 3 wks	
	Before Training	After Training	Before Detraining	After Detraining
LVEDD	48.7	52	51	46.3
LVPWT	9.4	10.1	10.7	8.0
$\dot{V}O_2$	52	60	62	57
Resting HR	70	63	57	64
EF	63%	63%	68%	63%

UCD Study (policemen)	Before Training	After Training
LVEDD	48	50
LVESD	30	29
LVPWT	9.1	10.1
Resting HR	69	63
$\dot{V}O_2$	36	41
EF	75%	80%
MVCFS	1.21	1.28

SUNY Downstate Medical Center Study	Before Training		After Training	
	rest	300 kpm	rest	300 kpm
LVEDD	47	46	50	50
LVESD	32	21	32	30
EF	70%	90%	73%	78%

Montreal Heart Institute (normal men $\simeq$ 40 yrs old)	Before Training	After Training
$\dot{V}O_2$	34	41
Septum	12.5	12.7
LVPWT	10	9.8
LVEDD	47.8	48.2
LVESD	33	33

Table IV continued

Salt Lake City Study (25 men exercised 3 mos, mean age 22 yrs)	Before Training	After Training
Resting HR	63	54
V̇O$_2$	49	56
% Body fat	17.2	13.7
R$_{v5}$	1.7 mV	2.0 mV
LVEDD	45.8	49.6
EF	62%	66%
LVPWT	10.9	10.3
LVESD	32.3	33.5

Washington University Rehab Study (9 post-MI patients, 1 yr of exercise)	Before Training	After Training
LVEDD	51	56
LVPWT	9	10
V̇O$_2$	26	35
R$_{v5}$	1.7 mV	2.0 mV

LVEDD = left ventricular end-diastolic dimension; LVPWT = left ventricular posterior wall thickness; V̇O$_2$ = maximal oxygen consumption; HR = heart rate; EF = ejection fraction; LVESD = left ventricular end-systolic dimension; MVCFS = mean ventricular circumferential fiber shortening. All dimensions are in millimeters, HR in beats/minute, oxygen consumption in ml of O$_2$/kg-min, and MVCFS in circ/sec.

and after 11 weeks of endurance exercise training. Training consisted of a walk-run program at 70% maximal heart rate for one hour four days a week. The subjects were participating in a program of endurance physical conditioning as part of training for the Sacramento Police Academy. The group, 15 men and 11 women, ranged in age from 20 to 34 years (mean 26 years). After training, they exhibited an increased left ventricular end-diastolic dimension, a decreased end-systolic dimension, and both an increased stroke volume and shortening fraction. An increase in mean fiber-shortening velocity was observed, as were increases in left ventricular wall thickness, electrocardiographic voltage, and left ventricular mass. The increase in left ventricular shortening fraction and calculated stroke volume suggests enhanced cardiac performance. However, other parameters of hemodynamic functions including cardiac output, blood pressure, and peripheral vascular resistance at rest were not altered following conditioning. Hemodynamics in the posttraining period were characterized by a maintenance of the same cardiac output at a reduced heart rate and an increased stroke volume, which was accomplished by an augmented left ventricular diastolic volume, shortening fraction, and contraction velocity. Peripheral resistance was unchanged.

Stein and colleagues at the State University of New York Downstate Medical Center studied the effects of exercise training on ventricular dimensions at rest and during supine submaximal exercise. Fourteen healthy students were studied using M-mode echocardiography at rest and in the third minute of 300 kpm of supine bicycle exercise. They were studied before and after a 14-week training program that resulted in a 30% increase in maximal O_2 consumption. Eleven nontrained students acted as controls and showed no changes. Ejection fraction was calculated by the cube technique. The authors concluded that exercise training is associated with an increased stroke volume mediated by the Frank-Starling effect and enhanced contractility.

Parrault and colleagues at the Montreal Heart Institute studied 14 subjects (40 ± 3 years of age) with a chest x-ray, electrocardiogram, vectorcardiogram, and echocardiogram before and after five months of training. Maximal oxygen consumption increased 20%. There was a slight increase in left precordial voltage, but no change in the heart size from the chest x-ray. The echocardiograms showed no significant changes, in contrast to the studies in younger subjects. Wolfe and colleagues performed a similar study in 12 men with a mean age of 37 who exhibited 14% and 18% increases in aerobic capacity after three and six months of training, respectively. They concluded that resting end-diastolic volume and stroke volume were increased but that left ventricular structure and resting contractile status are not altered by six months of jogging in healthy, previously sedentary men.

Frick and colleagues studied the effects of moderate physical training on heart volume using biplane chest x-rays, on blood volume by ^{131}I-tagged human albumin, and on left ventricular wall thickness by ultrasound. Twenty normal men (19 to 20 years of age) participated in a moderate physical training program for two months. This training increased physical working capacity by 13% and maximal oxygen consumption by 6%. Heart and blood volumes remained essentially unchanged. There was no significant change in left ventricular wall thickness. A study by Thompson and colleagues in young men failed to find any changes in cardiac dimensions after 11 weeks of aerobic training.

The Salt Lake City research group led by Yanowitz noninvasively studied the effects of an aerobic training program on the hearts of healthy college-age men (25 experimental subjects and 11 controls with a mean age of 22 years). Echocardiographic, electrocardiographic, and oxygen consumption measurements were obtained before and after a three-month exercise program. The exercise program consisted of 50 minutes of jogging five days a week at 85% of maximal heart rate. Compared with the control group, echocardiography after training showed an increase in left ventricular end-diastolic dimension, but no change in wall thickness or in ejection fraction. Electrocardiographic measurements revealed a decrease in resting heart rate and an increase in R-wave voltage in leads V_5 and V_6. Measured oxygen consumption increased by 16%. Although there was no change in myocardial wall thickness, the increase in end-diastolic dimension resulted in a calculated increase in left ventricular mass.

Ehsani and colleagues reported their results after 12 months of intense aerobic exercise training in a highly selected group of ten patients with coronary heart disease. The patients, ranging in age from 44 to 63 years, were the first to complete 12 months in a high-level exercise program. Nine had sustained a single myocardial infarction, and one had severe three-vessel coronary artery disease. All ten had asymptomatic exercise-induced ST-segment depression. Eight similar men were considered as controls. After three months of exercise training at a level of 50% to 70% of maximal oxygen consumption, the level of training increased to 70% to 80%, with two to three intervals at 80% to 90% interspersed throughout the exercise session. Patients exercised three times a week during the first three months and four to five times a week for the next nine months. The duration was initially 30 minutes and later increased to 60 minutes.

Since none of these men developed symptoms during exercise testing, a true maximal oxygen consumption could be measured. The maximal amount of reported ST-segment depression was .30 mV, but most had .20 mV of depression, which was less at repeat testing one year later in spite of a higher double product, greater treadmill work load, and a 38% increase in maximal oxygen consumption. In addition, 0.1 mV of ST-segment depression occurred at a higher double product after the year of training. A weight loss from a mean of 79 kg to 74 kg occurred. The sum of SV_1 and RV_5 increased by 15%. Both left ventricular end-diastolic dimension and posterior wall thickness were significantly increased after training. This resulted in an increase in left ventricular mass from 93 to 135 g/m^2.

One wonders if ST-segment depression in Z was included since the specific lead with ST-segment depression was not given. In Z, ST depression is really ST elevation anteriorly and is probably not due to ischemia. Also, how many of these asymptomatic men with coronary disease actually had false-positive ST-segment abnormalities, that is, depression not due to ischemia?

Though these results are exciting, it is questionable that they can be generalized. These ten men are a highly selected group, all with asymptomatic ST-segment depression and able to exercise at levels often difficult for younger men. If applied to most patients with ischemic heart disease, this intensity certainly could lead to a high incidence of orthopedic and cardiac complications.

At the University of California, San Diego, echocardiograms were obtained in 14 coronary patients before and after an average of 7 months (range 3 to 14 months) of supervised arm and leg exercise. Each echocardiogram was interpreted jointly by two blinded observers, using three different measurement conventions and a semiautomated method of analysis to minimize errors of interpretation. Exercise training led to subjective improvement in all 14 patients and to an objective increase in functional capacity in 13 of 14 patients, as evidenced by an increase in maximal oxygen consumption estimated from symptom-limited treadmill testing (9 and 11 METs before and after training, respectively, $P < .01$). However, this functional improvement was not accompanied by any significant change in left ventricular end-diastolic diameter, posterior wall thickness, or interventricular septal thickness. Likewise, left ventricular cross-sectional area (CSA), an index of left ventricular mass (Figure 1) that corrects for altered ventricular volume and theoretically reflects directional changes in mass despite nonuniform wall thickness, did not change significantly after training by any measurement convention (Figure 2). The left ventricular cross-sectional area was 18.0 ± 6.5 and 17.6 ± 6.5 cm^2 before and after training, respectively, determined by American Society of Echocardiography measurement standards. These data suggest that improved functional capacity after exercise training in patients with ischemic heart disease is not due to exercise-induced left ventricular hypertrophy.

Discussion. Despite technical and theoretic limitations related to transducer angulation, beam-width distortion, and endocardial surface recognition, echocardiographic measurements of left ventricular posterior wall thickness and internal dimensions closely correspond to similar measurements determined by left ventriculography. Several echocardiographic methods of estimating left ventricular mass have been demonstrated to reflect accurately true anatomic mass. The usefulness of left ventricular cross-sectional area in evaluating myocardial mass has been previously reported. Since this index is relatively independent of changes in ventricular volume, cross-sectional area is a

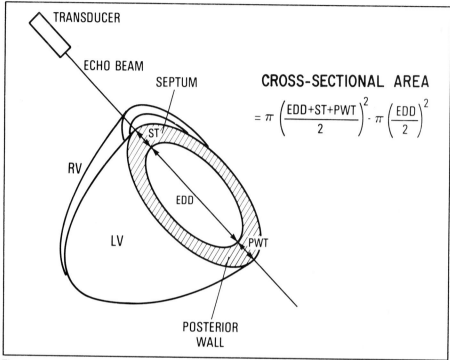

Figure 1. Illustration shows left ventricular cross-sectional area—an index of left ventricular mass. RV = right ventricle; LV = left ventricle; EDD = end-diastolic diameter; ST = interventricular septal thickness; PWT = posterior wall thickness. (With permission of the Am Heart J.)

more reliable means of assessing serial changes in left ventricular mass than is either interventricular septal or posterior wall thickness alone. Furthermore, whereas echocardiographic estimates of absolute left ventricular mass would be of questionable accuracy in the presence of nonuniform wall thickness, directional changes in cross-sectional area remain theoretically valid indices of changes in actual mass if measurements are derived from an area that includes at least some viable myocardium and if myocardial hypertrophy is uniform in distribution. For example, in a patient with septal scarring due to prior infarction, any change in ventricular mass should be reflected in cross-sectional area by changes in posterior wall thickness (corrected for altered ventricular volume). Although such changes would not necessarily be quantitatively accurate (because any regional area of nonviable myocardium could potentially reduce the magnitude of change in cross-sectional area disproportionately, when compared with its influence on changes in ventricular mass as a whole), directional changes in both cross-sectional area and total mass would remain concordant.

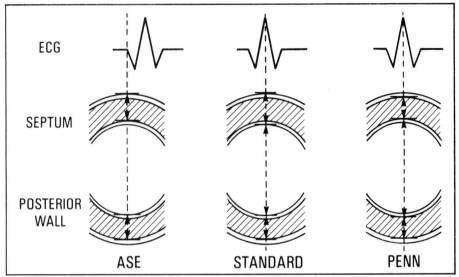

Figure 2. The three different measurement conventions for determining left ventricular wall thickness are shown. ASE = convention recommended by the American Society of Echocardiography; STANDARD = standard convention; PENN = Penn convention.

The subjective nature of echocardiographic interpretation presents a further problem in terms of quantitative analysis. Special precautions are necessary to minimize subjective errors of interpretation and to ensure reproducibility. Foremost among these precautions is the elimination of echocardiograms on which chamber dimensions and wall thickness are not clearly defined. Although echocardiograms performed in nearly all of the coronary patients who entered our cardiac rehabilitation program during the period of this study were considered adequate for clinical purposes, less than half had both pretraining and posttraining studies of sufficient quality to justify more detailed analysis. Although this yield is lower than usually reported, a relatively strict approach was taken in an attempt to reduce interpretative errors. In addition, joint interpretation by two observers and a semiautomated analysis system were utilized both to limit the individual subjectivity inherent in echocardiographic interpretation and to ensure accuracy in calibration and arithmetic manipulation. Furthermore, potential bias due to the use of a single, arbitrary measurement convention was excluded by demonstrating concordance among results obtained by three widely recommended conventions. Even so, our individual estimates of cross-sectional area were not perfectly reproducible. However, there was a good overall correlation between repeated measurements, and directional changes in mean values before and after training were the same. Furthermore, the same conclusions were supported by both sets of measurements. Two-dimensional (2-D) echocardiography has theoretic advantages, particularly in patients with regional disease, but endoepicardial measurements are even more tenuous. Perhaps digital enhancement of echocardiographic images will improve this situation.

Summary. M-mode echocardiography has been utilized to evaluate cardiac adaptations to exercise training in both cross-sectional and longitudinal studies. Reported cardiac changes secondary to endurance training in young subjects have included increased ventricular mass, wall thickness, volume, and function. The echocardiographic studies have failed to yield consistent and conclusive results, probably because of the subjective nature of echocardiographic measurements. However, increases in left ventricular mass may not occur in younger subjects unless higher levels of exercise are used and may never occur in older subjects.

EXERCISE ELECTROCARDIOGRAPHIC STUDIES

Since abnormal ST-segment shifts in coronary patients are most likely secondary to ischemia, lessening of such shifts would be consistent with improved myocardial perfusion. For purposes of comparison, only similar myocardial oxygen demands can be considered, therefore, it is necessary only to compare ST segments at matched exercise heart rate–systolic blood pressure products. The product of heart rate times systolic blood pressure is the best noninvasive estimate of myocardial oxygen demand during exercise. The following describes the studies of the effect of an exercise program on the exercise electrocardiogram.

Costill and colleagues entered 24 men who demonstrated ST-segment depression in lead CM_5 during treadmill testing three months into an exercise program. A second group of men with coronary heart disease and ST depression were reexamined at the same interval but were not trained. A third group of men with low physical fitness and no ST-segment depression were trained at the same relative intensity as the trained group with coronary disease. After 12 weeks of training, maximal oxygen consumption was increased by approximately 25% in the trained groups. Training produced a lowering of heart rate for all submaximal exercise levels, permitting the men to perform more work before the onset of angina or ST-segment depression (which occurred at the same heart rate before and after training) or both. Training had no effect on the amount of exercise-induced ST-segment depression.

Salzman and colleagues analyzed the exercise electrocardiograms of 100 coronary patients with a mean age of 48 years before and after an average of 33 months of cardiac rehabilitation. The exercise electrocardiogram improved in 31 subjects, did not change in 41, and deteriorated in 28. Improvement in the exercise electrocardiogram was more likely to occur in the group who showed improvement in physical fitness, whereas deterioration was more likely in the group who showed a worsening of physical fitness. Improvement in the exercise electrocardiogram occurred in 80% of subjects with initial borderline or abnormal exercise electrocardiograms and who had an improvement in physical fitness. Deterioration of the exercise electrocardiogram occurred in 70% of the patients with initially normal exercise electrocardiograms who had a worsening of physical fitness. They concluded that improvement of the exercise electrocardiogram was directly related to improved physiologic function, but these findings could be due to selection.

Kattus and colleagues identified 30 subjects with abnormal ST-segment depression in response to exercise testing and without anginal pain in a screening study. All 30 of the abnormal responders were invited to enter a supervised exercise program. Two refused further participation, and 15 found it impossible to participate in the training program but agreed to return for a repeat treadmill test in the future. Thirteen of the abnormal responders participated in a supervised exercise program that led to an increased exercise capacity. Four of these 13 subjects (13%) had reversion of their ST-segment depression to normal. Among those abnormal responders who did not train, there was no improvement of exercise capacity, yet two of the 15 (13%) subjects normalized their electrocardiographic patterns.

Detry and Bruce measured symptom-limited maximal oxygen uptake and electrocardiographic response to treadmill testing before and after three months of exercise training in 14 patients with coronary heart disease. ST-segment responses were measured by computer averaging of 100 beats/sample of lead CB_5, which was recorded on magnetic tape during the last two minutes of each exercise level. ST measurements were made 50 to 70 msec after the nadir of the S wave. There was less ST-segment depression at submaximal exercise, along with a lower double product. However, at maximal exercise both depression and double product were greater. The quantitative relationship of ST-segment depression to exercise heart rate, to the product of heart rate and systolic blood pressure (double product), or to rate-pressure product (heart rate times mean blood pressure) was unaffected by the exercise program. Maximal oxygen consumption increased by 21%, and the product of heart rate and systolic blood pressure at symptom-limited maximal exercise increased by 10% in the angina patients. Apparently, the only electrocardiographic changes were due to changes in the heart rate and blood pressure response to exercise rather than due to improved coronary circulation.

Raffo and colleagues studied 24 patients with stable angina and exercise-induced ST depression who were randomized into two groups. The 12 patients in group I followed the Canadian Air Force exercise program and the 12 patients in group II were controls. Exercise testing on a bicycle ergometer was performed at entry and six months later. Heart rate at the same level of ST-segment depression in CM_5 and the duration of the test increased in those in the exercise program, whereas heart rate at submaximal work loads decreased. These studies are summarized in Table V.

At the University of California, San Diego, we have studied 14 patients with stable coronary heart disease using computerized exercise electrocardiography before and after six months of an exercise program. Eleven patients had myocardial infarctions, and three had stable angina pectoris.

Before and after training, supine bicycle exercise testing was performed to evaluate the training effect. A multistage maximal supine bicycle exercise test was performed on an imaging table (Uniwork 845T, Quinton) because scintigraphic images were also obtained. The end point of testing was usually fatigue, though several patients were stopped due to angina pectoris, ST-segment depression of up to 0.3 mV, or both. During exercise testing, blood pressure was taken at the end of each stage, and continuous electrocardiographic and vectorcardiographic data were recorded.

Electrocardiographic data acquisition was quality controlled by visualizing the recorded data on the strip-chart recorder as it was entered on the floppy disk. The data were digitized with 12-bit resolution at 250 samples/sec. A MAC I Data Logger (Marquette Electronics) was used; it utilizes a Motorola 6800 microprocessor as the central processing unit and a Motorola bus to communicate with the peripheral devices. Date, patient identification, and blood pressure were entered on the floppy disks by the digi-switches on the Data Logger. Electrocardiographic and vectorcardiographic data were collected using the Mason-Likar exercise adaptation of the 12-lead electrocardiogram and the Mayo Clinic adaptation of the Frank vectorcardiographic leads so that 14 electrodes were used to derive 15 leads. The Dalhousie square was used to assure consistent electrode placement. Three leads were recorded and digitized simultaneously in time-coherent fashion as follows: at rest, 5 seconds each for I, II, III; R, L, F; V_1, V_2, V_3; and V_4, V_5, V_6, and 10 seconds for X, Y, Z; during exercise and recovery the acquisition durations were

TABLE V
STUDIES PERFORMED WITH EXERCISE ELECTROCARDIOGRAPHIC ANALYSIS
BEFORE AND AFTER AN EXERCISE PROGRAM

Principal Investigator	Number Trained	Number of Controls	Length of Exercise Program	ECG Lead Monitored	Description of Subjects	Exercise ECG Results
Costill Salzman	24 100	— None	3 mos 33 mos	CM$_5$ C$_4$V, CH$_6$	Three groups (see text) MI, angina, and/or abnormal exercise ECG	No change in ST-segment response ST-segment changes correlated to changes in functional capacity
Kattus	13	15	5 mos	CA$_5$	Asymptomatic with abnormal exercise ECG	Similar ST-segment improvement rate in control subjects
Detry	14	None	3 mos	CB$_5$	MI and/or angina	No change in computerized ST-segment measurements at matched DP
Raffo	12	12	6 mos	CM$_5$	Angina with abnormal exercise ECG	Higher heart rate for same amount of ST depression
Watanabe Ehsani	14 10	None 8	6 mos 12 mos	XYZ V$_{4-6}$	Mixed coronary disease 9 post-MI > 4 mos; 1 with 3-VD; all with asymptomatic ST depression	Changes only in spatial analysis Less ST-segment depression at matched DP and at maximal exercise; higher DP at ischemic ST threshold (0.1 mV flat)

MI = myocardial infarction; DP = double product (SBP × HR); VD = vessel disease; ECG = electrocardiogram.

doubled. The data were stored on soft sector, single-sided double-density floppy disks for off-line processing. Digital electrocardiographic data for the waveform analysis were processed by a Burroughs computer using software developed at the University of California, San Diego, and based on Vectan II and USAFSAM programs. Digital data for each group of three leads transferred from floppy disks to magnetic tape were read, and then absolute spatial vector velocity (ASVV) and coincidence function (CF) were calculated for the detection of the QRS complex. CF lessens the impact of noise on the estimation of an accurate fiducial point. The detection of the QRS complex was performed by setting a threshold for ASVV and CF, which was 30% of the maximal ASVV and 15% of the maximal CF. At the point just beyond both thresholds, a window was opened and the peak on each beat in ASVV was searched for by moving backward 20 msec and forward 80 msec. Then 90% of the peak value after the peak was used as the temporary fiducial point.

The isoelectric line was estimated as the 16 msec segment of least activity between 20 msec and 120 msec of ASVV prior to the fiducial point. The mean value of this segment was computed in each lead. For the correction of baseline drift, the modified cubic spline mathematical technique was applied for consecutive PR segments or nodes. Smooth electrocardiographic baseline was obtained by subtracting the estimated baseline drift from the uncorrected electrocardiogram. QRS complexes with a prior RR interval less than 80% of the mean RR interval were eliminated to exclude premature beats.

To classify each beat, product-moment correlation coefficient (r) was used. The r was calculated for ASVV in a 200-msec region for a beat, while the next beat was moved back and forth by a maximum of plus and minus 10 msec in steps of 2 msec from the temporary fiducial point. The point of maximum correlation was used to align the beats and mark the final fiducial point. The first beat was called template 1. When the r between template 1 and the ASVV of the second beat was less than 0.9, the beat was classified as a new template, or template 2, and so on. Usually the number of templates was limited to three, and consecutive beats, except those discarded, were classified into a maximum of three templates. The QRS complex in each lead was aligned according to the fiducial points found in ASVV.

The QRS complexes in the dominant template in each lead were averaged and filtered. A low-pass nonrecursive filter (35 coefficient) with a cut-off frequency of 40 Hz was used. The ASVV was rederived from averaged, filtered beats, and the waveform recognition program was applied. The detection of QRS beginning and end was performed on the ASVV by a threshold set at 5% of maximal ASVV with a 10-msec window. PQ interval was located as a 15-msec interval, with minimum activity defined by the lowest value summing seven consecutive points of ASVV in a 50-msec segment before the beginning of QRS. The average value for this interval in each lead was used as the isoelectric baseline.

T-wave beginning and end were similarly detected on the ASVV by a threshold set at 20% of maximal ASVV attained within a segment between 50 msec after the end of QRS and the end of the averaged beat (maximum of 660 msec, or 55% of the RR interval, after the fiducial point). If the estimated QT interval was greater than 550 msec, the threshold was incremented by 10% until the QT interval was less than 550 msec.

The P-wave end and beginning were determined in a manner similar to the onset and offset of QRS, starting from QRS onset, moving backward, and defining the end and the beginning of P wave. Twenty percent of the maximal ASVV found between QRS onset to a point 450 msec (or 45% of the RR interval) before the fiducial point was used as a threshold. Measurements were made on the scalar Frank leads, on lead groupings V_4, V_5, V_6, and also on the Eigenleads derived from the Frank leads. The Eigenleads consisted of U (the narrow width), V (the length), and W (the thickness) of the Eigenloop. Spatial, or Eigenplane-derived, leads were based on the concept of containment of maximum energy of the QRS complex in a single plane. The maximum energy is concentrated at the peak amplitude, i.e., in about half to two thirds of the QRS interval. Usually, more than 70% to 80% of the QRS energy is contained in this middle portion of the QRS complex, and it predominantly defines the Eigenvectors and Eigenplane. A flow diagram of our program is shown in Figure 3.

In each lead, ST-segment amplitude was measured at the J junction (QRS end) and at 60 msec after J junction (ST 60). The ST-segment slopes were measured between the J junction and 60 msec after the J junction. ST integral, ST index, and time-normalized ST segment were also available. Spatial vector length was calculated as the amplitude of $\sqrt{X^2 + Y^2 + Z^2}$ at any point.

Electrocardiographic and vectorcardiographic data of pretraining and posttraining were analyzed during supine rest, maximal exercise, the highest matched heart rate during exercise, and at three minutes into recovery. Segments of the exercise electrocardiogram and vectorcardiogram were classified by heart rate as follows: 70 to 90, 91 to 110, 111 to 130, 131 to 150, and 151 or greater. The electrocardiographic and vectorcardiographic segments from

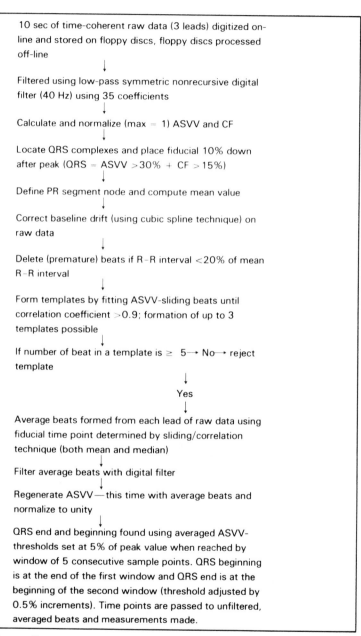

10 sec of time-coherent raw data (3 leads) digitized on-line and stored on floppy discs, floppy discs processed off-line

↓

Filtered using low-pass symmetric nonrecursive digital filter (40 Hz) using 35 coefficients

↓

Calculate and normalize (max = 1) ASVV and CF

↓

Locate QRS complexes and place fiducial 10% down after peak (QRS = ASVV >30% + CF >15%)

↓

Define PR segment node and compute mean value

↓

Correct baseline drift (using cubic spline technique) on raw data

↓

Delete (premature) beats if R–R interval <20% of mean R–R interval

↓

Form templates by fitting ASVV-sliding beats until correlation coefficient >0.9; formation of up to 3 templates possible

↓

If number of beat in a template is ≥ 5 → No → reject template

↓

Yes

↓

Average beats formed from each lead of raw data using fiducial time point determined by sliding/correlation technique (both mean and median)

↓

Filter average beats with digital filter

↓

Regenerate ASVV — this time with average beats and normalize to unity

↓

QRS end and beginning found using averaged ASVV-thresholds set at 5% of peak value when reached by window of 5 consecutive sample points. QRS beginning is at the end of the first window and QRS end is at the beginning of the second window (threshold adjusted by 0.5% increments). Time points are passed to unfiltered, averaged beats and measurements made.

Figure 3. A flow diagram illustrates the University of California, San Diego, computerized exercise electrocardiographic analysis program. ASVV = absolute spatial vector velocity; CF = coincidence function.

pretraining and posttraining were chosen within the same range of heart rate but at the highest range. QRS duration, S-wave amplitude, QRS angles, and R-wave amplitude showed no significant change. No significant difference was found in the standard ST-segment depression and slope measurements in the most sensitive lead, V_5, or in any of the X, Y, and Z Frank leads that view the heart three-dimensionally. The mean response to the exercise test both pretraining and posttraining was an abnormal ST-segment depression in X, Y, and V_5. ST-segment depression and R waves were of greater amplitude in V_5 than in the Frank X lead.

ST-segment amplitude at 60 msec after QRS end (ST 60) was analyzed because Simoons has demonstrated it to be the optimal criterion for ischemia. No significant difference was found in the ST-60 mean measurement pretraining and posttraining in the X, Y, and Z leads. However, a statistically significant improvement in ST-60 posttraining was found in the Eigenplane V lead. Using either absolute values or the mean calculations, there appeared to be less ST-segment displacement after the exercise program in the Eigenplane.

The finding of significant differences in ST-segment displacement in three-dimensional space is an interesting observation. In 1962, Pipberger reported studying the vectorcardiogram in its own frame of reference. He noted that nearly 95% of the electrical energy generated by the heart could be localized to a plane in space called the Eigenplane. How the ellipsoid heart maintains most of its electrical energy in a plane is unknown. One could hypothesize that the disarray of electrical conduction secondary to fibrosis or myocardial ischemia could increase the amount of nonplanar energy. The mean value in our population was only 3% of the electrical energy out of the Eigenplane at rest, which increased to 4% with exercise, but there was no difference after the exercise program. No matter what the explanation, Eigenplane values must be considered in looking for changes in serial observation of the exercise electrocardiogram.

CONCLUSION

An exercise program cannot be said to lessen exercise-induced ischemia as assessed indirectly by ST-segment depression in most cardiac patients. Randomized studies are essential to such investigations because those patients who spontaneously improve are likely to be selected by an exercise program. More specific indications of myocardial ischemia than ST-segment depression are needed before it can be concluded that there is no effect of exercise on ischemia.

REFERENCES
CHAPTER III

ANIMAL STUDIES OF THE EFFECTS OF CHRONIC EXERCISE

Aldinger EE: Effects of digitoxin on the development of cardiac hypertrophy in the rat subjected to chronic exercise. Am J Cardiol 25:339, 1970.

Aldinger EE, Sohal RS: Effects of digitoxin on the ultrastructural myocardial changes in the rat subjected to chronic exercise. Am J Cardiol 26:369, 1970.

Arcos JC, Dohal RS, Sun SC, et al: Changes in ultrastructure and respiratory control in mitochondria of rat heart hypertrophied by exercise. Exp Mol Pathol 8:49, 1968.

Banister EW, Tomanek RJ, Cvorkov N: Ultrastructural modifications in rat heart—Responses to exercise and training. Am J Physiol 220:1935, 1971.

Barnard R, Duncan H, Baldwin K, et al: Effects of intensive exercise training on myocardial performance and coronary blood flow. J Appl Physiol:Respirat Environ Exercise Physiol 49:444, 1980.

Bershon MM, Scheuer J: Effects of physical training on end-diastolic volume and myocardial performance of isolated rat hearts. Circ Res 40:510, 1977.

Bershon MM, Scheuer J: Effect of ischemia on the performance of hearts from physically trained rats. Am J Physiol 234:H215, 1978.

Bloor CM, Pasyk S, Leon AS: Interaction of age and exercise on organ and cellular development. Am J Pathol 58:185, 1970.

Burt JJ, Jackson R: The effects of physical exercise on the coronary collateral circulation of dogs. J Sports Med Phys Fitness 4:203, 1965.

Carew TE, Covell JW: Left ventricular function in exercise-induced hypertrophy in dogs. Am J Cardiol 42:82, 1978.

Carr DB, Bullen BA, Skrinar GS: Physical conditioning facilitates the exercise-induced secretion of beta-endorphin and beta-lipotropin in women. N Engl J Med 305:560, 1981.

Crews J, Aldinger EE: Effect of chronic exercise on myocardial function. Am Heart J 74:536, 1967.

Dowell RT, Cutilletta AF, Rudnik MA, et al: Heart functionl responses to pressure overload in exercised and sedentary rats. Am J Cardiol 230:199, 1976.

Dowell RT, Stone HL, Sordahl LA, et al: Contractile function and myofibrillar ATPase activity in the exercise-trained dog heart. J Appl Physiol 43:977, 1977.

Eckstein RW: Effect of exercise and coronary artery narrowing on coronary collateral circulation. Circ Res 5:230, 1957.

Froelicher VF: Animal studies of the effects of chronic exercise on the heart and atherosclerosis: A review. Am Heart J 84:496, 1972.

Guski H: The effect of exercise on myocardial interstitium: An ultrastructural morphometric study. Exp Mol Pathol 18:141, 1980.

Hakkila J: Studies of the myocardial capillary concentration in cardiac hypertrophy due to training. Ann Acad Sci Fenn [Exp Biol] 33(suppl 10):1, 1955.

Heaton WH, Marr KC, Capurro NL, et al: Beneficial effect of physical training on blood flow to myocardium perfused by chronic collaterals in the exercising dog. Circulation 57:575, 1978.

Holloszy JO: Morphological and enzymatic adaptations of training—A review, in Larsen OA, Malmborg RO (eds): Coronary Heart Disease and Physical Fitness. Baltimore, University Park Press, 1971, p 147.

Kaplinsky E, Hood WB Jr, McCarthy B, et al: Effects of physical training in dogs with coronary artery ligation. Circulation 37:556, 1968.

Kerr A Jr, Bommer WJ, Pilato S: Coronary artery enlargement in experimental cardiac hypertrophy. Am Heart J 75:144, 1968.

Kiessling KH, Piehl K, Lundquist CG: Number and size of skeletal muscle mitochondria in trained sedentary men, in Larsen OA, Malmborg RO (eds): Coronary Heart Disease and Physical Fitness. Baltimore, University Park Press, 1971, p 143.

Laks MM, Morady F, Swan HJ, et al: Presence of widened and multiple intercalated discs in the hypertrophied canine heart. Circ Res 27:391, 1970.

Leon AS, Bloor CM: Exercise effects on the heart at different ages (abstract). Circulation 41 & 42(suppl 3):50, 1970.

Leon A: Comparative cardiovascular adaptation to exercise in animals and man and its relevance to coronary heart disease, in Bloor CM (ed): Comparative Pathophysiology of Circulatory Disturbances. New York, Plenum, 1974, p 143.

Ljungqvist A, Unge G: Capillary proliferative activity in myocardium and skeletal muscle of exercised rats. J Appl Physiol 43:306, 1978.

Malik AB: Coronary vascular adjustments in exercise training. Cardiovasc Med 2:1137, 1977.

McElroy CL, Gissen SA, Fishbein MC: Exercise-induced reduction in myocardial infarction size after coronary artery occlusion in the rat. Circulation 57:958, 1978.

Moskowitz RM, Burns JJ, DiCarlo EF, et al: Cage size and exercise affects on infarct size in rat after coronary artery cauterization. J Appl Physiol:Respirat Environ Exercise Physiol 47:393, 1979.

Neil A, Oxedine R: Do collaterals improve perfusion during exercise? Circulation 60:1501, 1979.

Oscai LB, Mole PA, Holloszy JO, et al: Cardiac growth and respiratory enzyme levels in male rats subjected to a running program. Am J Physiol 220:1238, 1971.

Oscai LB, Mole PA, Holloszy JO: Effects of exercise on cardiac weight and mitochondria in male and female rats. Am J Physiol 220:1944, 1971.

Penpargkul S, Scheuer J: The effect of physical training upon the mechanical and metabolic performance of the rat heart. J Clin Invest 49:1859, 1970.

Petren T, Sylven B, Sjostrand T: Der Einfluss des Trainings and die Haufigkeit der Capillaren in Herz and Skeklettmuskatur. Arbeitsphysiologica 9:376, 1936.

Poupa O, Rakusan K, Ostadal B: The effect of physical activity upon the heart of vertebrates, in Brunner D (ed): Medicine and Sport, Vol 4. Baltimore, University Park Press, 1970, p 202.

Ritzer TF, Bove AA, Care RA: Left ventricular performance characteristics in trained and sedentary dogs. J Appl Physiol:Respirat Environ Exercise Physiol 48:130, 1980.

Sanders M, White FC, Peterson TM, et al: Effects of endurance exercise on coronary collateral blood flow in miniature swine. Am J Physiol 234:H614, 1978.

Schaible T, Scheuer J: Cardiac function in hypertrophied hearts from chronically exercised female rats. J Appl Physiol:Respirat Environ Exercise Physiol 50:1140, 1981.

Scheel K, Ingram L, Wilson J: Effects of exercise on the coronary and collateral vasculature of beagles with and without coronary occlusion. Circ Res 48:523, 1981.

Scheuer J, Kapner L, Stringfellow CA, et al: Glycogen, lipid, and high energy phosphate stores in hearts from conditioned rats. J Lab Clin Med 75:924, 1970.

Scheuer J, Tipton CM: Cardiovascular adaptations to physical training. Ann Rev Physiol 39:221, 1977.

Stevenson JA, Feleki V, Rechnitzer P, et al: Effect of exercise on coronary tree size in the rat. Circ Res 15:265, 1964.

Stone HL: Coronary flow, myocardial oxygen consumption and exercise training in dogs. J Appl Physiol:Respirat Environ Exercise Physiol 49:759, 1980.

Tepperman J, Pearlman D: Effects of exercise and anemia on coronary arteries of small animals as revealed by the corrosion-case technique. Circ Res 9:576, 1961.

Tibbits G, Barnard R, Baldwin K, et al: Influence of exercise on excitation-contraction coupling in rat myocardium. Am J Physiol 240:H472, 1981.

Tibbits G, Koziol BJ, Roberts NK, et al: Adaptation of the rat myocardium to endurance training. J Appl Physiol:Respirat Environ Exercise Physiol 44:85, 1978.

Tomanek RJ: Effects of age and exercise on the extent of the myocardial capillary bed. Anat Rec 167:55, 1970.

Tomanek RJ, Taunton CA, Liskop KS: Relationship between age, chronic exercise, and connective tissue of the heart. J Gerontol 27:33, 1972.

Wexler BC, Greenberg BP: Effect of exercise on myocardial infarction in young vs old male rats: Electrocardiographic changes. Am Heart J 88:343, 1974.

Wikman-Coffelt J, Parmley W, Mason D, et al: The cardiac hypertrophy process analyses of factors determining pathological vs physiological development. Circ Res 45:697, 1979.

Wyatt HL, Chuck L, Rabinowitz B, et al: Enhanced cardiac response to catecholamines in physically trained cats. Am J Physiol 234:H608, 1978.

Effects on Atherosclerosis and Risk Factors

Carlson LA: Lipid metabolism and muscular work. Fed Proc 26:1755, 1967.

Faris AW, Browning FM, Ibach JD: The effect of physical training upon total serum cholesterol levels and arterial distensibility of male white rats. J Sports Med 11:24, 1971.

Goodrick CL: Effects of long-term voluntary wheel exercise on male and female Wistar rats. Gerontol 26:22, 1980.

Kobernick SD, Niawayama G, Zuehlewski AC: Effect of physical activity on cholesterol atherosclerosis in rabbits. Proc Soc Exp Biol Med 96:623, 1957.

Kramsch DM, Aspen AJ, Abramowitz BM, et al: Reduction of coronary atherosclerosis by moderate conditioning exercise in monkeys on an antherogenic diet. N Engl J Med 305:1483, 1981.

McAllister FF, Bertsch R, Jacobson J, et al: The accelerating effect of muscular exercise on experimental atherosclerosis. Arch Surg 80:54, 1959.

Mehta J, Mehta P: Comparison of platelet function during exercise in normal subjects and coronary artery disease patients: Potential role of platelet activation in myocardial ischemia. Am Heart J 103:49, 1982.

Myasnikov AL: Influence of some factors on development of experimental cholesterol atherosclerosis. Circulation 17:99, 1958.

Pedersoli WM: Physical exercise, atherogenic diet, and serum lipids in swine. Cur Therap Res 23:464, 1978.

Rasmussen EW, Hostmark AT: Age-related changes in the concentration of plasma cholesterol and triglycerides in two groups of rats with inherited widely different levels of spontaneous physical activity. Circ Res 42:598, 1978.

Tipton CM, Matthes RD, Callahan A, et al: The role of chronic exercise on resting blood pressure of normotensive and hypertensive rats. Med Sci Sports 9:168, 1977.

Warnock NH, Clarkson RB, Stevenson R: Effect of exercise on blood coagulation time and atherosclerosis of cholesterol-fed cockerels. Circ Res 5:478, 1957.

Changes in Peripheral Blood Flow in Response to Acute Exercise

Fixler DE, Atkins JM, Mitchell JH, et al: Blood flow to respiratory, cardiac, and limb muscles in dogs during graded exercise. Am J Physiol 231:1515, 1976.

Tomoike H, Franklin D, McKown D, et al: Regional myocardial dysfunction and hemodynamic abnormalities during strenuous exercise in dogs with limited coronary flow. Circ Res 42:487, 1978.

HEMODYNAMIC STUDIES OF THE EFFECTS OF AN EXERCISE PROGRAM

Studies of Normal Subjects

Ekblom B: Effect of physical training on oxygen transport system in man. Acta Physiol Scand (suppl 328):1, 1969.

Froelicher VF: The hemodynamic effects of physical-conditioning in healthy young, and middle-aged individuals, and in coronary heart disease patients, in Naughton J, Hellerstein H (eds): Exercise Testing and Exercise Training in Coronary Heart Disease. New York, Academic Press, 1973, p 63.

Hanson JS, Tabakin BS, Levy AM: Comparative exercise-cardiorespiratory performance of normal men in the third, fourth, and fifth decades of life. Circulation 37:345, 1968.

Hanson JS, Tabakin BS, Levy AM, et al: Long-term physical training and cardiovascular dynamics in middle-aged men. Circulation 38:783, 1968.

Hartley LH, Grimby G, Kilbom A, et al: Physical training in sedentary middle-aged and older men. Scand J Clin Lab Invest (III)24:335, 1969.

Holmgren A: Vasoregulatory asthenia, in Larson OA, Malmborg RO (eds): Coronary Heart Disease and Physical Fitness. Baltimore, University Park Press, 1971, p 34.

Kilbom A, Hartley LH, Saltin B, et al: Physical training in sedentary middle-aged and older men. Scand J Clin Lab Invest (I)24:315, 1969.

Longhurst JC, Kelly AR, Gonyea WJ, et al: Chronic training with static and dynamic exercise: Cardiovascular adaptation, and response to exercise. Circ Res 48:171, 1981.

Orenstein DM, Franklin BA, Doershuk CF, et al: Exercise conditioning and cardiopulmonary fitness in cystic fibrosis—The effects of a three-month supervised running program. Chest 80:392, 1981.

Rerych S, Scholz P, Sabiston D, et al: Effects of exercise training on left ventricular function in normal subjects: A longitudinal study by radionuclide angiography. Am J Cardiol 45:244, 1980.

Saltin B, Blomqvist G, Mitchell JH, et al: Response to exercise after bed rest and after training. Circulation 38:1, 1968.

Saltin B, Hartley LH, Kilbom A, et al: Physical training in sedentary middle-aged and older men. Scand J Clin Lab Invest (II)24:323, 1969.

Tabkin BS, Hanson JS, Levy AM: Effects of physical training on the cardiovascular and respiratory response to graded upright exercise in distance runners. Br Heart J 27:205, 1965.

Studies of Coronary Heart Disease Patients

Bergman H, Varnauskas E: The hemodynamic effects of physical training in coronary patients, in Jokl E, Brunner D (eds): Medicine and Sport, vol 4. Baltimore, University Park Press, 1970, p 138.

Bruce RW, Kusumi F, Frederick R: Differences in cardiac function with prolonged physical training for cardiac rehabilitation. Am J Cardiol 40:597, 1977.

Carter CL, Amundsen LR: Infarct size and exercise capacity after myocardial infarction. J Appl Physiol 42:782, 1977.

Clausen JP: Effects of physical conditioning, a hypothesis concerning circulatory adjustment to exercise (a review). Scand J Clin Lab Invest 24:305, 1969.

Clausen JP, Lassen NA: Muscle blood flow during exercise in normal man studied by the Xenon 133 clearance method. Cardiovasc Res 5:245, 1971.

Clausen JP, Trap-Jensen J: Effects of training on the distribution of cardiac output in patients with coronary artery disease. Circulation 42:611, 1970.

Clausen JP, Trap-Jensen J, Lassen NA: Evidence that the relative exercise bradycardia induced by training can be caused by extra cardiac factors, in Larsen OA, Malmborg RO (eds): Coronary Heart Disease and Physical Fitness. Baltimore, University Park Press, 1971, p 27.

DeBusk RF, Houston N, Haskell W, et al: Exercise training soon after myocardial infarction. Am J Cardiol 44:1223, 1979.

Detry JR, Rousseau M, Vandenbroucke W, et al: Increased arteriovenous oxygen difference after physical training in coronary heart disease. Circulation 44:109, 1971.

Ferguson RJ, Petitclerc R, Choquette G, et al: Effect of physical training on treadmill exercise capacity, collateral circulation and progression of coronary disease. Am J Cardiol 34:764, 1974.

Foster GL, Reeves TJ: Hemodynamic responses to exercise in clinically normal middle-aged men and in those with angina pectoris. J Clin Invest 43:1758, 1964.

Frick MH, Katila M: Hemodynamic consequences of physical training after myocardial infarction. Circulation 37:192, 1968.

Frick MH, Katila M, Sjogren AL: Cardiac function and physical training after myocardial infarction, in Larsen OA, Malmborg RO (eds): Coronary Heart Disease and Physical Fitness. Baltimore, University Park Press, 1971, p 43.

Frick MH, Konttineen A, Sarajas HS: Effects of physical training on circulation at rest and during exercise. Am J Cardiol 12:142, 1963.

Lee AP, Ice R, Blessey R, et al: Long-term effects of physical training on coronary patients with impaired ventricular function. Circulation 60:1519, 1979.

Letac B, Cribier A, Desplanches JF: A study of LV function in coronary patients before and after physical training. Circulation 56:375, 1977.

Nolewajka AJ, Kostuk WJ, Rechnitzer PA, et al: Exercise and human collateralization: An angiographic and scintigraphic assessment. Circulation 60:114, 1979.

Paterson DH, Shephard RK, Cunningham D: Effects of physical training on cardiovascular function following myocardial infarction. J Appl Physiol 47:482, 1979.

Sim DN, Neill WA: Investigation of the physiological basis for increased exercise threshold for angina pectoris after physical conditioning. J Clin Invest 54:763, 1974.

Sylvester R, Camp J, Canmarco M: Effects of exercise training or progression of documented coronary arteriosclerosis, in Milvy P (ed): The Marathon: Physiological, Medical, Epidemiological and Psychological Studies. New York, New York Academy of Sciences, 1977, p 495.

Varnauskas E, Bergman H, Houk P, et al: Haemodynamic effect of physical training in coronary patients. Lancet 2:8, 1966.

Varnauskas E, Bjorntorp P, Fahlen M, et al: Effects of physical training on exercise blood flow and enzymatic activity in skeletal muscle. Cardiovasc Res 4:418, 1970.

ECHOCARDIOGRAPHIC STUDIES OF THE EFFECTS OF AN EXERCISE PROGRAM

Cross-Sectional Studies Comparing Echocardiographic Measurements of Normals and of Athletes

Gilbert CA, Nutter DO, Felner JM, et al: Echocardiographic study of cardiac dimensions and function in the endurance-trained athlete. Am J Cardiol 40:528, 1977.

Morganroth J, Maron BJ, Henry WL, et al: Comparative left ventricular dimensions in trained athletes. Ann Intern Med 82:521, 1975.

Parker BM, Londeree BR, Cupp GV, et al: The noninvasive cardiac evaluation of long-distance runners. Chest 73:376, 1978.

Paulsen W, Boughner DR, Patrick KO, et al: Left ventricular function in marathon runners: Echocardiographic assessment. J Appl Physiol 51:881, 1981.

Roeske WR, O'Rourke RA, Klein A, et al: Noninvasive evaluation of ventricular hypertrophy in professional athletes. Circulation 53:286, 1976.

Echocardiography Before and After an Exercise Program

Adams TD, Yanowitz FG, Fischer AG, et al: Noninvasive evaluation of exercise training in college-age men. Circulation 64:958, 1981.

Clark P, Glasser S: Diagnostic insights—problem: Cardiomegaly in a 60-year-old runner. Cardiovasc Med 4(4):441, 1979.

DeMaria AN, Neumann A, Lee G, et al: Alterations in ventricular mass and performance induced by exercise training in man evaluated by echocardiograpy. Circulation 57:237, 1978.

Ditchey RV, Watkins J, McKirnan, MD, et al: Effects of exercise training on left ventricular mass in patients with ischemic heart disease. Am Heart J 101:701, 1981.

Ehsani AA, Hagberg JM, Hickson RC: Rapid changes in left ventricular dimensions and mass in response to physical conditioning and deconditioning. Am J Cardiol 42:52, 1978.

Ehsani AA, Heath GW, Hagberg JM, et al: Noninvasive assessment of changes in left ventricular function induced by graded isometric exercise in healthy subjects. Chest 80:51, 1981.

Frick MH, Sjogren AL, Paraslo J, et al: Cardiovascular dimensions and moderate physical training in young men. J Appl Physiol 29:452, 1970.

Parrault H, Peronnet F, Cleroux J, et al: Electro- and echocardiographic assessment of left ventricle before and after training in man. Can J Appl Sports Sci 3:180, 1978.

Schieken RM, Clarke WR, Mahoney LT, et al: Measurement criteria for group echocardiographic studies. Am J Epidemiol 110:504, 1979.

Stein RA, Michielli D, Fox EL, et al: Continuous ventricular dimensions in man during supine exercise and recovery. Am J Cardiol 41:655, 1978.

Thompson P, Lewis S, Areskog N, et al: Generalized training effects without changes in cardiac performance. Med Sci Sports 10:1, 1978.

Wolfe L, Cunningham D, Rechnitzer P, et al: Effects of endurance training on left ventricular dimensions in healthy men. J Appl Physiol:Respirat Environ Exercise Physiol 47:207, 1979.

Zeldis SM, Morganroth J, Rubler S: Cardiac hypertrophy in response to dynamic conditioning in female athletes. J Appl Physiol:Respirat Environ Exercise Physiol 44:849, 1978.

Exercise Electrocardiographic Studies

Bhargava V, Watanabe K, Froelicher VF, et al: Computer techniques for assessing serial changes in the ECG/VCG response to exercise testing and training. Computers in Cardiology 335, September 1979.

Costill DL, Branam GE, Moore JC, et al: Effects of physical training in men with coronary heart disease. Med Sci Sports 6:95, 1974.

Detry J, Bruce RA: Effects of physical training on exertional S-T-segment depression in coronary heart disease. Circulation 44:390, 1971.

Ehsani AA, Heath GW, Hagberg JM, et al: Effects of 12 months of intense exercise training on ischemic ST-segment depression in patients with coronary artery disease. Circulation 64:116, 1981.

Kattus AA, Jorgensen CR, Worden RE, et al: ST segment depression with near-maximal exercise: Its modification by physical conditioning. Chest 62:678, 1972.

Pipberger HV, Carter TN: Analysis of the normal and abnormal vectorcardiogram in its own reference frame. Circulation 15:827, 1962.

Raffo JA, Luksic IY, Kappagoda CT, et al: Effects of physical training on myocardial ischaemia in patients with coronary artery disease. Br Heart J 43:262, 1980.

Salzman SH, Hellerstein HK, Radke JD, et al: Quantitative effects of physical conditioning on the exercise electrocardiogram of middle-aged subjects with arteriosclerotic heart disease, in Blackburn H (ed): Measurements in Exercise ECG. Springfield, Ill, Charles C Thomas, 1969, p 388.

Sidney KH, Shephard RJ: Training and electrocardiographic abnormalities in the elderly. Br Heart J 39:1114, 1977.

Watanabe K, Bhargava V, Froelicher V: Computerized approach to evaluating rest and exercise-induced ECG/VCG after cardiac rehabilitation. Clin Cardiol 5:27, 1982.

CHAPTER

IV

Exercise in the Prevention and Management of Coronary Heart Disease

Since most animal, clinical, and pathologic studies have not shown exercise to be directly related to the atherosclerotic process, one must conclude that physical inactivity does not have a direct effect on atherosclerosis. Instead, the effects of regular exercise enable the body to better tolerate ischemia and lessen the manifestations of coronary heart disease. In addition, it can possibly alter other risk factors for atherosclerosis. The potential beneficial actions of regular exercise are multifactorial, which makes physical inactivity a complex risk factor to assess. Some of the difficulties in studying physical inactivity as a risk factor will be discussed, along with many of the studies that have been performed.

Does exercise protect from coronary artery disease rather than select out those with less coronary artery disease who are better able to tolerate being physically active? Exercise can be related to other risk factors or risk markers, and often studies have not considered the selection of these factors. Particularly in a modern, mechanized society, there is usually only a small gradient of activity between different jobs. An important consideration is that people often leave active jobs with onset of the first symptoms of heart disease, even without realizing the cause of the symptoms. That is, there is a premorbid transfer from an active job to a less active job, biasing the relationship of inactivity to coronary heart disease. Also, individuals are often selected for active jobs or for life-styles of physical activity. There are other difficulties in studying this question, including the uncertainty of what type and quantity of exercise is protective.

Although the most accurate way of assessing the physiologic effect of an activity level would be an exercise test, few studies have had this luxury. Job title or class has often been used and in some instances was quite accurate. However, consideration of off-the-job activity is important. Questionnaires have been used, but their reproducibility and accuracy are often doubtful. Parameters such as vital capacity, handgrip strength, and dietary assays have obvious limitations.

The methods of diagnosing coronary artery disease have included death certificates, rest and exercise electrocardiograms, medical records, medical evaluations, and autopsy. Even an autopsy has distinct limitations since it is usually not done using standardized methods. The death certificate is often coded with the most common cause of death in the community rather than an accurate description of the cause of death. Also, multiple causes of death confuse the actual cause of death. Certainly, physicians functioning as clinicians or pathologists do not feel the same need for accuracy and precision in completing these forms and records as do epidemiologists.

Many different types of populations have been used for epidemiologic studies. There are three basic types of epidemiologic studies: retrospective, prevalence, and prospective studies. Retrospective studies involve populations in which data have been obtained in the past not specifically for epidemiologic purposes. Prevalence, or cross-sectional, studies consist of screening a population for the current manifestations of a disease. Prospective, or longitudinal, studies involve a cohort of individuals specifically chosen and studied for the purpose of following them over a period of time for the development of disease.

RETROSPECTIVE STUDIES OF PHYSICAL INACTIVITY AS A RISK FACTOR

This group of retrospective studies includes three large population studies that have utilized death certificate and population data from an entire city, state, or country. Activity level was judged from the occupation listed on the death certificate, and the end point was coronary artery disease listed on death certificates.

Morris has presented the data from the occupational-mortality records in England and Wales, interpreting the information as support for the hypothesis that occupational physical inactivity is a risk factor for coronary artery disease. Social class as used in these studies was based on the grading of occupation by its level of skill and role in production, and its general standing in the community. Social class ranged from class 1, which includes professions such as physicians and stockbrokers, to class 5, which includes unskilled workers such as railroad porters and builders' helpers. The level of activity was based on the independent evaluation of the occupations by several industrial experts. The activity level of the last job held was found to be inversely related to the mortality from coronary artery disease, as determined from death certificates. Some of the limitations of this study include imprecise diagnostic criteria and bias due to the selection of the sick for less active jobs.

Stamler and associates analyzed the mortality statistics in Chicago for the years 1951 and 1953. Both the cause of death and occupation were obtained from the death certificates, and the occupations were broken down into five categories: (1) professional and semiprofessional workers, proprietors, managers, and officials; (2) clerical and sales people; (3) craftsmen, foremen, and operatives; (4) service workers; and (5) laborers. These categories were also combined as white-collar workers (categories 1 and 2) and blue-collar workers (categories 3, 4, and 5). The authors found no significant occupational group differences in age-specific coronary artery disease death rates for white males 45 to 64 years of age.

Breslow and Buell compared groups with similar general mortality to make apparent the protective effect of physical activity, in agreement with the previously mentioned British studies. They analyzed census and death certificate data in California from 1949 to 1951. They found inconsistencies, however, in the records as to whether the last, the usual, or longest held occupation was reported. Nonetheless, they felt that the data revealed a gradient of decreasing mortality rate from coronary heart disease with increasing physical activity, but only when occupational groups of similar general mortality were considered.

The following retrospective studies involved analysis of data from a specific population with activity level assessed by job classification, or questionnaire, or both and with coronary artery disease listed on the death certificate or reported symptoms of coronary artery disease used as end points.

Morris and co-workers presented data from a sequence of epidemiologic studies to support the hypothesis quoted here. "Men in physically active jobs have a lower incidence of coronary heart disease than men in physically inactive jobs. More important, the disease is not so severe in physically active workers, tending to present first in them as angina pectoris and other relatively benign forms and to have a smaller early case fatality and a lower early mortality rate." The first study dealt with the drivers and conductors of the London transport system. Thirty-one thousand white males, 35 to 64 years of age, were included for analysis over a period of 18 months from 1949 to 1950. The end points were coronary insufficiency, myocardial infarction, and angina as reported on sick-leave records and listing of coronary artery disease on death certificates. The age-adjusted total incidence was 1.5 times higher in the driver group as compared with the conductor group, and the sudden and three-month mortality were two times higher. The authors suggested that these findings could be explained by differences in constitution, mental stress, or physical activity. The difference in physical activity was only inferred from knowing that one group drove the buses, whereas the other group conducted on the double-decker vehicles. No attempt was made to quantitate the activity difference or to measure differences in off-the-job activity. In their original study, the authors did not investigate differences in selection in the two groups but proceeded to a similar study with postmen and clerks, which also resulted in numbers that agreed with their hypothesis. Interestingly, though, in 1956 Morris published a paper subtitled "The Epidemiology of Uniforms," which reported that the drivers had greater girth than the conductors. A later study in 1966 by Morris also showed that the drivers had higher serum cholesterol levels and higher blood pressures than did the conductors. Also, a study by Oliver documented that for some unknown reason, even the recruits for the two jobs differed in lipid level and in weight. These differences put the drivers at increased risk to coronary artery disease for reasons other than an approximated difference in physical activity.

Zukel and colleagues analyzed data from a population of 106,000 individuals living in six counties in North Dakota. From the 20,000 men aged 35 years or more greater within this population, they found 228 men with coronary artery disease that became manifest during 1957. The data were obtained from reviewing death certificates or from office visits or hospital admissions reported by local doctors for acute myocardial infarctions, coronary ischemia, congestive heart failure due to coronary artery disease, or angina. Farmers had slightly less total coronary artery disease and one half the infarctions and death from coronary artery disease. The authors did not relate this result directly to differences in physical activity since they were aware of socioeconomic and environmental differences between the two groups. Physical activity was related to coronary artery disease based on a questionnaire of physical activity administered to survivors of infarction and to matched controls. Unfortunately, interview information on physical activity is very unreliable. By dividing hours of heavy physical work into 0, 1 to 6, and 7 or more, only a 51% agreement was found for 273 men in whom replicate information was obtained. Moreover, there was a tendency for men to report less heavy physical work in their usual occupation after their heart attack than before.

Brunner has surveyed Jews of European origin living in kibbutzim, or collective settlements, in Israel over the period of 1946 to 1961, with 5,279 men aged 40 to 69 years in the group as of 1961. Coronary heart disease was determined from medical records of myocardial infarction, angina pectoris, and sudden death due to coronary artery disease. Sedentary workers, defined as those who spent 80% or more of their time at work sitting, had 2.5 to 4.0 times the incidence of coronary artery disease as the nonsedentary workers (all others). Although Brunner believes that this population is ideal for study because their mode of life eliminates socioeconomic differences, no investigation of differences in risk factors was reported. Characteristics of the sedentary group other than physical activity could equally account for differences in the incidence of coronary artery disease.

These next retrospective studies involve data obtained from specific occupational groups with the activity level assessed by the standardized job title and with coronary artery disease listed as the cause of death in the industrial records as the end point.

In a mortality study, Adelstein compared white South Africans working for South African railroads as officers (clerks, administrators, high-paid executives) with railroad employees (ranging from unskilled laborers to skilled artisans). Mortality among these employees, secondary to coronary artery disease during 1954 to 1959, when age adjusted, did not differ from the general population. The categories of artisans, semiskilled and others, were analyzed with the physical demand of work within each group determined on a scale of one to five by four experienced, industrial health inspectors, and mean ratings were used. Again, no significant differences were found in mortality from coronary artery disease and level of physical activity.

Taylor and colleagues have reported on the mortality of white males employed by the United States railroad industry. The employees were separated by job title into three groups representing three levels of physical activity. Death certificates for the years 1955 and 1956 were analyzed by these groupings, and the following age-adjusted rates were obtained: (1) clerks, light activity, 5.7 deaths per 1,000 man-years; (2) switchmen, moderate activity, 3.9 deaths per 1,000 man-years; and (3) section men, heavy activity, 2.8 deaths per 1,000 man-years. They concluded that the data were consistent with the hypothesis that men in sedentary occupations have more coronary heart disease than do those in occupations requiring moderate to heavy physical activity.

In planning a prospective study, the authors discovered a number of important points that pertained to their mortality study. They found that the groups were not clearly separated by occupation as to the level of physical activity. Work analyses and further questioning revealed that some clerks consumed as many calories per day as did section men, who presumably were working more vigorously. The most important finding was that men with coronary artery disease withdrew from the ranks of switchmen at a greater rate than from the ranks of sedentary clerks. It then became apparent that this bias in job transfers and in retirement could explain the difference in mortality between the groups, rather than any protective influence exerted by physical activity.

Kahn gathered information from federal employee records to analyze mortality data on men who were appointed to positions in the Washington, D.C., Post Office from 1906 to 1940. Of 2,240 men so identified, 93% were determined as either dead or alive as of January 1962. The mortality data of sedentary clerks were compared with active mail carriers. Kahn noted that the records showed that the carriers transferred to clerk positions much more frequently than clerks switched jobs. He adjusted for this effect by considering a subsample of men who did not change jobs. The data from this preselected group suggested that the clerks had 1.4 to 1.9 times the mortality from coronary artery disease than the carriers. It is entirely possible that the differences observed were only coincidentally related to physical activity differences.

The following retrospective studies represent specific populations in which the activity level was assessed by occupation or questionnaire; diagnosis of acute myocardial infarction served as the end point.

Frank and associates have studied 55,000 men aged 25 to 64 years enrolled in the Health Insurance Plan of Greater New York (HIP). In this group, 301 men were identified as having had an initial myocardial infarction between November 1, 1961, and April 30, 1963. An index for on-the-job and off-the-job activities was obtained by patient completion of a questionnaire during a personal interview after the infarction by the patients or by the wives of those who had died. The men were divided into three categories: least active, intermediate, and most active. The authors concluded that inquiry about customary physical activities on and off the job permitted delineation of a group of least active men who were much more likely to experience a clinically severe episode and die within four weeks of its onset than were men who were relatively more active.

There are a number of inherent difficulties in this study. Many of the 301 men who provided incidence data on infarction were ill prior to infarction. Twenty-two percent had manifestations of coronary artery disease, 19% had high blood pressure, and 10% were diabetic, and it would be expected that these people would be less active. Being less active and at high risk for acute MI, they represent a statistical bias for inactivity and subsequent MI as well as for the severity of the infarction. Another difficulty was that widows tended to underestimate the physical activity of their dead husbands.

Shanoff and colleagues studied a group of men with documented myocardial infarction, randomly selected from the files of the Toronto Veterans Administration Hospital, and matched to a group, also from the hospital files, of patients admitted with nonchronic illnesses. Within both groups, there were approximately 25 individuals for each decade from the fourth through seventh decades of life for a total of 100 individuals per group. The individuals were questioned as to lifelong activity, and physical activity in childhood, youth, and adult life was assessed. This type of questioning made available additional information because the two groups did not differ as to present activity or occupation but did differ as to habitual activity. In this study, coronary artery disease was not associated with habitual physical inactivity.

Forssman and Lindegard organized a study in Malmo, a Swedish town of about 200,000 people. The city is served by one hospital, and the study group was comprised of all male survivors of an acute myocardial infarction admitted to the hospital from 1948 to 1955 and whose age at the time of the study examination in 1956 was 55 or less. This group included 66 men for whom healthy similarly aged controls were randomly selected from the town. Occupational physical activity was determined by knowledge of the job rather than by personal questioning. No difference in occupational physical activity between the controls and postinfarction group were determined.

PREVALENCE STUDIES OF PHYSICAL INACTIVITY AS A RISK FACTOR

The following three prevalence, or cross-sectional, studies represent a modification of the retrospective, or case history, approach. The main advantage is that the statistics on the studied disease are gathered at the time of the study. Thus, the end points can be well defined, and the methods for diagnosis standardized. Unfortunately, selection continues to be a problem.

In 1958, 1,465 male employees of a utility company in Chicago were evaluated. Prevalence of coronary heart disease was determined by reviewing industrial health records for diagnostic electrocardiographic changes or for history consistent with coronary artery disease. There was little difference in major risk factors between the activity level groups. Prevalence of coronary artery disease was lower in the blue-collar workers than in the white-collar workers and lower in the nonsedentary than in the sedentary. These data were confounded by such factors as differential rates of retirement among blue- and white-collar workers, and shifts from blue-collar to white-collar jobs after a coronary artery disease episode.

In 1957 to 1959, a sample of 3,049 railroad men were randomly selected for study of the prevalence of risk factors in coronary artery disease. Active switchmen and sedentary clerks and executives were included to have two different activity groups for comparison. Extensive screening was performed, and the manifestations of coronary artery disease were well defined. The data on the 1948 men that submitted to the evaluation suggested that the switchmen had less coronary artery disease. However, occupational mobility of the switchmen with coronary disease was greater than that of clerks. The majority of the factors affecting observed prevalence rates operated to exaggerate any true protective influences of physical activity.

In 1960, the population of Evans County, Georgia, was studied for the prevalence of coronary heart disease. Coronary artery disease was defined as angina pectoris, history of a myocardial infarction, or diagnostic electrocardiographic findings. Definite and probable cases, according to defined standards, were used for statistical analysis. The study group included 1,062 men consisting of almost equal numbers of high social class whites, low social class whites, and blacks. Within the study group there were 52 cases of coronary artery disease. Social class and occupational comparison among black males was not possible because they were predominantly of low social class and in physically active occupations. Among white males, distribution of coronary artery disease by occupation suggested that those with high activity had less prevalence of coronary artery disease. White males had three times the coronary artery disease as the black males, whereas high social class white males had two times as much disease as low social class white males and five times as much as black males. Black males were felt to be more active by analysis of occupation and caloric consumption, but they also were thinner and had lower serum cholesterol levels. The authors concluded that physical activity appeared to be a major determinant of coronary artery disease prevalence. A seven-year prospective study in Evans County found the incidence of coronary artery disease to be lower among professionals (94/1,000) and highest among manual laborers and clerks (184/1,000). This contradictory result is interesting, especially since the two other prevalence studies were felt to be influenced by a bias that favored the physical activity hypothesis.

PROSPECTIVE STUDIES OF PHYSICAL INACTIVITY AS A RISK FACTOR

In 1958, Stamler and colleagues began a prospective study of 1,241 apparently healthy male employees of the Peoples Gas Company in Chicago. By 1965, there were 39 deaths due to coronary artery disease among the groups. They found that the coronary artery disease mortality was higher in blue-collar workers (37 deaths per 1,000 men) who had an estimated higher habitual activity at work than in the white-collar workers (20 deaths per 1,000). Stamler felt these findings were consistent with the hypothesis that groups of men with similar findings with respect to the cardinal risk factors (hypertension, hypercholesterolemia, cigarette smoking, and excessive weight) will experience similar incidences and mortality rates for coronary heart disease irrespective of habitual physical activity at work. However, the population in general had a low level of physical activity, and lack of a gradient of physical activity limits the possibility of demonstrating an association of mortality and physical activity.

From 1956 to 1960, 687 healthy London busmen were examined for risk factors and coronary artery disease. In 1965, they were reexamined and 47 cases of coronary artery disease were diagnosed, including sudden deaths, myocardial infarction, electrocardiographic changes, and angina. Incidence rates per 100 men over five years were 4.7 for conductors and 8.5 for drivers. However, the drivers were found to have significantly higher blood pressure and serum cholesterol levels than the conductors. Furthermore, classifying the conductors as an activity-protected group was inconsistent because they had an incidence of CAD similar to sedentary London physicians.

Taylor studied the effects of occupational activity differences among railroad men in the U.S. Thirty groups of men were randomly selected from a population of 3,049 men working for 20 northwestern railroads. Of this group, there were 860 sedentary clerks, 251 executives, and 837 active switchmen, 40 to 59 years of age, when first examined from 1957 to 1959. Energy expenditure was estimated by activity and dietary analysis. It was found that the switchmen expended 600 to 1,200 calories a day more than the sedentary groups. The groups did not differ by any of the major risk factors. After five years of follow-up, no difference in coronary incidence rates between the two different activity levels was found.

In 1957, 1,719 white men aged 40 to 55 years were randomly selected from the 20,000 employees of the Hawthorne Electric Works in Chicago. After eight years of follow-up, there were 24 deaths due to coronary artery disease, 53 acute myocardial infarctions with survival, and 80 patients with the diagnosis of angina pectoris. Activity off the job was assessed by a personal interview. Approximate differences in caloric expenditure and intensity of work were determined for shop workers and office workers, and also with special means for two different classes of shop workers. No difference was found in coronary artery disease among the different levels of activity.

In 1949, 1,403 healthy white men with a median age of 47 years were randomly chosen from 20,200 civil servants in Los Angeles. After an initial examination in 1951, periodic follow-up examinations and yearly questionnaires were completed. By 1962, a total of 177 new events of coronary artery disease as manifested by myocardial infarction, sudden death, angina pectoris, or coronary insufficiency were diagnosed. No differences in the incidence of coronary heart disease was observed according to socioeconomic class or to level of physical activity as determined from job title.

The Western Electric collaborative group study was initiated in 1961 with emphasis on psychologic patterns. Annual follow-up studies were obtained through 1965 on 3,182 men, initially aged 35 to 59 years and healthy at the onset. New coronary heart disease as manifested by symptomatic myocardial infarction, angina, and electrocardiographic changes was observed in 133 individuals. The customary exercise habits of each participant were determined by personal interview. Nine hundred sixty subjects were classified as exercising with reasonable regularity, i.e., daily or almost daily they performed some calisthenics, walking exercise, athletics, or equivalent physical activity. The remaining 2,222 subjects admitted to only occasionally engaging in some form of physical activity. No differences in age or risk factors in these two groups were apparent, except that the exercising group had slightly lower triglyceride and cholesterol measurements. After 4 1/2 years of follow-up, the annual incidence of coronary heart disease was 10/1,000 for men without regular exercise habits, compared with 7.4/1,000 in men with such habits. This difference was due to symptomatic myocardial infarction, since no difference was observed in the incidence of silent infarction, angina, or recurring infarction. Fatal myocardial infarction occurred in 2/1,000 men without regular exercise habits compared with 0.5/1,000 men with such habits.

The Seven Countries Coronary Artery Disease Study consists of collaborative groups from Japan, Yugoslavia, United States, Finland, Italy, the

Netherlands, and Greece. This study minimized self-selection, rendering complete examination coverage to all men aged 40 to 59 years in the geographically defined areas. The examinations and definitions were rigidly standardized and coordinated at facilities at the University of Minnesota. Individuals were classified as sedentary, moderately active, or very active, as determined by a questionnaire for evaluating total physical activity. Data from 200,000 man-years observed showed no difference in coronary artery disease incidence between physically active and sedentary men.

In 1963, Werko and co-workers began a study on a cohort consisting of one third of all men born in 1913 in the industrial Swedish town of Gothenburg. This cohort consisted of 834 males 50 years of age without signs or symptoms of coronary artery disease. Over the next four years, there were 23 acute myocardial infarctions, 18 individuals with angina pectoris, and 9 individuals with diagnostic electrocardiographic changes of a myocardial infarction. The symptomatic infarction group was questioned to assess retrospectively activity level on and off the job one year prior to their infarction. Activity levels were categorized as light, moderate, or heavy. A random sample of healthy men of a comparable age were questioned as to activity in a similar fashion, and in comparison, this sample group was more active than those with infarctions.

Epstein, Morris, and colleagues studied the relationship of vigorous exercise during leisure time to the resting electrocardiogram. From 1968 to 1970, approximately 17,000 middle-age male executive civil servents on a randomly selected Monday morning recorded their leisure-time activities over the previous weekend. Their work was sedentary. In 1971, a sample of 509 of these men completed further questionnaires for medical, social, and smoking history; at that time, the 509 had a resting electrocardiogram, serum cholesterol level, and other physiologic parameters recorded. Vigorous exercise in leisure time had previously been reported by 25% of the men. As a group, these active men had significantly fewer electrocardiographic abnormalities than the men not reporting vigorous exercise. The electrocardiographic abnormalities included changes consistent with myocardial ischemia, ectopic beats, and sinus tachycardia. This difference was maintained when all men with any history suggestive of cardiovascular disease were excluded from the analysis. Blood pressure, serum cholesterol, and smoking habits were examined along with vigorous exercise in relation to the electrocardiogram. The only relation found was increased electrocardiographic abnormalities with increasing blood pressure. Even among men with higher blood pressures, those reporting vigorous exercise had fewer electrocardiographic abnormalities. An 8 1/2-year follow-up of this population has demonstrated a

50% lower incidence of coronary events in those maintaining rigorous activity on the weekend.

Morris and colleagues reported the results of following 337 healthy middle-age Englishmen. During 1956 to 1966, these men participated in a seven-day dietary survey. By the end of 1976, 44 of them had developed clinical coronary disease that showed two relationships to diet. Men with a high-energy intake, as assessed by diet, had a lower rate of disease. Independently of this fact, men with a high intake of dietary fiber from cereals also had a lower rate of disease. A high-energy intake reflects physical activity and supports the exercise hypothesis.

Members of the Fellowship of Cycling Old-Timers (FCOT) were chosen arbitrarily and studied by means of a questionnaire. The club was formed in 1965 for cyclists over 50 years of age. There was a 90% response to 329 questionnaires sent to members living in England. The pattern of activity was 5,000 to 10,000 miles cycled per year, which declined to 2,000 miles as the member got older. At the time of the study, 75% of members were still cycling regularly throughout the year, and 54% of those over 70 were cycling once a week or more throughout the year. A decrease in the incidence of myocardial infarction and ischemic heart disease was found in all cyclists, but the tenfold decrease in incidence of all ischemic heart disease in the over 75 age group was striking. Details of the cause of death were obtained from death certificates. The average age of death was high (79 years) but expected because membership was restricted to those age 50 or older.

Costas and colleagues reported a prospective study involving 8,171 urban and rural men 45 to 64 years old participating in the Puerto Rico Heart Program. The 2 1/2-year incidence of coronary heart disease was examined in relation to serum cholesterol, triglycerides, physical activity, and relative weight. A physical activity index was based on the number of hours spent at five different levels of physical activity as assessed by questionnaire. Coronary disease end points included myocardial infarction, death, and angina pectoris. A slight increase in risk was found in the least active group of urban men. The physical activity index was too crude, and the level of physical activity was not related to the incidence of coronary heart disease.

In an attempt to evaluate the exercise hypothesis, investigations at the Aerobic Center in Dallas have used treadmill performance to quantitate physical fitness. In a cross-sectional study of 3,000 men, treadmill performance was found to be inversely related to body weight, percent body fat, lipids, glucose, and systolic blood pressure. In a longitudinal study, men who were treadmill tested both before and after an elective exercise program were analyzed to determine if their performance had improved. Those men who reached the upper quartile of improved aerobic fitness exhibited decreases in lipids, diastolic blood pressure, serum glucose, uric acid, and weight. This study demonstrates that regular exercise resulting in increased aerobic capacity can decrease other risk factors.

Cross-sectional studies found runners to have higher levels of high-density lipoprotein (HDL) cholesterol, and prospective studies found high levels of HDL cholesterol to be protective from coronary disease. The main carriers of cholesterol in the blood are the beta lipoproteins (low-density lipoproteins or LDL) and the alpha lipoproteins (high-density lipoproteins). The low-density lipoproteins carry the majority of cholesterol; however, HDL levels are important because HDL acts as a vehicle to transport cholesterol from the body. HDL appears to be important for transporting cholesterol from the intimal cells of arteries to the serum and eventually to the bile for excretion from the body. A person with a serum cholesterol level of 240 mg/100 ml and HDL cholesterol of 90 mg/100 ml can have a low risk, whereas if the HDL cholesterol is only 20 mg/100 ml he can have a high risk for coronary disease. The ratio of total cholesterol to HDL cholesterol helps to estimate risk. There is an average risk with a ratio of 5, a high risk with a ratio of 10, and a low risk with a ratio of 3 or 4. Runners often exhibit a ratio of 3, but ratios below 2.5 are not physiologically possible. There are two apoproteins in HDL, the A1 fraction and the A2 fraction. The A1 fraction, which is found in higher levels in runners, appears to be more important than the A2 in removing cholesterol from the intima of arteries. Leanness, high social status, and being female are also related to high HDL levels. Regular, moderate alcohol consumption may increase HDL levels and decrease coronary risk.

Paffenbarger and colleagues have reported numerous analyses of epidemiologic data from the San Francisco longshoremen. Work on the waterfront has been performed at relatively high activity levels under conditions well governed and documented by the longshoremen union. Longshoremen tend to enter the industry in youth and remain active in it for many years. Paffenbarger analyzed a 22-year follow-up of the longshoremen, from 1951 to 1972, for 59,401 man-years of energy expenditure on the job. One third of this experience was classified as high-energy work and the rest as low-energy work by analyzing the energy output for various longshoremen jobs. High-energy jobs required 5 to 7 kcal/min (approximately 2 METs).

Multiphase screening performed in 1951 assessed the men for obesity, smoking habits, blood pressure levels, and prior history of heart disease.

TABLE I
POTENTIAL RATE REDUCTION OF FATAL HEART ATTACKS (THE THEORETICAL EFFECT OF INTERVENTION) WITH THE ELIMINATION OF SPECIFIC RISK FACTORS OR COMBINATIONS OF RISK FACTORS*

	Reduction
Increase physical activity	50%
Stop heavy smoking	30%
Lower systolic blood pressure	30%
Any two above	65%
All three	88%

*Study of longshoremen in San Francisco.

Serum cholesterol was measured in 1961. An annual accounting was taken of job transfers so that the data on energy expenditures could be correlated to the occurrence of fatal heart attack. Deaths from heart attacks were assigned to the category in which the deceased had been employed six months prior to death to avoid selective bias due to premorbid job transfers (e.g., transfers to less active jobs secondary to illness). Age-adjusted frequencies of other risk factors among longshoremen were compared between the two energy expenditure groups, and little difference was found. Three parameters were found to put longshoremen at increased risk for fatal heart attacks—low-energy work output, smoking more than one pack of cigarettes a day, and an elevated systolic blood pressure (equal to or greater than the mean). Each of these factors posed an approximate twice-normal risk. Potential reduction in rates of fatal heart attacks (theoretical effect of intervention), with the elimination of specific combinations of these risk factors, are listed in Table I. Paffenbarger concluded that physical activity is protective (a cause of reduced fatal myocardial infarction) and not selective (i.e., not an effect of premorbid job transfers or other biases). The threshold of 5 kcal/min seemed to hold for strenuous bursts rather than for sustained activity.

Paffenbarger performed another population study, one involving 36,000 Harvard University alumni who entered college between 1916 and 1950. Records of their physical activity were gathered from their student days and later during middle age. Alumni offices and questionnaires were used to obtain information on adult exercise habits, morbidity, and mortality. A 6- to 10-year follow-up during the period of 1961 to 1972 totaled 117,680 man-years of observation after the first questionnaire, and apparently healthy men were classified with specific measures of energy expenditure. They remained under study until heart attack occurrence, death from any cause, age 75, or the end of observation in 1972. Validation of the questionnaire showed the sensitivity and specificity of responses for coronary heart disease and hypertension to be quite acceptable at 80% and 99%. Weekly updating of death lists by the alumni office provided the means to obtain official death certificates. A physical activity index was devised to provide a composite estimate of total energy expenditure from stairs climbed, blocks walked, and sports played. This index was scaled in kcal/wk, and was divided at 2,000 kcal/wk, which produced a 60% to 40% division of man-years of observation into low- and high-energy categories.

During the 6- to 10-year follow-up period, 572 men had their first myocardial infarction. Men with a physical activity index below 2,000 kcal/wk were at 64% higher risk than were classmates with a higher activity index. Varsity athletic status implied selective cardiovascular fitness, and such selection alone was insufficient to explain a lower heart attack risk in later adult years. Former varsity athletes retained a lower risk only if they maintained a high physical activity index as alumni.

Three high-risk characteristics were identified in this study: low physical activity index (less than 2,000 kcal/wk), cigarette smoking, and hypertension. Presence of any one characteristic was accompanied by a 50% increase in risk, and the presence of two characteristics tripled risk. Maintenance of a high physical activity index could possibly have reduced heart attack risk by 26%.

The study of Harvard alumni found levels of energy output characteristic of the life-style of each individual. The results support the role of vigorous exercise in reducing the risk of heart attack. Innate or early acquired cardiovascular endowment may distinguish hardy from less vigorous individuals or the naturally more active from the less active. It would be an oversimplification to assume that early selection accounted for all the observed differences in heart attack risk.

In Framingham, Massachusetts, approximately 5,000 men and women, 30 to 62 years and free of clinical evidence of coronary artery disease at the onset, have been examined regularly since 1949. Coronary heart disease mortality was subsequently found to be higher in cohorts with indices or measurements consistent with sedentary life-style. However, physical inactivity did not have the predictive power of the three cardinal risk factors. Recently, Kannel and Sorlie reanalyzed the Framingham data for the effects of physical activity on overall mortality and cardiovascular disease mortality. The effect on mortality of being sedentary was rather modest compared with the other risk factors but persisted when these other factors were taken into account. A low correlation was noted between physical activity level and the major risk factors.

POSTMORTEM STUDIES OF PHYSICAL INACTIVITY AS A RISK FACTOR

The results of 207 consecutive autopsies of otherwise healthy white men aged 30 to 60 years who died suddenly and unexpectedly from accident, homicide, or suicide were reported by Spain and Bradess. The autopsies were done in the medical examiners office of Westchester County, New York. All major branches of the coronary arteries were examined in cross-section at 3-mm intervals. The estimated amount of reduction in luminal diameter by atherosclerotic lesions was used as the basic criterion for grading the degree of coronary atherosclerosis. The occupation of the individuals was determined from available information. All individuals who had a history or autopsy evidence of disease influencing atherosclerosis were excluded. They were separated by occupational title as active or sedentary, with approximately 100 in each group. The authors found no significant differences in the degree of coronary atherosclerosis between those engaged in sedentary occupations and those engaged in physically active occupations.

Mitrani and colleagues reported the results of consecutive specialized cardiovascular autopsies on 172 European-born Jews who were victims of traumatic death. According to personal documents and some information obtained from relatives, 93 had led a sedentary life and 79 were manual workers. Each coronary artery was cross-sectioned at 1-cm distances to measure internal and external diameters. The percentage of narrowing of the vessels was calculated using these measurements. There was no significant difference between the active and inactive groups.

Morris and Crawford sent out requests to approximately 200 British pathologists to complete a standard questionnaire on a series of autopsies performed on men 45 to 70 years of age. The pathologists were asked to give macroscopic estimates of the degree of coronary atheroma and fibrosis of the left ventricle and interventricular septum. The last occupation of the deceased was requested and estimated to involve light, active, or heavy physical activity on the basis of job title. In this manner, the results of 3,800 autopsies on individuals dying of causes other than coronary artery disease were gathered from 1954 to 1956. Ischemic myocardial fibrosis and complete coronary occlusion was more common in lighter work occupations, but coronary atheromas and diameter narrowing were of equally high prevalence in all occupational groups.

Measurements were made from radiographs of injected coronary arteries obtained from two necropsy studies at the Radcliff Infirmary, Oxford, England. Ninety-two cases without postmortem evidence of myocardial infarction were used as controls, whereas a group of 79 had evidence of acute or healed infarction. The right coronary artery was measured in à nondiseased segment, approximately one half the distance between its origin and the right heart border, and was assumed to reflect the diameter of all the coronary arteries. The physical activity of the last occupation, as determined by job title, was described as light, active, or heavy. The diameter of the right coronary artery in normal subjects increased with age, but the infarction group showed a smaller diameter of the right coronary artery in each age group. In normal subjects coronary artery diameter increased with activity of work, whereas in the infarction group it decreased with the activity of work. These differences were not statistically significant, and no determination of the degree of atherosclerosis was made.

MARATHON HYPOTHESIS

Currens and White presented the cardiovascular autopsy results of Clarence DeMar, a famous long-distance runner who died of rectal carcinoma. He was still actively involved in long-distance running until shortly before his death at age 70. His coronary arteries were found to be two to three times normal size, with some atherosclerotic involvement but no narrowing.

Recent reports have disproved the hypothesis that marathon running provides absolute protection against death from atherosclerosis. Waller and Roberts reported autopsy results of five conditioned runners, aged 40 or over. All had severe coronary atherosclerosis, and it was concluded that coronary disease is a major killer of conditioned runners age 40 and older who die while running. They also suggested that chest trauma during a football game resulted in rupture of a coronary plaque and the subsequent death of a young man. Thompson and associates studied the circumstances of death based on medical and physical activity histories of 18 individuals who died during or immediately after jogging. Superior physical fitness did not guarantee protection against exercise-induced death. Also, exercise poses a risk for orthopedic disability and heatstroke.

Koplan investigated the question, What is the expected level of cardiovascular deaths on the basis of chance alone in runners while running? This question is important because when a person dies of cardiovascular causes during recreational running it is frequently assumed that exercise caused the death. Koplan used data from the National Center of Health Statistics and found that approximately 100 cardiovascular deaths per year are predicted on a purely temporal basis in runners in the United States. This prediction certainly exceeds the actual number of deaths reported.

CARDIAC REHABILITATION STUDIES

Early Ambulation after Acute Myocardial Infarction. Prior to 1960, patients with acute myocardial infarction were thought to require prolonged restriction of their physical activity. Patients were often kept at strict bed rest for two months with all activities performed by nursing personnel. The concern was that physical activity would lead to ventricular aneurysm formation, cardiac rupture, congestive heart failure, dysrhythmias, reinfarction, or sudden death. Hospitalization could last for three to four months, with limitation of activities for at least one year. This approach was based on pathologic studies that showed at least six weeks were required for necrotic myocardium to form a firm scar and based on the increased prevalence of cardiac rupture reported among patients who infarcted in mental hospitals where bed rest could not be enforced.

A revolutionary approach to treatment occurred when chair treatment was recommended for the postinfarction patient in the 1940s. The benefits of the sitting versus supine position included increased peripheral venous pooling and decreased preload on the myocardium. Such a reduction would decrease resting left ventricular wall tension and hence reduce myocardial oxygen demand. This approach also lessened the risk of thrombosis and pulmonary embolism, and others recommended the use of the bedside commode to avoid the Valsalva maneuver. The latter, which is common when an individual strains with a bowel movement, can lead to deleterious elevations of systemic blood pressure early after infarction. Physiologic studies have documented the hemodynamic alterations caused by deconditioning. After prolonged bed rest, tachycardia and hypotension are common on standing, most likely owing to alterations of vasomotor reflexes and to hypovolemia, which occurs with bed rest. It is now recommended to begin progressive activities as soon as possible in the coronary care unit.

In 1961 Cain and colleagues reported the use of a progressive activity program for acute myocardial infarction patients. They had difficulty having this report accepted for publication because the approach was considered dangerous. They reported 335 patients with an uncomplicated myocardial infarction who were at least 15 days postinfarction. The patients had been restricted to bed, chair, and commode. The electrocardiogram was monitored after the patient performed activities such as climbing stairs and walking up a grade. They concluded that electrocardiographic monitoring of early activity was a more reliable means of ascertaining the presence of coronary insufficiency than were physical signs or symptoms. They explained that they were not advising early ambulation for all patients, but only those who responded favorably.

In 1964 Torkelson reported the results achieved in ten patients with an uncomplicated myocardial infarction. On the sixth week of his inhospital rehabilitation program, a low-level exercise treadmill test was performed using 1.7 mph at a 10% grade. He concluded that the treadmill test was a valuable procedure for the documentation of the specific exercise response of patients recovering from an acute myocardial infarction. He felt that consideration of the response to a treadmill test made possible the appropriate progression of an exercise program.

Most later publications do not include electrocardiographic monitoring as part of progressive ambulation. Instead, generalized statements as to the activities on each postinfarct day are made for all patients, rather than individualized activity progression. Recently, Sivarajan, Bruce, and colleagues have returned to the approach of Cain and Torkelson. They reported 12 patients with an acute myocardial infarction whose symptoms, signs, and hemodynamic and electrocardiographic responses during and after three activities were assessed. These activities included sitting upright, walking to the toilet, and walking on a treadmill. Studies of these activities were done at three, six, and ten days after infarction. They concluded that successful performance of these three activities provided useful criteria for discharge of the patient with a myocardial infarction. If a patient has an abnormal response, such as a systolic blood pressure drop, severe chest pain, marked ST changes, or dysrhythmias, his or her progressive ambulation program and discharge from the hospital are delayed until the responses are acceptable. This approach constitutes optimal care of the postinfarct patient.

It is well known that morbidity and mortality in postinfarction patients who have complicated courses are much higher than in those with uncomplicated infarcts. The criteria for a complicated infarct are listed in Table II. Certainly, early ambulation is not appropriate for the patient with a complicated infarct. The progressive ambulation program should be held up until such individuals reach an uncomplicated status, and even then progressive ambulation should be slower.

TABLE II
CRITERIA FOR A COMPLICATED ACUTE MYOCARDIAL INFARCTION

Continued cardiac ischemia (pain, late enzyme rise)
Left ventricular failure (congestive heart failure, new murmurs, x-ray changes)
Shock (blood pressure drop, pallor, oliguria)
Significant cardiac arrhythmias (premature ventricular contractions > 6/min, atrial fibrillation)
Conduction disturbances (bundle branch block, atrioventricular block, hemiblock)
Severe pleurisy or pericarditis
Complicating illnesses
Marked creatine kinase rise without a noncardiac explanation

Note: If these criteria are not present, rapid progressive ambulation and early discharge are appropriate.

There has been some controversy over the relative long-term risk of subendocardial versus transmural myocardial infarction. Some of this difficulty has been due to terminology. Traditionally, an infarct with evolving Q waves on the electrocardiogram has been called transmural and considered to be large, whereas an infarction with only ST- and T-wave changes has been called subendocardial and considered to be small. Estimation of the severity of a myocardial infarction requires consideration of clinical findings and test results other than the electrocardiogram to judge a patient's risk and infarct size. The presence of Q waves does not prove the occurrence of a transmural myocardial infarction, and a transmural infarction can occur with only ST- and T-wave changes. The severity of an infarction should be judged by clinical findings, hemodynamic monitoring, the level of creatinine kinase elevation, and the presence of congestive heart failure or shock, or both. The concept that a subendocardial infarction is "uncompleted" and poses an increased postdischarge risk has not been substantiated; however, the risk is surprisingly similar to a Q-wave or transmural infarction. Q-wave infarcts and anterior wall infarcts have a higher inhospital morbidity and mortality, as do multiple infarcts indicated by history.

Hayes and colleagues studied 189 patients with an uncomplicated myocardial infarction selected at random for early or late mobilization and discharge from the hospital. Patients were admitted to the study after 48 hours in a coronary care unit if they were free of pain and showed no evidence of heart failure or significant dysrhythmias. One group of patients was mobilized immediately and discharged home after a total of 9 days in the hospital, and the second group was mobilized on the 9th day and discharged on the 16th day. Outpatient assessment was carried out six weeks after admission.

No significant differences were observed between the groups in terms of morbidity or mortality, as reflected by the incidence of recurrent chest pain or myocardial infarction, heart failure, dysrhythmia, or venous thrombosis detected either clinically or by radionuclide scanning.

In a strictly randomized controlled study, Bloch and colleagues studied the effects of early mobilization after uncomplicated myocardial infarction. One hundred fifty-four patients under 70 years of age who were hospitalized for an acute myocardial infarction and had no complications on day 1 or day 2 were randomly assigned to two treatment groups. In the early mobilization group, patients were treated by a physiotherapist with a progressive activity program that began on day 2 or day 3 after infarction. In the control group, the patients underwent the traditional hospital regimen of strict bed rest for three or more weeks. The mean duration of hospitalization was 21 days for active patients and 33 days for the control group. The follow-up period ranged from 6 to 20 months, with an average of 11 months. There were no significant differences between the two groups with regard to hospital or follow-up mortality, to rates of reinfarction, dysrhythmias, heart failure, angina pectoris, ventricular aneurysm, or to the results of an exercise test. On follow-up examination, there was actually greater disability in the control than in the active group.

Sivarajan and colleagues have reported a study of the effects of early supervised exercises in preventing deconditioning after an acute myocardial infarction. Eighty-four patients were randomized to a control group, 174 to an exercise group. The exercise program began at an average of 4.5 days after admission. The mean discharge was ten days after admission for both groups. There were no differences between the two groups in the clinical, hemodynamic, or electrocardiographic responses to a low-level treadmill test performed on the day before hospital discharge. Nor was there any significant difference between the two groups for the incidence of complications or death. This well-designed and accomplished study was probably an anachronism. That is, by the time the study was funded, the standard of community medical care in Seattle included early ambulation and discharge. Therefore, the control group received treatment that was hardly different from the exercise group. Also, for safety reasons the sicker patients who most needed rehabilitation were excluded from this study. Six patients needed cardiac surgery prior to discharge in the exercise group, but none required it in the control group, which can be explained by chance distribution (failure of randomization) rather than by the mild exercises employed. These three randomized studies of patients with an uncomplicated infarction have demonstrated that the risks of early ambulation are minimal and that progressive mobilization during the early stages of an acute myocardial infarction is recommended.

Prognostic Indicators. Shephard analyzed the experience of the Ontario Multi-Center Exercise Trial to determine the recurrence of myocardial infarction in an exercising population. The study followed 751 men postmyocardial infarction; comparison was made between the 50 participants who sustained a recurrence and the 701 participants who did not. Reinfarction was more likely with a history of multiple previous infarctions but was unrelated to such indicators of infarction severity as symptoms, electrocardiographic abnormalites, enzyme changes, cardiac arrest, dysrhythmias, or hypotension. Features noted on admission to the study suggesting an adverse prognosis included smoking history, disability, shortness of breath, and angina. The main physiologic warning sign was a low and decreasing cardiac output at submaximal work loads, with a widening of the AV O_2 difference. None of the adverse findings was of sufficient consistency to be of value when advising individual patients.

Kavanagh and colleagues evaluated prognostic indices in 610 patients, beginning eight months after myocardial infarction and lasting approximately three years, in a vigorous exercise-centered rehabilitation program. Over this period, 23 had a fatal and 21 a nonfatal recurrence of myocardial infarction. The most significant prognostic feature was noncompliance with the exercise program, but this was due to self-selection of those with symptoms or signs. Patients who dropped out of the exercise program had a reinfarction rate of approximately 50%, whereas those who stayed in the exercise program had only about a 2% recurrence rate. Risk ratios of 2 were observed for patients with persistent angina, aneurysm, enlarged heart, elevated serum cholesterol and for those who persisted in smoking cigarettes. ST-segment depression during the exercise test carried a risk ratio of greater than 3, whereas multiformed exercise-induced premature ventricular contractions had a risk ratio of less than 2. There was a low yearly fatality rate of 1.2% in the 610 patients and of only 0.7% in those without exercise-induced ST-segment depression. A combination of ST-segment depression and high serum cholesterol yielded a risk ratio of greater than 4. The prognosis for patients with these risk markers, however, remained at least as good as for comparable patients not receiving exercise training. Patients with the high-risk prognostic features had less lowering of their risk, but their prognosis remained more favorable than that of subjects who did not exercise. The high risk of being a dropout certainly is due to bias—the sickest could not tolerate the program.

Intervention Studies. Kallio and colleagues were part of a World Health Organization project to assess the effects of a comprehensive rehabilitation and secondary prevention program on morbidity, mortality, return to work, and various clinical, medical, and psychosocial factors after a myocardial infarction. The study included 375 consecutive patients under 65 years of age treated for acute myocardial infarction from two urban areas in Finland between 1973 and 1975. General advice on rehabilitation and secondary preventive measures was given to all patients who were discharged from the hospital. On discharge, the patients were randomly allocated to an intervention or to a control group, both of which were followed for three years.

Patients in the control group were followed by their own physicians and were seen by the study team only once a year during the three-year follow-up. The program for the intervention group was started two weeks after hospital discharge. An exercise program was determined from a bicycle test, and for most patients it was supervised.

After the three-year follow-up, the cumulative coronary mortality was significantly smaller in the intervention group than in the controls (18.6% versus 29.4%). This difference was mainly due to a reduction of sudden deaths in the intervention group (5.8% versus 14.4%). The reduction was greatest in the first six months after infarction. Of the intervention group and the controls, 18.1% and 11.2%, respectively, presented with nonfatal infarctions. These results suggest that cardiac rehabilitation during the first six months after an acute infarction can result in a significant reduction in the number of sudden deaths. Total mortality was 21.8% in the intervention group and 29.9% in the control group. Two weak points of this study are that more patients in the intervention group than in the control group took antihypertensives and beta blockers and that the functional capacity measured at one, two, and three years after acute infarction was similar in both groups.

The National Exercise and Heart Disease Project (NEHDP) included 651 postmyocardial infarction men enrolled in five centers in the United States. It was a randomized three-year clinical trial on the effects of a prescribed supervised exercise program starting two to 36 months after a myocardial infarction (80% were more than 8 months postinfarction). In this study 323 randomly selected patients underwent exercise three times a week that was designed to increase their heart rate to 85% of their individual maximal heart rate achieved during treadmill testing, and 328 patients served as controls. This study was carefully performed by experts who took two years to design the protocol. An initial low-level exercise session in both groups to exclude the faint of heart who would not comply with an exercise program was surprisingly effective in improving performance.

The three-year mortality rate was 7.3% (24 deaths) in the control group versus 4.6% (15 deaths) in the exercise group. Deaths from all cardiovascular causes (acute myocardial infarction, sudden death, arrhythmias, congestive heart failure, cardiogenic shock, and stroke) for the three-year follow-up were 6.1% (20 deaths) in the control group versus 4.3% (14 deaths) in the exercise group. Neither difference was statistically significant. However, when deaths due to acute myocardial infarction were considered as a separate category the exercise group had a significantly lower rate: one acute fatal myocardial infarction per three years (0.3%) in the exercise group versus eight fatal myocardial infarctions (2.4%) in the control group ($P < .05$). The rate of all recurrent myocardial infarctions per three years, fatal and nonfatal, did not significantly differ between groups: 23 cases (7.0%) in the control versus 17 cases (5.3%) in the exercise group. The number of rehospitalizations for reasons other than myocardial infarction were identical in the two groups (27.4% versus 28.5% per three years). The need for coronary artery sugrery was also equal in both groups—16 controls and 17 exercisers underwent surgery in the three-year period. This study suggests a beneficial effect of regular exercise postmyocardial infarction, but insufficient numbers of participants due to financial limitations and dropouts prevented a definitive conclusion.

Unfortunately, this study could not be definitive but instead has demonstrated the feasibility of resolving this important issue. It is most unfortunate that it was discontinued especially since the results are so encouraging. Only 1,400 patients would be required to demonstrate a statistically significant reduction in mortality rate in the exercise group if the reported trend persisted. The patients in the exercise group who suffered a recurrent myocardial infarction had a lower mortality rate, suggesting that an exercise program increases an individual's ability to survive a myocardial infarction.

The National Exercise and Heart Disease Project in the United States and the Ontario Exercise-Heart Collaborative Study found no significant difference in morbidity and mortality between the exercisers and the randomized controls. Both of these studies were limited by a sample size of only 700 men and by dropouts, which would make differences, other than very large ones, unlikely.

Complications of an Exercise Program. Haskell surveyed 30 cardiac rehabilitation programs in North America using a questionnaire to assess major cardiovascular complications. This survey included approximately 14,000 patients for 1.6 million exercise-hours. Of 50 cardiopulmonary resuscitations, 8 resulted in death, and of 7 myocardial infarctions, 2 resulted in death. Exercise programs resulted in four other fatalities occurring after hospitalization. Thus, there was one nonfatal event per 35,000 patient-hours and one fatal event per 160,000 patient-hours. The complication rates were lower in electrocardiographically monitored programs. The current programs reported a 4% annual mortality rate during exercise, which is a rate not different from that expected for such patients. Other programs have reported rates of cardiopulmonary resuscitations ranging from 1 in 6,000 to 1 in 25,000 man-hours of exercise. Such events are difficult to predict, can occur in patients with only single-vessel disease, and can occur at any time after being in a program.

The Georgia Baptist program in Atlanta reported a ventricular fibrillation rate of 1 in 13,000 gymnasium-hours, the Toronto program reported 1 in 15,000 gymnasium-hours, and the CAPRI program in Seattle reported the highest rate of 1 in 6,000 exercise-hours. Of 15 patients requiring defibrillation, the CAPRI group successfully resuscitated all of them. Eleven had angiography, which showed single-vessel disease in four patients and multivessel disease in seven. Subsequently, the CAPRI record has improved, and they have had experience with defibrillating two patients simultaneously; on another occasion, a physician monitoring an exercise class was defibrillated.

Fletcher and Cantwell reported five coronary disease patients resuscitated after ventricular fibrillation in an exercise program. Multivessel coronary disease that could be treated with bypass surgery was present in four of them. Resuscitation was required unexpectedly and at unpredictable times, occurring at any time 2 to 48 months after being in the exercise program. These two experienced cardiologists are now reluctant to graduate patients to exercise without medical supervision. Shephard and Kavanagh also agree that the potential victim of a cardiac arrest during exercise training cannot be identified. Even trained patients should avoid excessive and unusual exertion, particularly when it is associated with competition and emotional excitement. Patients should also learn to recognize dysrhythmias and angina and should moderate their activity if they sense ischemic prodromes, tension, or depression.

Summary. Exercise training can be effective in achieving the the physiologic, psychologic, and vocational goals of cardiac rehabilitation. However, the NEHDP, the Finnish WHO Project, and the Ontario Study, all of which are randomized controlled trials, have failed to demonstrate a beneficial effect on morbidity and mortality. Design problems, small sample size, and crossovers, including those to coronary bypass surgery, complicate this issue. Perhaps the greatest benefit of exercise is the increase in the anginal threshold and in functional capacity, which could be due to noncardiac adaptations. Changes in cardiac function and coronary blood flow secondary to exercise in humans remain unproved. However, initial studies in some patients have reported improvement in thallium exercise scans and in exercise ejection fraction using radionuclide ventriculography—improvements consistent with the hypothesis that exercise can result in beneficial cardiac changes (see Chapter 5). It is unlikely that exercise has a direct effect on the atherosclerotic process. The beneficial changes in hemodynamic measurements and work capacity secondary to an exercise program in patients with coronary disease could be due to changes in the peripheral circulation, the sympathetic nervous system, catecholamine levels, and skeletal muscles rather than due to cardiac alterations. Hemodynamic and work capacity changes that occur within several months of training in older subjects are most likely due to noncardiac peripheral changes, and longer periods of training are needed for cardiac alterations. In some instances, coronary artery bypass surgery is the optimal means of rehabilitation, but surgical patients often benefit from a cardiac rehabilitation program.

CONCLUSION

Though many of us exercise and prescribe exercise for health reasons, there is no definitive evidence that this is effective in the prevention or management of coronary heart disease. The association between physical inactivity and the underlying atherosclerotic process is modest compared with other factors such as serum cholesterol, cigarette smoking, and hypertension. An inversely proportional association between the level of activity and degree of atherosclerosis has not been demonstrated. Physical inactivity does not necessarily precede the atherosclerotic process. Many epidemiologic studies have been performed without finding physical inactivity to be a risk factor. Often physical inactivity was not determined to be an independent risk factor because other risk factors and markers concentrated in the inactive group. The capacity of physical inactivity to predict coronary events has not been reproducible when applied to different populations, nor has the consistency of the exercise hypothesis been documented in autopsy studies.

Recent studies of primary prevention support the life-style of regular physical activity: it most likely decreases one's risk for coronary heart disease and helps to decrease other risk factors. Cardiac rehabilitation is a proven modality for helping coronary heart disease patients manage their disease. If medically supervised, it has not been demonstrated to increase the risk of complications. The inclusion of regular moderate exercise in one's lifestyle makes good sense for many reasons. It can improve the quality of life by lessening fatigue and by increasing physical performance in those in whom such goals are important. The recommendation of a moderate exercise habit can help people pay attention to their health and make the changes necessary to lessen coronary risk factors. The most significant advances in public health have been in the prevention, not the treatment, of disease. The current public interest in physical fitness may be embarrassingly more effective than is the medical profession in making the public take responsibility for maintaining health.

REFERENCES
CHAPTER IV

RETROSPECTIVE STUDIES OF PHYSICAL INACTIVITY AS A RISK FACTOR

Adelstein AM: Some aspects of cardiovascular mortality in South Africa. Br J Prev Soc Med 17:29, 1963.

Breslow L, Buell P: Mortality from coronary heart disease and physical activity of work in California. J Chronic Dis 11:421, 1960.

Brunner D: The influence of physical activity on incidence and prognosis of ischemic heart disease, in Raab W (ed): Prevention of Ischemic Heart Disease. Springfield, Ill, Charles C Thomas, 1966, p 1.

Frank CW, Weinblatt E, Shapiro S, et al: Physical inactivity as a lethal factor in myocardial infarction among men. Circulation 34:1022, 1966.

Froelicher V, Battler A, McKirnan MD: Physical activity and coronary heart disease. Cardiology 65:152, 1980.

Froelicher VF, Brown P: Exercise and coronary heart disease. J Card Rehab 4:277, 1981.

Froelicher VF, Oberman A: Analysis of epidemiologic studies of physical inactivity as risk factor for coronary artery disease. Prog Cardiovasc Dis 15:41, 1972.

Hinkle LE, Whitney LA, Lehman EW, et al: Occupation, education, and coronary heart disease. Science 161:238, 1968.

Kahn H: The relationship of reported coronary heart disease mortality to physical activity of work. Am J Public Health 53:1058, 1963.

Kannel WB, Gordon T, Sorlie P, et al: Physical activity and coronary vulnerability: The Framingham Study. Cardiol Dig 28:28, 1971.

Keys A: Physical activity and the epidemiology of coronary heart disease, in Jokl E, Brunner D (eds): Medicine and Sport, vol 4. Baltimore, University Park Press, 1970, p 255.

Lilienfeld AM: Variation of mortality from heart disease. Public Health Rep 71:545, 1956.

Morris J: Health and social class. Lancet 1:303, 1959.

Morris J, Heady JA, Raffle PA, et al: Coronary heart disease and physical activity of work. Lancet 2:1111, 1953.

Morris J, Kagan A, Pattison DC, et al: Incidence and prediction of ischaemic heart disease in London busmen. Lancet 2:553, 1966.

Morris JN, Crawford MD: Coronary heart disease and physical activity of work. Br Med J 2:1485, 1958.

Morris JN: Epidemiology and cardiovascular disease of middle age (pts 1 and 2). Mod Concepts Cardiovasc Dis 29:625, 1960.

Morris JN, Heady JA, Raffle PA: Physique of London busmen. Lancet 2:569, 1956.

Oliver RM: Physique and serum lipids of young London busmen in relation to ischaemic heart disease. Br J Intern Med 24:181, 1967.

Paffenbarger RS, Laughlin ME, Gima AS, et al: Work activity of longshoremen as related to death from coronary heart disease and stroke. N Engl J Med 282:1109, 1970.

Pell S, D'Alonzo CA: Immediate mortality and five-year survival of employed men with a first myocardial infarction. N Engl J Med 270:915, 1964.

Pell S, D'Alonzo CA: A three-year study of myocardial infarction in a large employed population. JAMA 175:463, 1961.

Shanoff HM, Little JA: Studies of male survivors of myocardial infarction due to "essential" atherosclerosis: I. Characteristics of the patients. Can Med Assoc J 84:519, 1961.

Stamler J, Berkson DM, Lindberg HA, et al: Long-term epidemiologic studies on the possible role of physical activity and physical fitness in the prevention of premature clinical coronary heart disease, in Jokl E, Brunner D (eds): Medicine and Sport, vol 4. Baltimore, University Park Press, 1970, p 274.

Taylor HL, Blackburn H, Brozek J, et al: Railroad employees in the United States. Acta Med Scand 460:55, 1966.

Zukel WJ, et al: A short-term community study of the epidemiology of coronary heart disease. Am J Public Health 49:1630, 1959.

PREVALENCE STUDIES OF PHYSICAL INACTIVITY AS A RISK FACTOR

McDonough JR, Hames CG, Stulb SC, et al: Coronary heart disease among Negroes and whites in Evans County, Georgia. J Chronic Dis 18:443, 1965.

Stamler J, Kjelsberg M, Hall Y: Epidemiologic studies on cardiovascular-renal diseases: I. Analysis of mortality by age-race-sex-occupation. J Chronic Dis 12:440, 1960.

Taylor HL, Klepetar E, Keys A, et al: Death rates among physically active and sedentary employees of the railroad industry. Am J Public Health 52:1697, 1962.

PROSPECTIVE STUDIES OF PHYSICAL INACTIVITY AS A RISK FACTOR

Blackburn H, Taylor HL, Keys A: Coronary heart disease in seven countries. Circulation 41:154, 1970.

Castelli W, Poyle JT, Gordon T, et al: HDL cholesterol and other lipids in coronary heart disease: The Cooperative Lipoprotein Phenotyping Study. Circulation 55:767, 1977.

Chapman JM, Massey FJ: The interrelationship of serum cholesterol, hypertension, body weight, and risk of coronary disease. J Chronic Dis 17:933, 1964.

Cooper KH, Meyer BU, Blide R, et al: The important role of fitness determination and stress testing in predicting coronary incidence. Ann NY Acad Sci 301:642, 1977.

Costas R, Garcia-Palmieri MR, Nazario E, et al: Relation of lipids, weight and physical activity to incidence of coronary heart disease: The Puerto Rico Study. Am J Cardiol 42:653, 1978.

Epstein L, Miller GJ, Stitt FW, et al: Vigorous exercise in leisure time, coronary risk-factors, and resting electrocardiogram in middle-aged male civil servants. Br Heart J 38:403, 1976.

Kannel WB, Sorlie P: Some health benefits of physical activity: The Framingham Study. Arch Intern Med 139:857, 1979.

Miller NE, Forde OH, Thelle DS, et al: The Tromso Heart-Study: High-density lipoprotein and coronary heart-disease: A prospective case-control study. Lancet 1:965, 1977.

Morris JN, Marr JW, Clayton DG: Diet and heart: A postscript. Br Med J 2:1301, 1977.

Morris JN, Pollard R, Everitt MG, et al: Vigorous exercise in leisure-time: Protection against coronary heart disease. Lancet 2:1207, 1980.

Paffenbarger RS, Brand RJ, Sholtz RI, et al: Energy expenditure, cigarette smoking, and blood pressure level as related to death from specific diseases. Am J Epidemiol 108:12, 1978.

Paffenbarger RS, Wing AL, Hyde RT: Physical activity as an index of heart attack risk in college alumni. Am J Epidemiol 108:161, 1978.

Robertson HK: Heart disease in life-long cyclists. Lancet 2:1635, 1977.

Roseman RH: The influence of different exercise patterns on the incidence of coronary heart disease in The Western Collaborative Group Study, in Jokl E, Brunner D (eds): Medicine and Sport, vol 4. Baltimore, University Park Press, 1970, p 267.

Stamler J: Lifestyles, major risk factors, proof and public policy. Circulation 58:3, 1978.

Stamler J, Lindberg HA, Berkson DM, et al: Prevalence and incidence of coronary heart disease in strata of the labor force of a Chicago industrial corporation. J Chronic Dis 11:405, 1960.

Wood PD, Klein H, Lewis S, et al: Plasma lipoprotein concentration in middle aged runners. Circulation 50:111, 1974.

POSTMORTEM STUDIES OF PHYSICAL INACTIVITY AS A RISK FACTOR

Mitrani Y, Karplus H, Brunner D: Coronary atherosclerosis in cases of traumatic death, in Jokl E, Brunner D (eds): Medicine and Sport, vol 4. Baltimore, University Park Press, 1970, p 241.

Morris JN, Crawford MD: Coronary heart disease and physical activity of work. Br Med J 2:1485, 1958.

Rose G, Prineas RJ, Mitchell JR: Myocardial infarction and the intrinsic calibre of coronary arteries. Br Heart J 29:548, 1967.

Spain DM, Bradess VA: Occupational physical activity and the degree of coronary atherosclerosis in "normal" men. Circulation 22:239, 1960.

MARATHON HYPOTHESIS

Currens JH, White PD: Half a century of running. N Engl J Med 265:988, 1961.

Hartung G, Farge E, Mitchell R: Effects of marathon running, jogging, and diet on coronary risk factors in middle-aged men. Prev Med 10:316, 1981.

Hellerstein HK: Limitations of marathon running in the rehabilitation of coronary patients: Anatomic and physiologic determinants. Ann NY Acad Sci 301:484, 1978.

Koplan JP: Cardiovascular deaths while running. JAMA 242:2578, 1979.

Noakes TD, Opie LH, Rose AG, et al: Autopsy-proved coronary atherosclerosis in marathon runners. N Engl J Med 301:86–91, 1979.

Thompson PD, Stern MP, Williams P, et al: Death during jogging or running. JAMA 242:1265, 1979.

Waller BF, Roberts WC: Sudden death while running in conditioned runners aged 40 years or over. Am J Cardiol 45:1291, 1980.

CARDIAC REHABILITATION STUDIES

AHA Committee Report: Statement on exercise. Circulation 64:1327A, 1981.

Bloch A, Maeder JP, Haissly JC, et al: Early mobilization after myocardial infarction. Am J Cardiol 34:152, 1974.

Convertino V, Hung J, Goldwater D, et al: Cardiovascular responses to exercise in middle-aged men after 10 days of bedrest. Circulation 65:134, 1982.

DeBusk RF, Houston N, Haskell W, et al: Exercise training soon after myocardial infarction. Am J Cardiol 44:1223, 1979.

Duke M: Bed rest in acute myocardial infarction: A study of physician practices. Am Heart J 82:486, 1971.

Frick MH, Katila M, Sjogren AL: Cardiac function and physical training after myocardial infarction, in Larsen OA, Malmborg RO (eds): Coronary Heart Disease and Physical Fitness. Baltimore, University Park Press, 1971.

Groden B: The management of myocardial infarction: A controlled study of the effects of early mobilization. Card Rehab 1:13, 1971.

Harpur J, Kellet R, Conner W, et al: Controlled trial of early mobilization and discharge from hospital in uncomplicated myocardial infarction. Lancet 2:1331, 1971.

Hayes MJ, Morris GK, Hamptom JR: Comparison of mobilization after two and nine days in uncomplicated myocardial infarction. Br Med J 3:10, 1974.

Hossack KF, Bruce RA, Kusumi F: Altered exercise ventilatory responses by apparent propranolol-diminished glucose metabolism: Implications concerning impaired physical training benefit in coronary patients. Am Heart J 102:378, 1981.

Hutter AM Jr, Sidel VW, Shine KL, et al: Early hospital discharge after myocardial infarction. N Engl J Med 288:1141, 1973.

Kallio V, Hamalainen H, Hakkila J, et al: Reduction in sudden deaths by a multifactorial intervention programme after acute myocardial infarction. Lancet 2:1091, 1979.

Kavanagh T, Shephard RJ: Exercise for postcoronary patients: An assessment of infrequent supervision. Arch Phys Med Rehabil 61:114, 1980.

Kavanagh T, Shephard RJ, Chisholm AW, et al: Prognostic indexes for patients with ischemic heart disease enrolled in an exercise-centered rehabilitation program. Am J Cardiol 44:1230, 1979.

Kennedy CC, Spiekerman RE, Linsay MI, et al: One-year graduated exercise program for men with angina pectoris. Mayo Clin Proc 51:231, 1976.

Kentala E: Physical fitness and feasibility of physical rehabilitation after myocardial infarction in men of working age. Ann Clin Res (suppl 9), 1972.

Levine SA, Lown B: "Armchair" treatment of acute coronary thrombosis. JAMA 148:1365, 1952.

Malinosw M: Regression of atherosclerosis in humans: Fact or myth? Circulation 64:1, 1981.

Mayou R, MacMahon D, Sleight P, et al: Early rehabilitation after myocardial infarction. Lancet 2:1399, 1981.

McNeer JF, Wagner GS, Ginsburg PB, et al: Hospital discharge one week after acute myocardial infarction. N Engl J Med 298:229, 1978.

McNeer JF, Wallace AG, Wagner GS, et al: The course of acute myocardial infarction: Feasibility of early discharge off the uncomplicated patient. Circulation 51:410, 1975.

Oberman A: Cardiac rehabilitation. Circulation 62:909, 1980.

Oldridge NB, Wicks JR, Hanley C, et al: Noncompliance in an exercise rehabilitation program for men who have suffered a myocardial infarction. Can Med Assoc J 118: 361, 1978.

Palatsi I: Feasibility of physical training after myocardial infarction and its effect on return to work, morbidity and mortality. Acta Med Scand 88:599, 1976.

Pratt CM, Welton DE, Squires WG, et al: Demonstration of training effect during chronic β-adrenergic blockade in patients with coronary artery disease. Circulation 64:1125, 1981.

Rahe RH, Ward HW, Hayes V: Brief group therapy in myocardial infarction rehabilitation three- to four-year follow-up of a controlled trial. Psychosom Med 41:229, 1979.

Rechnitzer PA: The effect of exercise prescription on the recurrence rate of myocardial infarction in men. Am J Cardiol 47:419, 1981.

Grande P, Pedersen A, Schaadt O, et al: Cardio-specific serum enzyme CK-MB follow physical exercise and acute myocardial infarction. Eur J Cardiol 11:161, 1980.

Sanne H: Readaptation after Myocardial Infarction. New York, World Rehabilitation Fund, 1979.

Scalzi CC, Burke LE, Greenland S: Evaluation of an inpatient educational program for coronary patients and families. Heart Lung 9:846, 1980.

Siegel AJ, Silverman LM, Holman BL: Elevated creatine kinase MB isoenzyme levels in marathon runners. JAMA 246:2049, 1981.

Sivarajan E, Bruce R, Almes M, et al: In-hospital exercise after myocardial infarction does not improve treadmill performance. N Engl J Med 305:357, 1981.

Wenger N, Hurst J: Coronary bypass surgery as a rehabilitative procedure. Cardiac Rehabilitation Quarterly 11:1, 1980.

Wilhelmsen L, Sann H, Elmfeldt D, et al: A controlled trial of physical training after myocardial infarction. Prev Med 4:491, 1975.

Complications of an Exercise Program

Fletcher GF, Cantwell JD: Ventricular fibrillation in a medically supervised cardiac exercise program. JAMA 238:2627, 1977.

Fogoros RN: "Runner's trots." JAMA 243:1743, 1980.

Gibbons L, Cooper K, Meyer B, et al: The acute cardiac risk of strenuous exercise. JAMA 244:1799, 1980.

Graboys TB: The economics of screening joggers. N Engl J Med 30:258, 1979.

Hanson PG, Zimmerman SW: Exertional heatstroke in novice runners. JAMA 242:154, 1979.

Haskell WL: Cardiovascular complications during exercise training of cardiac patients. Circulation 57:920, 1978.

Jelinek V: Exercise induced arrhythmias: Their implications for cardiac rehabilitation programs. Med Sci Sports 12:223, 1980.

Maron B, Roberts W, McAllister H, et al: Sudden death in young athletes. Circulation 62:218, 1980.

Mead WF, Pyfer HR, Trombold JC, et al: Successful resuscitation of near simultaneous cases of cardiac arrest with a review of fifteen cases occurring during supervised exercise. Circulation 53:187, 1976.

Morales A, Romanelli R, Boucek R: The mural left anterior descending coronary artery, strenuous exercise and sudden death. Circulation 62:230, 1980.

Norfray JF, Schlachter L, Kernahan WT, et al: Early confirmation of stress fractures in joggers. JAMA 243:1647, 1980.

Roberts W, Maron B: Sudden death while playing football. Am Heart J 102:1061, 1981.

Shephard RJ, Kavanagh T: Predicting the exercise catastrophe in the "post coronary" patient. Can Fam Physician 24:614, 1978.

CHAPTER

V

The Use of Exercise Radionuclide Testing To Evaluate Cardiac Rehabilitation

Noninvasive nuclear techniques for imaging the heart are a new and exciting means of evaluating the effects of exercise on the heart. Shortly after intravenous injection, thallium-201 accumulates in the myocardium in approximate proportion to coronary artery blood flow and can be used to detect myocardial damage and ischemia. Technetium-99m labeled human serum albumin or red blood cells allows imaging of left ventricular contraction. The latter technique has been demonstrated to reproducibly measure ejection fraction at rest and during exercise. There should be an agreement with Q waves or bundle branch block, redistribution thallium defects, and decreased resting ejection fraction since all are consistent with myocardial damage. Likewise, there should be agreement with exercise-induced ST-segment depression, reversible thallium defects, and a flat or decreasing ejection fraction response to exercise since they are all manifestations of myocardial ischemia.

These radionuclide techniques are applicable to studies before and after an intervention because they produce minimal radiation exposure. They can be used to categorize disease severity and provide a baseline for exercise training. In addition, they can identify patients for whom disease worsens and thus need other treatment modalities.

Our group at the University of California, San Diego, has been systematically applying these techniques for this purpose for the past four years. We started by using the techniques in all patients being treated for coronary heart disease and by trying to correlate results and validate our analysis techniques. Next, we repeated the radionuclide studies in a small group of patients after a median of six months of exercise training. At present, we are performing a randomized trial called PERFEXT (Perfusion and Perform-ance Exercise Trial), sponsored by the National Institutes of Health, with radionuclide studies performed initially and then repeated after one year. This chapter summarizes the design of PERFEXT and our preliminary find-ings.

INITIAL CORRELATIVE AND VALIDATION STUDIES

All patients referred for cardiac rehabilitation or for cardiac evaluation were studied with three noninvasive techniques: electrocardiography, thalli-um imaging, and radionuclide ventriculography, all three at rest and during exercise. Studies using contrast angiography and radionuclide ventriculogra-phy have reported that most normal subjects increase ejection fraction dur-ing exercise, whereas most individuals with coronary heart disease show no change or a decrease in ejection fraction. The profiles of the ejection fraction response to supine exercise are discussed in Chapter 2. The response of coronary heart disease patients is due to ischemia developing with exercise, which causes cardiac dysfunction, or possibly due to inadequate cardiac re-serve secondary to myocardial damage. It is important to study cardiac func-tion and perfusion during exertion since that may be the only time in which cardiac changes secondary to an exercise program can be detected. In regard to thallium, redistribution defects seen at four or more hours following injec-tion during exercise can represent severe ischemia, but they usually are due to scar. The presented analyses are based on the first 85 patients studied.

In comparing the physiologic, symptomatic, and electrocardiographic re-sults of the two radionuclide exercise studies, several differences were ap-parent (Table I). The maximal heart rate was higher, the systolic blood pressure was lower, and the double product, which is a good estimate of myocardial oxygen demand, was higher during treadmill testing. These dif-ferences were significant ($P < .001$), as was the estimated maximal oxygen consumption, which was one third higher during treadmill testing. A true maximal effort was not achieved during the bicycle test because the last work load had to be performed for three minutes in a relative steady state; however, both tests had angina and electrocardiographic responses that agreed by more than chance.

For analysis of exercise-induced electrocardiographic responses, the more sensitive treadmill test was utilized. Nearly all of the patients (93%) had abnormal rest or exercise electrocardiographic results including 11 who

TABLE I
PHYSIOLOGIC RESPONSES TO TWO EXERCISE TESTS IN 85 PATIENTS (MEAN ± 1 SD)

	Treadmill	Supine Bicycle	× Difference (SD)
Systolic blood pressure	173.7	181.9	+ 8.1
(mm Hg)	(± 28.4)	(± 26.6)	(± 19.8)
Heart rate	146.4	130.9	− 15.5
(beats/min)	(± 25.8)	(± 23.6)	(± 16.8)
Heart rate × Systolic blood	25.5	24.2	− 1.3
pressure × 10³	(± 6.8)	(± 6.0)	(± 4.2)
Estimated V̇O₂	31.9	20.0	− 11.9
(ml O₂/kg-min)	(± 9.0)	(± 6.0)	(± 6.4)
Percent with angina as end point	22%	22%	
Percent with abnormal ECG response	80%	70%	

Note: By using the paired t-test, all of the hemodynamic measurements are significantly different ($P <$ .001); however, angina and electrocardiographic (ECG) responses agreed to a degree not explained by chance alone ($P < .02$).

only had borderline treadmill tests. Q waves and myocardial scarring could appear independently as predicted by previous electrocardiographic-pathologic correlations. Though thallium imaging was comparable to the electrocardiogram in identifying scarring, it detected ischemia half as often as did the exercise electrocardiogram or the ejection fraction response to exercise. One third of our patients had abnormal ejection fractions at rest, and of these nearly one third had aneurysms demonstrated. Only one patient had a normal resting ejection fraction and a ventricular aneurysm. Eighty-one percent of our patients had abnormal rest or exercise ejection fractions. Follow-up studies are necessary to see if the ejection fraction response to exercise can improve the prognostic capacity of resting ejection fraction and other noninvasive screening criteria. A practicing physician should consider that a completely normal electrocardiogram is highly predictive of a normal resting ejection fraction and excellent prognosis.

Static categorization of the patients was done according to whether or not they had (1) a history of myocardial infarction, (2) Q waves on the electrocardiogram, (3) thallium redistribution defect, or (4) an abnormal resting ejection fraction (less than 50%). With no method of verifying scarring, we compared the results of these tests (Table II and Figure 1). As can be seen at the top of Table II, when all three studies were normal, a previous

TABLE II
COMPARISON OF RESTING RESULTS AND CLINICAL HISTORY OF INFARCTION

	Q wave or BBB	^{201}Tl Scar	ABNL EF	History of Q-wave Infarct (N = 49)	History of ST Infarct (N = 13)	No History of Infarct (N = 23)	Total (N = 85)
Combined	no	no	no	6	6	18	30
study results	yes	no	no	6*	1÷	5÷	12
	no	yes	no	1	2	—	3
	no	no	yes	—	1	—	1
	yes	yes	no	11	1	—	12
	yes	no	yes	2	—	—	2
	no	yes	yes	4	1	—	5
	yes	yes	yes	19*	1	—	20
Cumulative	yes	—	—	38	3	5	46
abnormalities	—	yes	—	35	5	—	40÷
	—	—	yes	25	3	—	28

Q wave or BBB = Q wave or bundle branch block on resting electrocardiogram; ^{201}Tl Scar = defect does not fill in by 4 hr postexercise; ABNL EF = resting ejection fraction less than 50%.
*One left bundle branch block included.
÷One right bundle branch block included.
‡Prevalences of electrocarodiographic abnormalities $\left(\frac{46}{85} = 54\%\right)$; ^{201}Tl Scar $\left(\frac{40}{85} = 47\%\right)$ and abnormal EF $\left(\frac{28}{85} = 33\%\right)$
Note: By using the Kappa test, all pairs of studies agreed by more than expected due to chance alone ($P < .02$).

myocardial infarction associated with a Q wave (QMI) was unlikely. When all three tests were abnormal, most of the patients had a history of myocardial infarction. Whereas most patients with a history of QMI had an abnormal electrocardiogram or thallium redistribution defect, only half had an ejection fraction less than 50%. Nearly a third of the patients without a history of myocardial infarction had Q waves on their resting electrocardiogram, whereas none had an abnormal thallium defect or ejection fraction less than 50%. The most frequently abnormal resting study was the electrocardiogram (slightly more than half), next the thallium redistribution defect (in almost half), and only one third had an ejection fraction less than 50% at

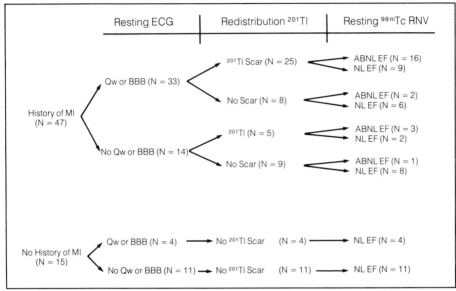

Figure 1. Stratification by the myocardial infarction history, resting electrocardiogram, redistribution thallium study, and resting radionuclide ejection fraction. MI = myocardial infarction; Qw = Q waves diagnostic of a myocardial infarction; BBB = bundle branch block; ^{201}Tl scar = persistent defect on thallium redistribution study; ^{99m}Tc RNV = technetium radionuclide ventriculography; ABNL/NLEF = abnormal or normal ejection fraction, respectively, at rest with the criterion for normal set at 50% or greater.

rest. Using the Kappa test, all pairs of these studies agreed by more than that expected due to chance alone ($P < .02$).

Figure 1 demonstrates the additional information gained over the history and the resting electrocardiogram by the two radionuclide studies. Patients could be further subdivided; i.e., those with Q waves and a history of a myocardial infarction could be divided into those with a thallium redistribution defect and an abnormal ejection fraction and into those with no scar and a normal ejection fraction. Certainly these two subgroups will have a different clinical course, prognosis, and potential for cardiac response to training.

Thallium redistribution defects were detected only in patients with a history of myocardial infarction, including five with a myocardial infarction associated with only ST changes. A normal resting electrocardiogram and no thallium redistribution defect were highly predictive of a normal resting ejection fraction. A completely normal resting electrocardiogram alone was highly associated with normal resting radionuclide studies. Thirty of 39 patients

TABLE III
COMPARISON OF THE EXERCISE TEST RESULTS

	ST ABNL	^{201}Tl Ischemia	EF ABNL	Total (N = 83)
Combined	no	no	no	8*
study results	yes	no	no	14
	no	yes	no	1
	no	no	yes	7÷
	yes	yes	no	6
	yes	no	yes	23
	no	yes	yes	1
	yes	yes	yes	23
Cumulative	yes	—	—	66
abnormalities	—	yes	—	31‡
	—	—	yes	54

ST ABNL = ST abnormality; EF ABNL = ejection fraction abnormality (less than 5% increase with exercise).

Two patients had left bundle branch block with uninterpretable ST segments. One had an abnormal % change EF. The second had both an abnormal % change EF and thallium-201 ischemia. Three patients had angina as an end point with a normal ST segment response. One had normal studies (*). The other two had abnormal % change EF with exercise (÷).

‡ Prevalences of ST abnormalities $\left(\frac{66}{83} = 80\%\right)$; ^{201} Tl ischemia $\left(\frac{31}{60} = 37\%\right)$; and abnormal EF response $\left(\frac{54}{85} = 65\%\right)$.

When using the Kappa test, the hypothesis of chance agreement was not rejected for ST abnormalities versus thallium or versus the EF response, however, the agreement of the results of the thallium and EF response was greater than due to chance (Kappa test, $P. < .01$).

without Q waves or bundle branch block had no thallium redistribution defects and normal resting ejection fractions.

Dynamic categorization of the patients was done according to whether or not they had (1) ischemia on the exercise thallium image, (2) exercise test-induced ST abnormalities, and (3) an abnormal ejection fraction response to exercise (Table III and Figure 2). With no method of verifying ischemia, we compared the results of these tests. Nearly all the patients had at least one abnormal exercise study. The test with the lowest percentage of

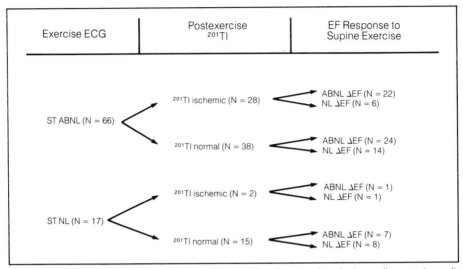

Exercise ECG	Postexercise ^{201}Tl	EF Response to Supine Exercise

Figure 2. Stratification by the exercise studies including the exercise electrocardiogram, immediately after exercise thallium scan, and the ejection fraction response to supine bicycle exercise. ST ABNL/NL = ST-segment depression abnormal or normal with a criterion set at 0.1 mV of horizontal or downsloping ST-segment depression; ^{201}Tl ischemic = thallium defect on immediate postexercise image; ABNL/NLΔEF = abnormal or normal change of ejection fraction, respectively, from rest to maximal supine bicycle exercise with the criterion for normal set at an increase of 10% or greater over the resting value.

abnormal exercise responses was thallium with 35%, compared with 78% with abnormal ST changes and 64% with abnormal ejection fraction responses. Both the ECG and the ejection fraction response to exercise were sensitive indices of exercise-induced ischemia, with a majority of patients being identified as ischemic by these tests. Using the Kappa test, it is apparent that whereas the radionuclide tests agree in their assessment of exercise-induced ischemia, the ST-segment response does not agree with either of them.

There was the possibility that only one third of the patients had thallium ischemia because they had completed myocardial infarctions without residual ischemia. However, thallium ischemia occurred in 34% of patients with completed QMI as compared with 38% of the remaining patients (P = NS).

Table III and Figure 2 show the subdivision that is possible by adding the exercise radionuclide studies to the exercise electrocardiogram. With exercise-induced ST abnormalities, patients were as diverse as those with thallium ischemia and an abnormal ejection fraction response and those with normal thallium and a normal ejection fraction response.

TABLE IV
COMPARISON OF SCAR AND ISCHEMIA BY EITHER THALLIUM IMAGING OR
ELECTROCARDIOGRAPHIC STUDIES AND LEFT VENTRICULAR DYSFUNCTION BY
RADIONUCLIDE VENTRICULOGRAPHY IN 83 PATIENTS

	Normal Resting EF		Abnormal Resting EF		
	EX EF NL	EX EF ABNL	EX EF NL	EX EF ABNL	Total
No Scar, no ischemia	4	6	1	—	11
No Scar, ischemia	6	16	—	—	22
Scar, no ischemia	6	3	3	3	15
Scar, ischemia	—	15	9	11	35
Total	16	40	13	14	83

EX EF = ejection fraction response to exercise; Scar = abnormal resting electrocardiogram or thallium redistribution defect or both; ischemia = abnormal exercise electrocardiogram or thallium exercise defect or both.
Note: Two patients with left bundle branch block were excluded.

Although all patients had coronary heart disease, eight had normal responses to all three exercise studies. Of these eight, coronary heart disease was documented by myocardial infarction in three, an abnormal coronary angiogram in two, and five had coronary artery bypass surgery. Fourteen patients had normal exercise radionuclide studies despite exercise-induced ST abnormalities. Of these 14, 9 had myocardial infarctions (2 with apical aneurysms), 7 had angiographic obstructions, 2 had coronary artery bypass surgery, and 1 was asymptomatic but at high risk for coronary heart disease.

Left ventricular aneurysms and exercise-induced ST elevation appear to be related and identify patients with severe myocardial damage. Only 8 of 20 patients with ST elevation had thallium ischemia, and only 2 of the 8 also had an aneurysm. Patients without resting aneurysms with exercise-induced ST elevation were most likely to develop dyskinetic areas only during exercise.

Table IV combines both the electrocardiogram and thallium for the identification of scar (Q waves, redistribution defects, or both) and ischemia (exercise-induced ST abnormality or exercise thallium defect) for comparison with radionuclide ventriculography. Sixty of the 83 patients (excluding the 2 with left bundle branch block) had scar or ischemia (by thallium or electrocardiogram) and abnormal heart function (abnormal resting or exercise ejection fraction).

The boxes on a diagonal line from upper left to lower right in Table IV represent 34 patients whose results agree. The patients in these boxes without scar or ischemia have a normal resting ejection fraction and a normal exercise ejection fraction and patients with a scar and no ischemia have an abnormal resting ejection fraction and a normal exercise ejection fraction. The major discrepancy rests in the 24 patients with a scar with a normal resting ejection fraction and in the 15 patients with ischemia with a normal exercise ejection fraction. Regional wall motion abnormalities can be present and still have normal global function. The size of the infarction and the amount of compensatory hypertrophy have an impact on global function. In addition, ST elevation does not always indicate the presence of ischemia and cannot be included with ST depression. A failure of the ejection fraction to rise with exercise could be the result fo inadequate cardiac reserve and not of ischemia. Future investigations will require phase and regional wall motion analysis.

This study was designed to evaluate myocardial scarring, ischemia, and function in patients with coronary heart disease using a combination of radionuclide techniques and the electrocardiogram during rest and exercise. The radionuclide techniques made it possible to subdivide patients according to the severity of their coronary heart disease in a more definite way than is possible from their history and electrocardiogram alone. Findings at rest included Q waves or bundle branch block in 54%, 47% had persistent thallium defects, and 33% had an abnormal ejection fraction (less than 50%). Of the 39 patients with normal electrocardiograms, 3l had no scars, and only one of these 3l (3%) had an abnormal ejection fraction. Abnormal ejection fractions or thallium redistribution defects did not occur in patients without a history of a myocardial infarction. Abnormal resting ejection fractions occurred in 63% of patients with abnormal thallium redistribution scans versus 7% of those with normal scans. Exercise test results included an abnormal ST-segment response in 80%, abnormal ejection fraction response in 65%, and a thallium ischemic defect in 37%. Twenty patients had exercise-induced ST elevation, and this phenomenon was related more to ventricular aneurysms than to ischemia. Thallium imaging, radionuclide ventriculography, and electrocardiography provide results regarding myocardial damage that agree by more than chance alone, whereas exercise-induced ST-segment changes did not agree with the radionuclide indications of exercise-induced ischemia.

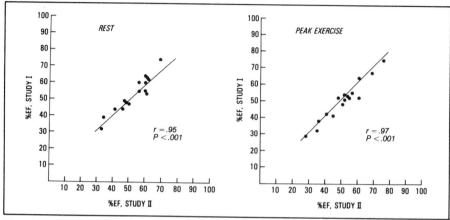

Figure 3. Results of repeating ejection fraction measurements for 16 stable patients at rest and during supine bicycle exercise, with the two studies separated by approximately two weeks.

The reproducibility of ejection fraction determined by equilibrium radionuclide angiography at rest, during supine bicycle exercise, and in the recovery period have been studied. Sixteen patients with stable, chronic coronary artery disease were studied twice within an average 15-day period. Following injection of 20 to 25 mCi of technetium-tagged human serum albumin, data were analyzed for two-minute periods at rest, during two to three stages of exercise (submaximal, maximal), and during 2- and 3-minute recovery and at 9- and 10-minute recovery. The patients reached similar heart rate–blood pressure products in both studies. As illustrated in Figure 3, the reproducibility of ejection fractions was excellent at rest, at peak exercise, and in the early recovery period, but less good during submaximal exercise and later after exercise. Maximal symptom-limited exercise was essential for obtaining reproducible exercise ejection fraction results.

To assess the reliability or agreement of human interpretation of analogue thallium myocardial perfusion images, four experienced observers interpreted 100 images on two separate occasions using a form designed to limit reader variability (Figure 4). A high intraobserver reliability (agreement by same observer at separate times) of 89% to 93% was found when films were interpreted as normal or abnormal (a dichotomous decision). Interobserver reliability (agreement between observers) for a majority grouping of observers (three or four) was 75% for an abnormal interpretation and 68% for a normal interpretation. Reliability ranged from 11% to 79%, however, when interpreters were asked to determine the anatomic location of

Patient Name: _____   Age: _____   Date: _____

Pretest Clinical History: Yes No   MI □ □   Hx Abnl TM   Yes No □ □   Chest Pain   Yes No □ □

Medications: Beta Blockers   Yes No □ □   Nitrates   Yes No □ □

Other _____

Max Effort   Yes No □ □   Angina   Yes No □ □   Test Endpoint: _____

Rest HR _____   Rest Blood Pressure _____   Maximum HR _____   Maximum Blood Pressure _____

Comments: _____

Background:

Lung Uptake   Normal □   Increased □

Visceral Uptake   Normal □   Increased □

Right Ventricle   Normal □   Increased □

Comments: _____

Heart:

Chamber Size   Normal   Small   Enlarged

Wall Thickness   Normal   Thin   Enlarged

Comments: _____

	ANT		LAO 45°-50°		LAO 60°-70°		LEFT LATERAL	
	Exercise	Delay	Exercise	Delay	Exercise	Delay	Exercise	Delay
Defect Size								
Defect Intensity								

Size: 1 = 10% of total myocardial area; 2 = 20%; 3 = 30%; 4 = 40%, 5 = 50%

Intensity: 1 = Normal; 2 = Just less than normal; 3 = Just greater than background; 4 = Background

Final Assessment:

Figure 4. Exercise thallium scintigraphy data collection form (Atwood et al, with permission of Circulation).

defects. Posterior and lateral wall defects were interpreted with the least amount of reliability. These findings are illustrated in Figure 5. Using a scale of 1 to 10 to grade the severity of a defect, correlations of .82 to .86 were found when reading defects in the lateral and anterior projections. Higher correlations ranging from .86 to .94 were found in left anterior oblique views. These results indicate that caution must be used when interpreting defect location.

In summary, best observer reliability or agreement was found when dichotomous judgments were used in describing images and the least reliability (most variability) occurred with more complex descriptions such as those for anatomic location of defects and for overlapping areas, e.g., the

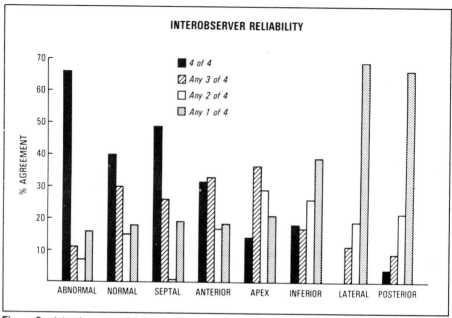

Figure 5.   Interobserver reliability, or percent agreement, based on 100 scans read by four experienced interpreters. (Atwood et al, with permission of Circulation.)

apical region. This lack of complete agreement is present in other areas of cardiology, and attempts should constantly be made to improve reliability as well as validity. Several possible modes for improving agreement include (1) simple dichotomous decisions, (2) standardized report forms, (3) multiple observers or one very experienced reader, (4) multiple blinded or unbiased interpretations, and (5) computer analysis. However, the grading system has given us a valid way to compare the severity of thallium defects before and after training using standard techniques.

PREEXERCISE AND POSTEXERCISE TRAINING STUDIES

A protocol consisting of radionuclide exercise testing to evaluate myocardial perfusion and function before and after a period of exercise training was approved by the Human Subjects Committee at University of California, San Diego, in 1978. Informed consent was obtained prior to each exercise study. Of the first 16 patients who consented to this protocol and had both the thallium treadmill and technetium supine bicycle tests before and after 3 to 12 months of exercise training, 5 patients were found to have improvement in both studies. Six of the pretraining and posttraining thallium images are shown in Figure 6. Though the top five images show subtle improvement, they were among 6 of 16 consistently chosen by blinded readers as indications of posttraining improvement. Of the remaining 10 patients, 2 had images that worsened (one of which is shown at the bottom of Figure 6, patient RP) and 8 showed no change. The treadmill data demonstrated a higher work load, greater myocardial oxygen demand, and no change in the exercise electrocardiogram after training.

The resting ejection fraction values were lower after training by 5% or more in two of the patients, but this is not consistent with the entire group of 16 who showed no significant change in resting ejection fraction (preexercise and postexercise: 58% $\pm$ 10% versus 56% $\pm$ 12%, respectively). Resting and exercise ejection fractions have been highly reproducible ($r \geq .94$) when studies are separated by two weeks or less, so the changes in resting ejection fractions seen in these five patients are best explained by technique variability over a longer time period. The percent change in ejection fraction is a more reliable estimate of alterations in myocardial function because the rest and exercise measurements are only separated by minutes. The entire group of 16 patients showed a statistically significant improvement in the exercise-induced percent change in ejection fraction after training (-3% $\pm$ 10% pretraining versus $+9\%$ $\pm$ 20% posttraining), with 9 normalizing their exercise ejection fraction response and 7 unchanged. When the first 19 patients were analyzed, a higher ejection fraction was found at matched submaximal work loads after six months of training. Consideration of medications such as propranolol and nitroglycerin is important since they can improve ejection fractions, but none of the patients had medication changes during the course of this study or had taken nitrates in proximity to testing.

Radionuclide techniques have enabled the noninvasive study of myocardial perfusion and function during exercise. Improvement of exercise thallium images in some patients following coronary artery bypass surgery and percutaneous transluminal coronary angioplasty has been reported. Also, Kent and colleagues demonstrated no change in resting ejection fraction after coronary artery bypass surgery, but they found an increased exercise ejection fraction in patients who clinically improved.

To improve analysis techniques, computer analysis of the thallium images has been applied. The first 17 consecutive coronary patients who underwent a thallium treadmill test and a radionuclide ejection fraction supine bicycle test before and after six months of an exercise program and who had

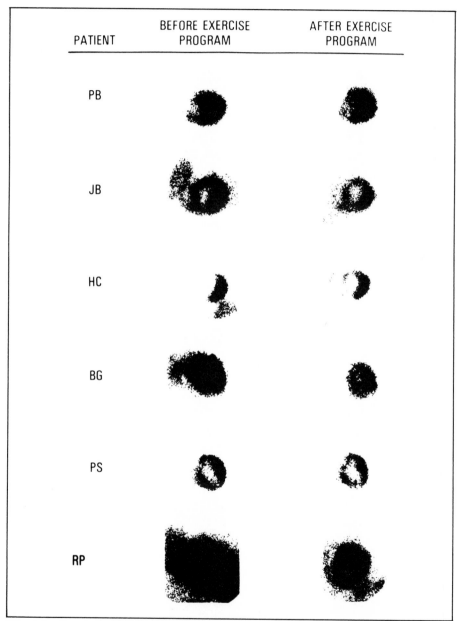

Figure 6.   Exercise thallium images of the five patients who showed improvement in both thallium image and ejection fraction response to supine bicycle exercise after six months of an exercise program. RP (bottom) is one of the 16 patients who showed worsening of both studies. He has done well after coronary artery bypass surgery.

data suitable for computer processing were analyzed. The thallium data were assessed both using analogue images and a computerized circumferential profile technique. Patients were exercised on the treadmill to a higher work load after the exercise program but achieved a similar rate-pressure product. When interpreting analogue thallium images, only 50% agreement was obtained for the assessment of changes before and after myocardial perfusion. The computer technique, however, had low interobserver and intraobserver variability (6%) and better agreement (90.5%). Using the circumferential profile program, five patients improved (a total of 11 regions) and one patient worsened (with 2 regions). Before the exercise program, the ejection fraction response to supine bicycle exercise was normal (an increase greater than 11%) in four, flat in seven, and severely abnormal (more than 4%) in six patients. After the exercise program, even though achieving similar or higher rate-pressure products, six patients improved their ejection fraction response, nine did not change, and two worsened. Of the five patients who improved their thallium images, one improved his ejection fraction response, two stayed normal, and two did not change. One of the latter increased his resting ejection fraction by 23%. One patient worsened both in the thallium study and in the ejection fraction response after the exercise program. Changes in thallium exercise images and the ejection fraction response to supine exercise occurred in the patients after an exercise program, but were not always concordant.

PERFEXT—A RANDOMIZED TRIAL OF THE EFFECTS OF EXERCISE ON HEART PERFUSION AND PERFORMANCE

Since September 1980, a randomized trial of the effects of a one-year exercise program on patients with stable coronary heart disease has been ongoing at the University of California, San Diego. The protocol for PERFEXT project (Perfusion and Performance Exercise Trial) is illustrated in Figure 7. Men 35 to 65 years of age who fulfill any one of the following criteria are accepted for entry into either an exercise group or a control group: (a) asymptomatic high-risk type, manifested by an abnormal treadmill test, abnormal coronary angiogram or both; (b) MI (four months or more prior to entry to trial); (c) typical stable angina pectoris, confirmated by angiography, radionuclide studies, or abnormal exercise test; and (d) coronary artery bypass surgery (four months or more prior to entry into the trial). Patients with a condition that might make their course unstable, such as CHF, life-threatening dysrhythmias, uncontrolled hypertension, or other medical, vascular, or orthopedic problems, are excluded. If candidates are on digoxin or beta blockers, only those stable enough to have medications stopped prior to initial and final exercise testing are included (two weeks for

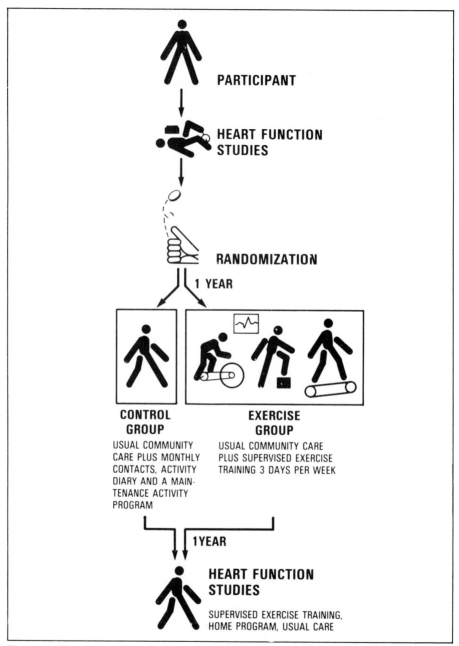

Figure 7. Illustration of the protocol followed for PERFEXT, a randomized trial sponsored by the NIH at the University of California, San Diego.

digoxin, three days for beta blockers). Nitrates are not taken in proximity to the time of testing to avoid their effect on performance. If CABS is performed during the study year, the participant is considered a dropout.

The specific purposes of the project are (a) determination of whether or not changes in cardiac function and exercise-induced myocardial ischemia can be detected in patients with coronary heart disease after one year of exercise training, compared with patients receiving usual community care; (b) development of new noninvasive techniques for identifying patients likely to respond or exhibiting a favorable cardiac response to exercise training, those unlikely to respond, and those at high risk for such a program who are better managed by other modalities; and (c) testing the hypothesis that computer-assisted rest and exercise electrocardiographic measurements can localize or quantitate changes in myocardial ischemia, asynergy, volume, function, and morphology.

During the one year of training, an attempt is made to wean patients in rehabilitation from digoxin and beta blockers when these are not clinically necessary. This attempt is made only after careful consideration of the impact that medication changes could have on the quality and quantity of each patient's life. Patients responding to exercise training can have their medications safely decreased and usually stopped. Beta blockers especially need to be discontinued because they may impede the attainment of a training effect and normalize the ejection fraction response to supine exercise testing; digitalis interferes with the accurate utilization of the ST segment as an indicator of myocardial ischemia. Though the effects of these drugs in relation to exercise training should be studied, in our study their interference with the effects of exercise training could invalidate results.

Patients who meet the above criteria and are referred for either cardiovascular evaluation or for cardiac rehabilitation undergo the initial series of tests. Afterward, they are randomized by a computer program to either routine community care or to University of California, San Diego, Cardiac Rehabilitation Program. Randomization occurs within the cells illustrated in Figure 8. This method improves the chances for balanced randomization and also guarantees equal numbers of trained versus control subjects within the subgroups of those with scarring versus no scarring, left ventricular dysfunction versus normal function, and ischemia versus absence of ischemia.

Those randomized to the control group understand that there is no scientific evidence to prove that exercise affects morbidity and mortality in patients with coronary disease and that we are evaluating the physiologic effect

		NORMAL RESTING EF $\geq 50\%$	ABNORMAL RESTING EF $< 50\%$
NO SCAR	NO ISCHEMIA BY ECG, THALLIUM OR ANGINA		
	ISCHEMIA		
SCAR (BY THALLIUM, HISTORY OF MI OR ECG)	NO ISCHEMIA		
	ISCHEMIA BY ECG, THALLIUM, OR ANGINA		

Figure 8. Matrix (4×2) of the cells in which patients in PERFEXT are classified prior to randomization.

of exercise training. They are offered medical treatment, risk factor modification, routine clinic follow-up, and a walking program as well as the opportunity to join our rehabilitation program after one year. Dropouts from the exercise group will not be used as controls.

Exercise Testing. Treadmill exercise and supine bicycle exercise studies are performed using a rest and exercise electrocardiographic digital data-acquisition system. Exercise is terminated with the occurrence of 0.3 mV or more of horizontal or downsloping ST-segment depression, 0.1 mV of ST-segment elevation, serious chest pain or dysrhythmias, an abnormal heart rate or blood pressure response, or fatigue. The patient's well-being is always maintained and supersedes all other end points.

Separate treadmill tests utilizing a modified Balke-Ware protocol are performed for the thallium imaging and the maximal oxygen consumption measurements. A redistribution study is done four hours after the thallium injection. Maximal oxygen consumption is measured, not estimated, using electronic gas-analysis equipment, and a microcomputer.

Electrocardiographic and Vectorcardiographic Techniques. After careful skin preparation, 14 electrodes are attached using the Mason-Likar exercise adaptation of the standard 12-lead and Frank lead system. Special small, nondisposable electrodes are used on the precordium so as not to interfere with radionuclide imaging. Consistent, proper electrode placement is accomplished with a Dalhousie square. The electrocardiogram is sampled at 250 samples/sec and collected on floppy disks in the specialized digital data-acquisition cart (Data Logger, Marquette Electronics). The floppy disks are processed off-line using a specially developed computer measurement program. The QRS complex and ST segment are analyzed spatially, and measurements of magnitude and direction are made.

Radionuclide Gated Left Ventricular Imaging. A15 mCi dose of technetium-labeled red blood cells is administered intravenously. A first-pass radionuclide ejection fraction is measured. Following equilibration, the activity within the blood pool is recorded in a right anterior oblique projection and, subsequently, in a modified left anterior oblique projection with a caudal tilt, which permits separation of the left ventricle. With the gamma camera in the modified left anterior oblique position, the patient performs graded supine bicycle exercise. The level of exercise is graded in two or three stages according to each patient's capacity. Stages will be matched pretraining and post-training for both submaximal work load and double product and finally for maximal effort.

Exercise Training. The Cardiac Rehabilitation Program at the University of California, San Diego, is divided into two phases. Phase I comprises continuously monitored exercise sessions for one hour, three times a week. The patients rotate between eight to ten exercise stations consisting of dynamic exercises for the upper and lower extremities—treadmill, bicycle ergometer, rowing, and arm crank. Patients exercise for approximately eight minutes at each station while an exercise specialist monitors a bipolar lead and ascertains that they can safely maintain 85% of their maximal heart rate. The training heart rate is determined from the maximal treadmill test. This phase lasts anywhere from eight weeks to an indefinite time for some patients at high risk for ventricular fibrillation. The decision to move a patient to phase II is determined by clinical assessment and by exercise testing. Phase II of the rehabilitation program is gymnasium or outdoor exercise supervised by an exercise specialist. Equipment for cardiopulmonary resuscitation is available, and intermittent patient electrocardiographic monitoring is done using "quick look" electrodes. These sessions last one hour, three times a week. All patients undergo periodic reevaluation and exercise testing to follow their progress and to optimize their exercise prescription. Perceived exertion scores of 13 to 15 are maintained during exercise sessions.

The noninvasive tests utilized in PERFEXT, including radionuclides and computerized electrocardiography, have had a great impact on cardiology in recent years. These techniques have not been optimally developed and thus have mainly been used for diagnostic purposes. They have had only limited application in evaluating cardiac changes and in cardiac rehabilitation—areas where they may possibly find their greatest value. In developing and comparing these techniques, it is possible that computer-assisted rest and exercise electrocardiographic analysis techniques, along with standard clinical assessment, will provide all the necessary clinical information. Radionuclide techniques may calibrate the resting and exercise electrocardiogram as has never before been possible. The approach documented here could become the major method for evaluating or categorizing patients regarding their response to exercise training and recognizing whether or not they are benefiting from it.

CONCLUSION

The results of our preliminary studies investigating the relationship of radionuclide techniques, the electrocardiogram, and clinical history have been described. The change in resting global ejection fraction secondary to coronary heart disease depends on the size of the scarring, the amount of compensatory hypertrophy, and the functional cardiac reserve; thus the problems with correlating the resting test results. In addition, ST-segment elevation over Q waves does not usually indicate exercise-induced ischemia, and therefore it should not be equated to ST depression. Also, an inadequate exercise ejection fraction response could be due to inadequate cardiac reserve rather than to ischemia; thus the problems with agreement among the different exercise test results. We now include wall motion and phase analysis of the ventriculograms, as well as circumferential profiling of thallium images in our randomized trial.

This chapter has reviewed only the experience at University of California, San Diego, using nuclear cardiology methods to evaluate patients with coronary heart disease and the subsequent effects of cardiac rehabilitation. Other institutions, particularly Duke University and Baylor University, have been active in this area and their work should be acknowledged. The Duke studies have been limited to the use of first-pass imaging with technetium during erect bicycle exercise, but the Baylor group has utilized thallium imaging as well. Nuclear cardiology offers exciting new techniques for determining disease severity and demonstrating the effects of any intervention on myocardial function and perfusion. PERFEXT, even now, is clarifying the strengths and limitations of nuclear techniques. Its main purpose, however, is to answer the question of whether or not exercise can improve the perfusion and function of a heart already diseased by coronary atherosclerosis.

REFERENCES
CHAPTER V

INITIAL CORRELATIVE AND VALIDATION STUDIES

Atwood JE, Jensen D, Froelicher V, et al: Agreement in human interpretation of analog thallium myocardial perfusion images. Circulation 64:601, 1981.

Battler A, Slutsky R, Karliner J, et al: Left ventricular ejection fraction and first third ejection fraction early after acute myocardial infarction: Value for predicting mortality and morbidity. Am J Cardiol 455:197, 1980.

Froelicher VF, Sebrechts C, Streitwiesser D, et al: Rest and exercise electrocardiograms and radionuclides in patients presenting for cardiac rehabilitation. Clin Cardiol 4:59, 1981.

Pfisterer ME, Battler A, Swanson SM, et al: Reproducibility of ejection-fraction determinations by equilibrium radionuclide angiography in response to supine bicycle exercise: Concise communication. J Nucl Med 20:491, 1979.

Pfisterer ME, Schuler G, Ricci D, et al: Profiles of left ventricular function by equilibrium radionuclide angiography during exercise and in recovery phase in normals and patients with heart disease. Cathet Cardiovasc Diagn 5:305, 1979.

Sullivan W, Vlodarer Z, Tuna N, et al: Correlation of ECG and pathologic findings in healed infarction. Am J Cardiol 42:724, 1978.

PREEXERCISE AND POSTEXERCISE TRAINING STUDIES

Atwood E, Jensen D, Froelicher V, et al: Radionuclide perfusion images before and after cardiac rehabilitation. Aviat Space Environ Med 51:892, 1980.

Froelicher VF, Jensen DG, Atwood E, et al: Evidence for improvement in myocardial perfusion and function after cardiac rehabilitation. Arch Phys Med Rehabil 61:517, 1980.

Gruntzig AR, Senning A, Siegenthaler WE: Nonoperative dilatation of coronary-artery stenosis: Percutaneous transluminal coronary angioplasty. N Engl J Med 301:61, 1979.

Iskandrian AS, Haaz W, Segal BL, et al: Exercise thallium 201 scintigraphy in evaluating aortocoronary bypass surgery. Chest 80:1, 1981.

Jensen D, Atwood JE, Froelicher V, et al: Improvement in ventricular function during exercise following cardiac rehabilitation. Am J Cardiol 46:770, 1980.

Kent KM, Borer JS, Green MV, et al: Effects of coronary-artery bypass on global and regional left ventricular function during exercise. N Engl J Med 298:1434, 1978.

Ritchie JL, Narahara KA, Trobaugh GB, et al: Thallium-201 myocardial imaging before and after coronary revascularization: Assessment of regional myocardial blood flow and graft patency. Circulation 56:830, 1977.

Tubau J, Witztum K, Froelicher V, et al: Reliability of radionuclide techniques in assessing changes in left ventricular perfusion and performance after cardiac rehabilitation. Am Heart J July 1982.

PERFEXT—A RANDOMIZED TRIAL OF THE EFFECTS OF EXERCISE ON HEART PERFUSION AND PERFORMANCE

Battler A, Ross J Jr, Slutsky R, et al: Improvement of exercise-induced left ventricular dysfunction with oral propranolol in patients with coronary heart disease. Am J Cardiol 44:318, 1979.

Gutmann MC, Squires RW, Pollock ML, et al: Perceived exertion–heart rate relationship during exercise testing and training in cardiac patients. J Cardiac Rehab 1:52, 1981.

Hindman MC, Wallace AG: Radionuclide exercise studies, in Cohen LS, Mock MB, Rinqvist I (eds): Physical Conditioning and Cardiovascular Rehabilitation. New York, John Wiley and Sons, 1981, p 33.

Slutsky R, Curtis G, Battler A, et al: Effect of sublingual nitroglycerin on left ventricular function at rest and during spontaneous angina pectoris: Assessment with radionuclides. Am J Cardiol 44:1365, 1979.

Verani MS, Hartung GH, Hoepfel-Harris J, et al: Effects of exercise training on left ventricular performance and myocardial perfusion in patients with coronary artery disease. Am J Cardiol 47:797, 1981.

Appendix: Exercise Testing and Cardiac Rehabilitation Forms

TESTING FORMS AND ILLUSTRATIONS

UNIVERSITY HOSPITAL
University of California
Medical Center, San Diego

**REPORT OF
TREADMILL EXERCISE TEST**
(PAGE ONE)

Rev. Code **750**

SEND REPORT TO							
				MD			*Patient Identification*
TMT NO.	AGE	SEX	WT (lbs)	HT (in)			
					Source	Request Date	Procedure No. 013 ☐

☐ INPATIENT   DATE (Mo., Day, Yr.)   24 HR. TIME   **CLINICAL REASONS FOR TEST**
☐ OUTPATIENT

DIAGNOSIS OF ATYPICAL SENSATION OR PAIN POSSIBLY DUE TO ASCVD (Explain)
☐

PREVIOUS TEST   HOURS SINCE LAST MEAL
☐ No   ☐ Yes, when:

MEDICATIONS | **EVALUATION OF ANGINA**
☐ DIGITALIS   ☐ NITRATES | ☐ TYPICAL   ☐ VARIANT   ☐ UNSTABLE
☐ BETA-BLOCKER   ☐ QUINIDINE/PRONESTYL | **DYSRHYTHMIA EVALUATION**
☐ ANTI-HBP   ☐ OTHER | ☐ PVCs   ☐ SVT   ☐ HB   ☐ SICK SINUS   ☐ OTHER

HYPERTENSION (>140/90) | **OTHER HEART DISEASE**   ☐ VALVULAR   ☐ HEART MUSCLE
HISTORY OF HYPER-TENSION   NOW ELEVATED   SERUM K+ (mEq/L) | ☐ MITRAL PROLAPSE   ☐ CONGENITAL   ☐ OTHER
☐ Yes   ☐ No   ☐ Yes   ☐ No | EVALUATION POST AMI   TIME SINCE LAST INFARCT

ACTIVITY STATUS | ☐   WEEKS   MONTHS   YEARS
☐ RECENT BED REST   ☐ SEDENTARY   ☐ ACTIVE   ☐ ATHLETIC | SCREENING ASYMPTOMATIC INDIVIDUAL   FUNCTIONAL CAPACITY EVALUATION
CIGARETTES | ☐   ☐

EVER SMOKE   CURRENTLY SMOKING | CORONARY BYPASS SURGERY   DATE OF SURGERY & TYPE
☐ Yes   ☐ No   ☐ Yes   ☐ No | ☐ PRE   ☐ POST

NUMBER YEARS AGO STOPPED   PACK-YEARS   PACKS/DAY | OTHER   ☐

RESTING ECG   DESCRIBE
☐ NORMAL   ☐ ABNORMAL

STAGE	MPH/ GRADE	~O₂ COST	MIN/SEC IN STAGE	HR (AT END OF STAGE)	BP	DESCRIBE: CHEST PAIN/DYSRHYTHMIA/ ST SLOPE/AMOUNT J-JCT UP OR DOWN/LEAD(S)
SUPINE						
HV FOR 30 SEC	3.5 CC/KG-MIN BASAL = 1 MET					
STAND						
1A	2.0/0%	7				
1B	3.3/0%	14				
2	3.3/5%	20				
3	3.3/10%	28				
4	3.3/15%	36				
5	3.3/20%	44				
6	3.3/25%	52				
IMMED	MAX SBP (_____) x					
2 MIN	MAX HR (_____) =					
5 MIN	___ ___ . ___ × 10³					
___ MIN	V̇O₂ max (est. = / mxed. =					

151-069 (8-77) SIC 600

WHITE - Medical Record   CANARY - Referring MD   PINK - Cardiology File   GREEN - Research File

UNIVERSITY HOSPITAL
University of California
Medical Center, San Diego
Rev. Code **750**

REPORT OF
TREADMILL EXERCISE TEST
(PAGE TWO)

Patient Identification

Source   Request Date   Procedure No. 013 ☐

PROBABILITY OF ASCVD BY HISTORY PRIOR TO TEST					EXPLAIN					
☐ Unlikely ☐ Possible ☐ Probable ☐ Very Probable										

PHYSICAL EXAM	PRE	YES / NO	S₃	YES / NO	S₄	MURMUR ☐ YES ☐ NO	TYPE			
	POST	YES / NO	S₃	YES / NO	S₄	SIGNS/SYMPTOMS CHF	MURMUR ☐ YES ☐ NO	TYPE		

REASONS FOR STOPPING 1 - Primary 2 - Secondary 3 - Tertiary	CHEST PAIN		DYSPNEA		FATIGUE/ WEAKNESS		CLAUDICATION	GENERAL APPEARANCE	CNS SYMPTOMS
	HYPER-TENSION		HYPO-TENSION		ST CHANGES		DYSRHYTHMIA	TECHNICAL PROBLEM	PHYSICAL DISABILITY
	POOR PATIENT COOPERATION		LEG PAIN		OTHER (Explain)				

ECG RESPONSE	DYSRHYTHMIA	NO EXPLAIN	OCC PVC	FREQ PVC	VT	SVT	AF
	ST SEGMENTS	NL EXPLAIN	BORDERLINE	ABNL	ELEVATE		NORMALIZE
	CONDUCTION	NL EXPLAIN	LBBB	RBBB	BLOCK		AXIS SHIFT

PATIENT RESPONSE	MAX HR ☐ NL ☐ HI ☐ LO		MAX SYSTOLIC BP ☐ NL ☐ HI ☐ LO		FUNCTIONAL CAPACITY ☐ NL ☐ HI ☐ LO	
	ANGINA ☐ YES ☐ NO	ATYPICAL CHEST PAIN ☐ YES ☐ NO	CHF ☐ YES ☐ NO	OTHER COMPLICATIONS ☐ YES ☐ NO	MAXIMAL EFFORT ☐ YES ☐ NO	

INTERPRETATION

INTERPRETED BY: _____ DATE: _____

APPROVED BY: _____ DATE: _____

UNIVERSITY HOSPITAL
University of California
Medical Center, San Diego

TREADMILL TEST WORKSHEET

PATIENT NUMBER	TAPE OR CASSETTE NUMBER	DATE (mo., day, yr.)	24 HOUR TIME

☐ Thallium ☐ Routine	AGE	SEX ☐ M ☐ F	WEIGHT (pounds)	HEIGHT (inches)	> 3 HOURS SINCE LAST MEAL ☐ Yes ☐ No

PRESCRIBED MEDICATIONS

Digitalis	☐ No ☐ Yes	amount _____ mg/day	stopped? ☐ No ☐ Yes	when? _____ (days)
Betablockers	☐ No ☐ Yes	amount _____ mg/day	stopped? ☐ No ☐ Yes	when? _____ (days)
Others	☐ No ☐ Yes	list:		

CLINICAL INFORMATION

			RESTING ECG

History of Angina   ☐ Yes ☐ No
Atypical CP   ☐ Yes ☐ No
MI   ☐ Yes ☐ No
date of last MI: __mo.__ __day__ __yr.__

CABS   ☐ Yes ☐ No
date: __mo.__ __day__ __yr.__

☐ Pre-Rehab   Mo. of Rehab ____   ☐ Post-Rehab

RESTING ECG:
☐ NL   ☐ ABNL   ☐ LBBB   ☐ RBBB   ☐ LVH with strain
☐ IVCD   ☐ LAD   ☐ PVC   ☐ NSSTW

	INF	ANT	LAT	POST
QW (Infarct)	☐	☐	☐	☐
ST Elevation	☐	☐	☐	☐
ST Depression	☐	☐	☐	☐
Inverted TW	☐	☐	☐	☐

POST TM	**NEW FINDINGS** ☐ S₃ ☐ S₄ ☐ Murmur ☐ Bulge

RESPONSES	SBP ☐ Normal ☐ Inadequate rise ☐ Drop	DBP ☐ Rise amount:

REASON(S) FOR STOPPING
☐ Angina   ☐ ST Changes   ☐ Fatigue   ☐ SOB   ☐ Claudication   ☐ Dysrhythmia

EXERCISE-INDUCED ECG CHANGES
☐ Normal   ☐ Abnormal:

DYSRHYTHMIA	☐ No ☐ Occ PVC ☐ Freq PVC ☐ VT ☐ SVT ☐ AF
	EXPLAIN

ST DEPRESSION (Amount in mm and slope)	INF	ANT	LAT	U = Upsloping D = Downward H = Flat
ST ELEVATION	INF	ANT	LAT	☐ RBBB ☐ LBBB ☐ LAD

PATIENT RESPONSE	ANGINA ☐ Yes ☐ No	ATYPICAL CHEST PAIN ☐ Yes ☐ No	CHF ☐ Yes ☐ No
	OTHER COMPLICATIONS ☐ Yes ☐ No		MAXIMAL EFFORT ☐ Yes ☐ No

STAGE	MPH/GRADE	~O₂ COST	MIN/SEC IN STAGE	HR	BP	ANGINA (1 - 4 +)	ECG CHANGES
					(AT END OF STAGE)		
SUPINE							
HV FOR 30 SEC	3.5 CC/KG-MIN BASAL = 1 MET						
STAND							
1A	2.0/0%	7					
1B	3.3/0%	14					
2	3.3/5%	20					
3	3.3/10%	28					
4	3.3/15%	36					
5	3.3/20%	44					
6	3.3/25%	52					
IMMED STD	MAX SBP (_____) x						
1 MIN SUPINE	MAX HR (_____) =						
5 MIN	____ ____ . ____ × 10³						
___ MIN	V̇O₂ max { est. = / mxed. = }						

INTERPRETATION

INTERPRETED BY	APPROVED BY

B178(7-80)6   ORIGINAL - Cardiac Rehab   COPY - Nuclear Medicine

TREADMILL FORM

NAME [   ]   PERFEXT # [   ]   UNIT # [   ]

DATE [   ]   24 HOUR TIME [   ]   TAPE/CASSETTE NUMBER [   ]

SOCIAL SECURITY # [   ]

[   ]   TEST TYPE   1 = VO_2; 2 = Thallium; 3 = Routine

[   ]   TEST PERIOD   1 = Initial; 2 = 3 Months; 3 = 6 Months;
                           4 = 1 Year; 5 = Other _____

[   ]   ON FLOPPIES   1 = No; 2 = Yes

[   ]   CURRENT MEDICATION STATUS:

```
0 = None                              NAME _____
1 = ON Digoxin                                 mg _____ x/day
NAME _____                 6 = ON Anti-Dysrhythmics
         mg _____ x/day             NAME _____
 2 = OFF Digoxin                              mg _____ x/day
LAST DOSE _____            7 = ON NTG
3 = ON Beta Blockers                  NAME _____
NAME _____                        mg _____ x/day
         mg _____ x/day             8 = OFF NTG
4 = OFF Beta Blockers 3 Days          LAST DOSE _____
LAST DOSE _____            9 = Other _____
5 = ON Anti-Hypertensives                     _____ mg _____ x/day
NAME _____
         mg _____ x/day
```

[   ]   RESTING ECG:

0 = NOT DONE; 1 = NL; 2 = ABNL; 3 = LBBB; 4 = RBBB; 5 = LVH; 6 = IVCD;
7 = LAD; 8 = PVC; 9 = NSSTW

	INF	ANT	LAT	POST
Q WAVE (INFARCT)	10	11	12	13
ST ELEVATION	14	15	16	17
ST DEPRESSION	18	19	20	21
INVERTED T WAVE	22	23	24	25

[   ]   REASON(S) FOR STOPPING:

0 = None; 1 = Angina; 2 = ST changes; 3 = Fatigue; 4 = SOB;
5 = Claudication; 6 = Dysrhythmias; 7 = Atypical Chest Pain; 8 = SBP Drop;
9 = Abnl SBP Rise; 10 = Leg Pain; 11 = Max Exercise; 12 = Other_____

[   ]   EXERCISE INDUCED CHANGES:

0 = None; 1 = Occ PVCs; 2 = Freq PVCs; 3 = VT; 4 = SVT; 5 = AF; 6 = RBBB;
7 = LBBB; 8 = LAD; 9 = ST; 10 = Angina

	INF	CODE	ANT	CODE	LAT	CODE
ST DEPRESSION (mm)						
ST ELEVATION (mm)						

CODES: 1 = Upsloping; 2 = Downward; 3 = Flat

STAGE	MPH/GRADE	O_2 COST	MIN/SEC STAGE	HR	BLOOD PRESSURE SBP/DBP	ANGINA (1-4+)	PE	COMMENTS
SUPINE								
STAND								
	2.0/0%	7			/			
	3.3/0%	14			/			
	3.3/5%	20			/			
	3.3/10%	28			/			
	3.3/15%	36			/			
	3.3/20%	44			/			
	3.3/25%	52			/			
RECOVERY: IMMEDIATE STANDING					/			
2 Min SUPINE					/			
5 Min SUPINE					/			
Min					/			

Max Ex SBP   [   ]

Max Ex HR   [   ]

VO$_2$ Max: Est [   ]

Measured   [   ]

INTERPRETATION:

Interpreted   Approved

UNIVERSITY HOSPITAL
University of California Medical Center
San Diego

THALLIUM²⁰¹ IMAGING DATA SHEET

B036(9-80)6

Tape/Cassette # _____ Tape/Cassette # _____ Tape/Cassette # _____

Magnetic Tape _____

NAME

UNIT NUMBER

DATE

MANUFACTURER

CAMERA

COLLIMATOR

MINS. EXERCISE POST INJ.

INJECTION TIME (EXACT)

(Start Timer)

FLOOD UNIFORMITY
☐ Yes ☐ No

DOSE

PHYSICIAN

IV SITE

ECG/NUC MED TECH

TIME EXERCISE STARTED

Technique and Positional Variants (state image number)

Interpretation

DELAYS (____ Hours)	IMMEDIATE DELAYS	IMMEDIATE

IMMEDIATE

LAO 45° Image # _____
ID Location _____
Position Comments (V-Lead and Origin) _____
Time Post Inj. _____
Camera Started _____
Acquisition Time _____
Total ID _____

ANTERIOR Image # _____
ID Location _____
Position Comments (V-Lead and Origin) _____
Time Post Inj. _____
Camera Started _____
Acquisition Time _____
Total ID _____

LAO 70° Image # _____
ID Location _____
Position Comments (V-Lead and Origin) _____
Time Post Inj. _____
Camera Started _____
Acquisition Time _____
Total ID _____

IMMEDIATE DELAYS

LAO 45° Image # _____
ID Location _____
Position Comments (V-Lead and Origin) _____
Time Post Inj. _____
Camera Started _____
Acquisition Time _____
Total ID _____

ANTERIOR Image # _____
ID Location _____
Position Comments (V-Lead and Origin) _____
Time Post Inj. _____
Camera Started _____
Acquisition Time _____
Total ID _____

LAO 70° Image # _____
ID Location _____
Position Comments (V-Lead and Origin) _____
Time Post Inj. _____
Camera Started _____
Acquisition Time _____
Total ID _____

DELAYS (____ Hours)

LAO 45° Image # _____
ID Location _____
Position Comments (V-Lead and Origin) _____
Time Post Inj. _____
Camera Started _____
Acquisition Time _____
Total ID _____

ANTERIOR Image # _____
ID Location _____
Position Comments (V-Lead and Origin) _____
Time Post Inj. _____
Camera Started _____
Acquisition Time _____
Total ID _____

LAO 70° Image # _____
ID Location _____
Position Comments (V-Lead and Origin) _____
Time Post Inj. _____
Camera Started _____
Acquisition Time _____
Total ID _____

UNIVERSITY HOSPITAL
University of California Medical Center
San Diego

RADIONUCLIDE IMAGING WORKSHEET

NAME		PERFEXT #	UNIT #		CASS OR TAPE #	MAG TAPE #		DATE

MASTER DISK	ON LINE TRANS?	PRODUCT AND MANUFACTURER						LOT #

AGE	HT	WT		BSA		CRIT		DATE OF CRIT

COLLIMATOR

POSITION
LAO _____ with Caudal Tilt

POSITIONAL VARIANTS

Patient Dose _____ mCi – in _____ ml

– Sur _____ mCi

= Act Inj _____ mCi

Standard Dose _____ mCi – in _____ ml

– Sur _____ mCi

= Act Inj _____ mCi

TIME OF INJECTION

TIME OF EXERCISE

EKG TECH	QUALITY OF STUDY	COMMENTS	COMMENTS Q	HR / BP	EF	ESV	EDV	ESC	EDC	e (t, 115)	FACE CPM	TRIPOD CPM	TIME COUNTED	TOTAL CTS	CTS FMS	NUMBER CYCLES	TIME FM	TIME DRAWN	STAGE
																			REST SITTING
																			REST SUPINE
NUC MED TECH																			EX – 1
PHYSICIAN																			

B082(11-80)6   WHITE - Nuclear Medicine   CANARY - Cardiac Rehab

NAME

PERFEXT #

DATE

Intensity was graded 1-4: 1=normal myocardial activity; 2=just less than normal; 3=just greater than background activity; and 4=equal to background activity.
Size was graded 1-5: 1= a lesion of at least 10% of the segment; 2=more than 20%; 3=more than 30%; 4=more than 40%; and 5=more than 50%.

Severity	Intensity paired with size
1	1,1; 1,2; 1,3; 1,4; 1,5
2	2,1
3	2,2; 3,1
4	2,3
5	3,2; 4,1
6	2,4; 3,3
7	4,2
8	2,5; 3,4; 4,3
9	3,5; 4,4
10	4,5

ANTERIOR   LAO-45   LAO-70

GRADE
SEGMENTS INVOLVED

DEFECTS

IMMEDIATE: INTENSITY
              SIZE

IMMED. DELAY: INTENSITY
              SIZE

DELAY: INTENSITY
              SIZE

ANTERIOR LATERAL INFERIOR SEPTAL APICAL

	3	7	6	9	1	9	4	2	5	8
IMMEDIATE:										
SEVERITY										
AVERAGE										
IMMED DELAY:	3	7	6	9	1	9	4	2	5	8
SEVERITY										
AVERAGE										
DELAY:	3	7	6	9	1	9	4	2	5	8
SEVERITY										
AVERAGE										

COMMENTS

LUNG UPTAKE SCALE 1 - 4
1 = NO UPTAKE   4 = SAME AS LV

IMMEDIATE
IMMEDIATE DELAY
DELAY

UNIVERSITY HOSPITAL
University of California
Medical Center, San Diego

**REPORT OF SUPINE BIKE
RADIONUCLIDE EXERCISE TEST**

(DATA PAGE)

SEND REPORT TO

_____ MD

TMT #	AGE	SEX	WT(lbs)	HT (in)			
					Source	Request Date	Patient Identification

☐ INPATIENT   DATE (mo./day/yr)   24 HOUR TIME
☐ OUTPATIENT

CLINICAL REASONS FOR TEST

MEDICATIONS

☐ DIGITALIS   ☐ NITRATES
☐ BETA-BLOCKER   ☐ QUINIDINE/PRONESTYL
☐ ANTI-HBP   ☐ OTHER

DIAGNOSIS OF ATYPICAL SENSATION OR PAIN POSSIBLY DUE TO ASCVD (Explain)
☐

EVALUATION OF ANGINA
☐ TYPICAL   ☐ VARIANT   ☐ UNSTABLE

HYPERTENSION (> 140/90)   > 3 HRS SINCE LAST MEAL

HISTORY OF HYPER-TENSION	NOW ELEVATED	☐ Yes ☐ No
☐ Yes ☐ No	☐ Yes ☐ No	

DYSRHYTHMIA EVALUATION
☐ PVCs   ☐ SVT   ☐ HB   ☐ SICK SINUS   ☐ OTHER

OTHER HEART DISEASE ☐ VALVULAR   ☐ HEART MUSCLE
☐ MITRAL PROLAPSE ☐ CONGENITAL   ☐ OTHER

ACTIVITY STATUS
☐ RECENT BED REST   ☐ SEDENTARY   ☐ ACTIVE   ☐ ATHLETIC

EVALUATION POST AMI TIME SINCE LAST INFARCT
☐   WEEKS   MONTHS   YEARS

CIGARETTES

EVER SMOKE   CURRENTLY SMOKING
☐ Yes   ☐ No   ☐ Yes   ☐ No

SCREENING ASYMPTOMATIC INDIVIDUAL   ABNORMAL ECG EXERCISE TEST
☐   ☐

NUMBER YEARS AGO STOPPED   PACK-YEARS   PACKS/DAY

CARDIAC SURGERY   DATE OF SURGERY & TYPE
☐ PRE ☐ POST

RADIOPHARMACEUTICAL   DOSE
                        mi Cu

OTHER
☐

RESTING ECG   DESCRIBE
☐ NORMAL   ☐ ABNORMAL

STAGE	KILOPONDS	MIN/SEC IN STAGE	HR	BP (AT END OF STAGE)	EF	WALL MOTION	LV VOLUME DIAS	LV VOLUME SYS	COMMENTS
SUPINE REST									
1									
2									
3									
Peak Exercise									

REASONS FOR STOPPING
☐ CHEST PAIN   ☐ DYSPNEA   ☐ ST CHANGES   ☐ DYSRHYTHMIA   ☐ TECHNICAL PROBLEMS
☐ PHYSICAL DISABILITY   ☐ LEG PAIN   ☐ POOR PATIENT COOPERATION   ☐ MAXIMAL EFFORT   ☐ OTHER:

☐ POST EXERCISE   ☐ POST INTERVENTION WITH:

	MINUTES								
1	___ TO ___								
2	___ TO ___								
3	___ TO ___								

WALL MOTION CODE: (1) Location: A = anterior I = inferior Ap = apical S = septal P = posterior
(2) Motion: N = normal R = reduced D = dyskinetic Ay = aneurysm Ak = akinetic

B 103 (9-78) SIC 600

BLUE · Medical Record   WHITE · Referring MD   PINK · Nuclear Medicine   CANARY · Exercise Lab

UNIVERSITY HOSPITAL
University of California
Medical Center, San Diego

REPORT OF SUPINE BIKE
RADIONUCLIDE EXERCISE TEST

(INTERPRETATION PAGE)

		Source		Request Date			Patient Identification	

		NO	OCC PVC	FREQ PVC	VT	SVT	AF
ECG RESPONSE	**DYSRHYTHMIA**	EXPLAIN					
		NORMAL	BORDERLINE	ABNORMAL	ELEVATE	NORMALIZE	
	ST SEGMENTS	EXPLAIN					

PATIENT RESPONSE	**ANGINA** ☐ YES ☐ NO	**ATYPICAL CHEST PAIN** ☐ YES ☐ NO	**CHF** ☐ YES ☐ NO	**OTHER COMPLICATIONS** ☐ NO ☐ YES **Describe:**

	RESTING	NORMAL	ABNORMAL:
EF RESPONSE	**EXERCISE**	NORMAL	ABNORMAL:
	INTERVENTION	NORMAL	ABNORMAL:

INTERPRETATION

INTERPRETED BY: _____   DATE: _____

APPROVED BY: _____   DATE: _____

B 103 (9-78) SIC 600

BLUE - Medical Record   WHITE - Referring MD   PINK - Nuclear Medicine   CANARY - Exercise Lab

DEPARTMENT OF MEDICINE

UNIVERSITY HOSPITAL

UNIVERSITY OF CALIFORNIA – SAN DIEGO

Exercise Heart Function Study

by Report

The Exercise Heart Function Study is an evaluation of the ventricle's response to exercise to aid in the detection of heart disease, usually coronary heart disease. The patient is informed of all aspects of the test, and consent is obtained before the procedure is begun.

This procedure is performed in the supine position with the patient's feet strapped to a bicycle ergometer. Blood pressure, electrocardiography (ECG), heart rate, and signs and symptoms are carefully monitored·throughout the entire test. The patient is asked to exercise to the point of: (a) chest pain, (b) noted ECG or blood pressure abnormalities, or (c) fatigue. The cardiologist present may elect to terminate the test· at any time.

During the exercise a nuclear scintillation camera is continually recording the small radioactivity that is being emitted from the patient. The radiopharmaceutical technetium-99m is used and introduced, using a small needle inserted in the arm vein, just prior to the start of exercise. Processing this information enables the referring physician to assess a patient's ventricular function, both at rest and during exercise. This information has been shown to be very sensitive in detecting heart disease as well as in helping to determine patient prognosis after myocardial infarction.

At all times during the procedure, the safety and well-being of the patient are of primary concern. Only trained personnel will participate and emergency equipment will always be available should the remote possibility of any untoward reaction occur.

The dose of radioactivity used is small and does not exceed approximately one-fifth of the permissible yearly dose for hospital workers using radioactive materials. This is considered to be a safe level.

It is understood that the patient may refuse to undergo this procedure at any time without affecting future care, reimbursement of expenses, employment status, or other entitlements. Similarly, the responsible physician may terminate the test at any time.

UNIVERSITY HOSPITAL
University of California
Medical Center, San Diego

EXERCISE HEART FUNCTION WORKSHEET

PATIENT NAME	PERFEXT NUMBER

UNIT NUMBER	TAPE OR CASSETTE NUMBER	DATE (mo., day,yr.)	24 HOUR TIME

AGE	SEX ☐M ☐F	WEIGHT (pounds)	HEIGHT (inches)	> 3 HOURS SINCE LAST MEAL ☐Yes ☐No

PRESCRIBED MEDICATIONS

Digitalis	☐No ☐Yes	amount _____ mg/day	stopped?	☐No ☐Yes	when? _____	(days)
Betablockers	☐No ☐Yes	amount _____ mg/day	stopped?	☐No ☐Yes	when? _____	(days)
Others	☐No ☐Yes	list:				

CLINICAL INFORMATION

History of Angina ☐Yes ☐No
  Atypical CP ☐Yes ☐No
MI ☐Yes ☐No
  mo. ___ day ___ yr. ___
  date of last MI:
CABS ☐Yes ☐No
  mo. ___ day ___ yr. ___
  date:

☐Pre-Rehab   Mo. of Rehab ___   ☐Post-Rehab

RESTING ECG

☐NL ☐ABNL ☐LBBB ☐RBBB ☐LVH with stain

☐IVCD ☐LAD ☐PVC ☐NSSTW

	INF	ANT	LAT	POST
QW (Infarct)	☐	☐	☐	☐
ST Elevation	☐	☐	☐	☐
ST Depression	☐	☐	☐	☐
Inverted TW	☐	☐	☐	☐

STAGE	WORK LOAD	STAGE LENGTH	HR	BP	LV VOLUMES EDV₁	EDV₂	ESV₁	ESV₂	EF	WALL MOTION	1 - 4+ ANGINA	Q̇	ECG/ COMMENTS
REST SIT													
REST SUPINE													

VOLUMES: 1 = UCSD   2 = J. Hopkins
WALL MOTION
  LOCATION: A = Anterior   I = Inferior   Ap = Apical   S = Septal   P = Posterior
  MOTION: N = Normal   H = Hypokinetic   Ak = Akinetic   D = Dyskinetic   An = Aneurysm

RESPONSES

SBP ☐Normal ☐Inadequate rise ☐Drop	DBP ☐Rise, amount:

REASON(S) FOR STOPPING
☐Angina   ☐ST Changes   ☐Fatigue   ☐SOB   ☐Claudication   ☐Dysrhythmia

EXERCISE-INDUCED ECG CHANGES

☐Normal ☐Abnormal:

DYSRHYTHMIA	☐No ☐Occ PVC ☐Freq PVC ☐VT ☐SVT ☐AF
	EXPLAIN

ST DEPRESSION (Amount in mm and slope)	INF	ANT	LAT	U = Upsloping D = Downward H = Flat
ST ELEVATION	INF	ANT	LAT	☐RBBB ☐LBBB ☐LAD

PATIENT RESPONSE	ANGINA ☐Yes ☐No	ATYPICAL CHEST PAIN ☐Yes ☐No	CHF ☐Yes ☐No
	OTHER COMPLICATIONS ☐Yes ☐No		MAXIMAL EFFORT ☐Yes ☐No

INTERPRETATION

INTERPRETED BY	APPROVED BY

B045(10-80)6   ORIGINAL - Cardiac Rehab   COPY - Nuclear Medicine

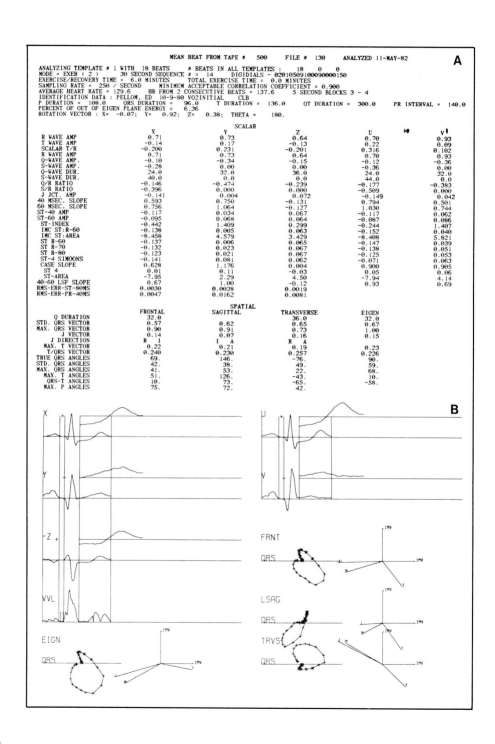

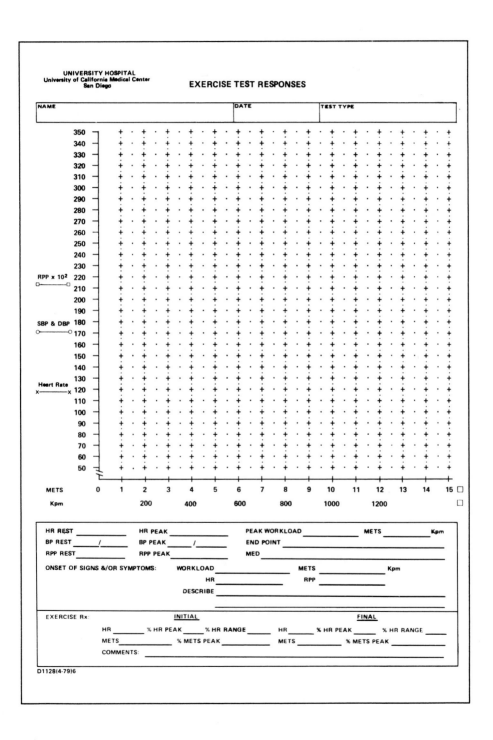

UNIVERSITY HOSPITAL
University of California Medical Center
San Diego

EXERCISE TEST RESPONSES

NAME	DATE	TEST TYPE

METS   0   1   2   3   4   5   6   7   8   9   10   11   12   13   14   15 □

Kpm   200   400   600   800   1000   1200   □

RPP x 10²   □———□   (220–210 region)

SBP & DBP   ○———○   (180–170 region)

Heart Rate   x———x   (120 region)

HR REST _____	HR PEAK _____	PEAK WORKLOAD _____ METS _____ Kpm
BP REST ____ / ____	BP PEAK ____ / ____	END POINT _____
RPP REST _____	RPP PEAK _____	MED _____

ONSET OF SIGNS &/OR SYMPTOMS: WORKLOAD _____   METS _____ Kpm

                                     HR _____   RPP _____

                                     DESCRIBE _____

EXERCISE Rx: **INITIAL**   **FINAL**

         HR _____ % HR PEAK _____ % HR RANGE _____   HR _____ % HR PEAK _____ % HR RANGE _____

         METS _____ % METS PEAK _____   METS _____ % METS PEAK _____

         COMMENTS: _____

D1128(4-79)6

WOMEN AND EXERCISE TESTING:
STUDIES EVALUATING THE SENSITIVITY AND SPECIFICITY
(THE LAST TWO ARE FOLLOW-UP STUDIES,
THE REST USED ANGIOGRAPHIC END POINTS)

Principal Investigator	Year	No.	Sensitivity (%)	Specificity (%)
Caru	1978	168	73	74
Cahen	1978	100	88	92
Sketch	1975	56	50	78
Detry	1977	45	89	63
Linhart	1974	98	71	78
Lesbre	1978	150	66	77
Broustet	1978	84	50	70
Barolsky	1979	92	60	68
Weiner	1979	580	76	64
Guiteras val	1982	112	79	66
Manca	1979	508	88	73
Bengtsson	1981	194	—	85

ANGIOGRAPHIC STUDIES USING COMPUTERIZED EXERCISE ELECTROCARDIOGRAPHY FOR DIAGNOSIS OF CORONARY HEART DISEASE

First Author	No. in Study	Mean Age	Computer Criteria for Ischemia	Standard Visual Analysis		Computer Analysis	
				Sensi-tivity (%)	Specific-ity (%)	Sensi-tivity (%)	Specific-ity (%)
McHenry	86 Patients	50	ST index	63	—	82	95
Sheffield	31 Patients 41 Normals	48 56	ST integral (using QRS end)	Not given		81	95
Sketch	107 Patients	48	ST integral (using R wave on Viagraph)	59	92	58	88
Turner	125 Patients	48	ST index (Quinton analog system)	Not given		82	83
Forlini	71 Patients 62 Normals	53 44	Isolated ST integral	Not given		85	90
Hollenberg	70 Patients 46 Normals	53 23	Treadmill score (Marquette CASE)	71	82	85	91
Simoons	Initial: 52 Patients 86 Normals	21–65	ST 60 with heart rate considered	50	94	85	91
	Test: 43 Patients 43 Normals	21–65		51	95	84	88

LEFT MAIN DISEASE AND EXERCISE TESTING:
STUDIES EVALUATING THE PREDICTIVE VALUE AND SENSITIVITY OF THE EXERCISE TEST FOR IDENTIFYING PATIENTS WITH LEFT MAIN CORONARY ARTERY DISEASE

Principal Investigator	Year	No. with Left Main Disease (total)	Criterion	Predictive Value (%)	Sensitivity (%)
Cheitlin	1975	11 (106)	0.2 mV depression	24	100
Goldschlager	1976	15 (410)	0.1 mV downsloping	8	67
McNeer	1978	108 (1,472)	0.1 mV in stage I or II	23	47
Nixon	1979	26 (115)	Angina or 0.1 mV depression at low work load	19 26	96 54
Levites, Anderson	1978	11 (75)	0.2 mV depression abnormal in stage I	50 24	82 63
Morris	1978	18 (460)	Extertional hypotension	14	17
Weiner	1981	35 (436)	"Markedly positive" Exertional hypotension	32 23	74 23
Blumenthal	1981	14 (40)	0.2 mV depression Anterior and inferior depression Exertional hypotension	38 57 75	100 93 21
Sanmarco	1980	29 (378)	0.3 mV only Exertional hypotension Both	15 15 27	24 28 35

Predictive value = % of those with abnormal response who have left main disease as defined by criteria; sensitivity = % of those with left main disease who have an abnormal response as defined by the investigators.

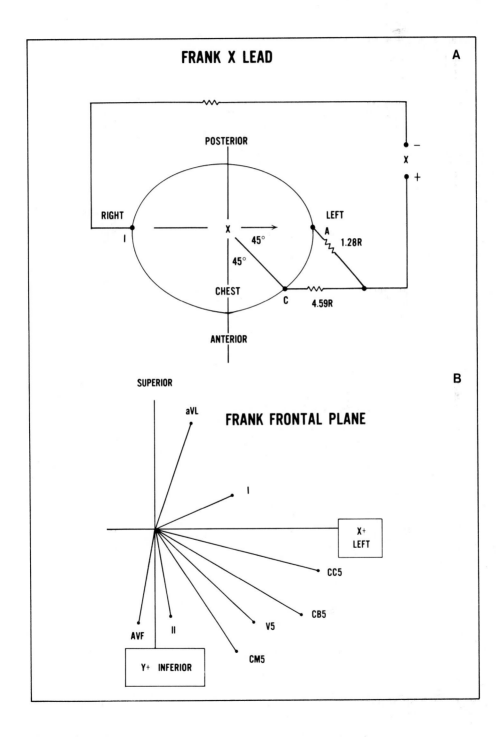

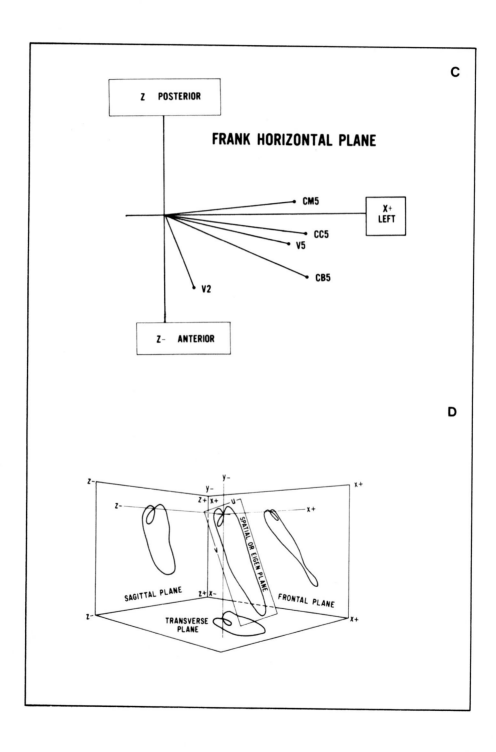

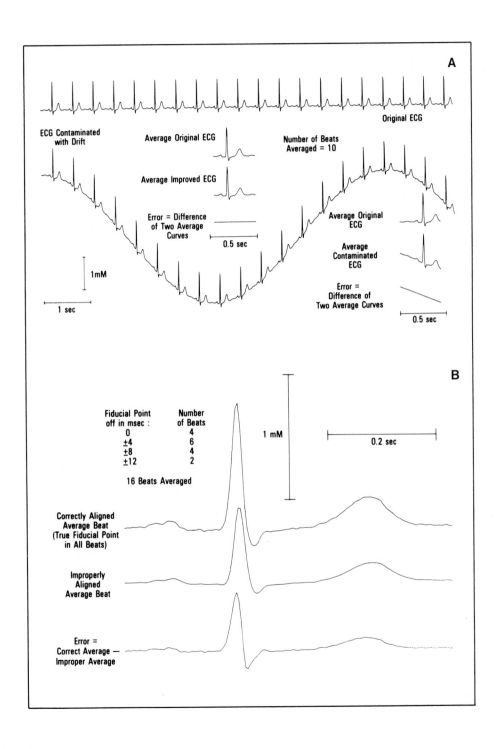

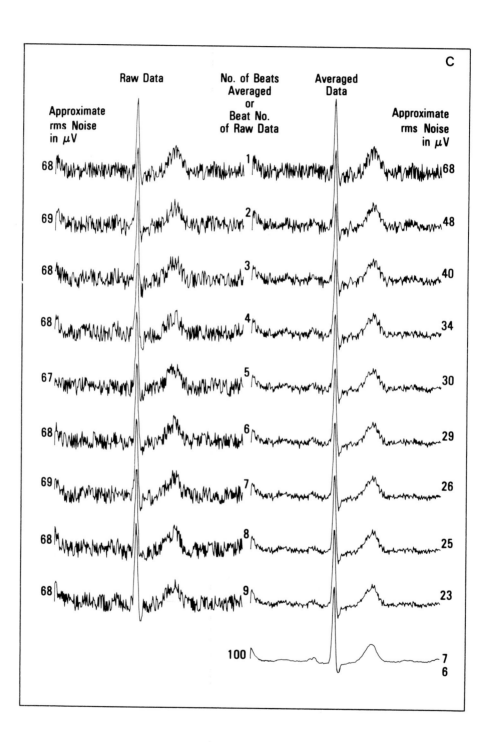

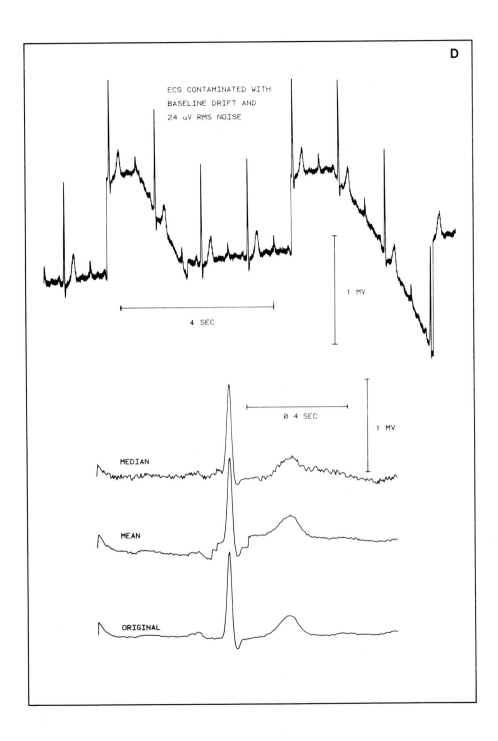

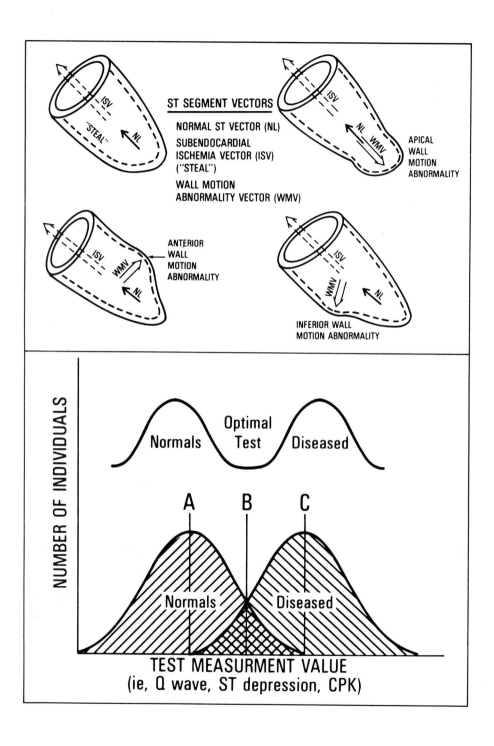

ST SEGMENT VECTORS

NORMAL ST VECTOR (NL)

SUBENDOCARDIAL
ISCHEMIA VECTOR (ISV)
("STEAL")

WALL MOTION
ABNORMALITY VECTOR (WMV)

APICAL
WALL
MOTION
ABNORMALITY

ANTERIOR
WALL
MOTION
ABNORMALITY

INFERIOR WALL
MOTION ABNORMALITY

NUMBER OF INDIVIDUALS

Optimal
Normals   Test   Diseased

A   B   C

Normals   Diseased

TEST MEASURMENT VALUE
(ie, Q wave, ST depression, CPK)

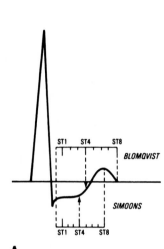

A ST amplitude at time-normalized ST midpoint.

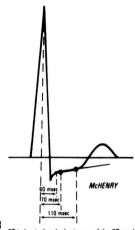

B ST index is the algebraic sum of the ST amplitude in mm (the average of two sample points at 60 msec and 70 msec) and the ST slope in mV/sec (measured between the two points at 70 msec and 110 msec after R peak).

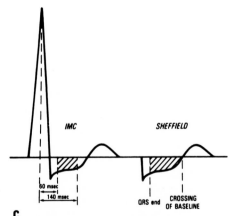

C ST integral calculated by the IMC system measures the area below the baseline from 60 msec to 140 msec beyond the peak of the R wave. Sheffield measures the area from the QRS end to the crossing of the baseline.

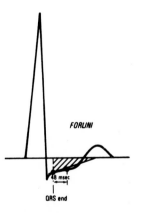

D The isolated ST integral is the area bounded by the isoelectric baseline and a line drawn from the QRS end to the baseline passing through a point 48 msec beyond the QRS end.

Appendix: Exercise Testing and Cardiac Rehabilitation Forms

TRAINING FORMS

UNIVERSITY HOSPITAL
University of California
Medical Center, San Diego

**CARDIOVASCULAR
REHABILITATION
HISTORY QUESTIONNAIRE**

INSTRUCTIONS: Answer questions in sections 1-5 only when response is "Yes".

ADMINISTERED BY

Patient Identification

AGE	SOCIAL SECURITY NO.		TELEPHONE: HOME/WORK
		Source Date	

1) The patient has been hospitalized for ischemic episode(s):
(specify type)

☐ Yes   ☐ No

☐ Myocardial infarct   ☐ Angina
☐ Unstable angina   ☐ "Rule out" infarct or uncertain

a) Hospital records or ECGs suggest the following
(give month and year)
1. Unstable preinfarction angina: _____

2. Transmural infarction (Q waves): _____
   circle location(s): anterior, inferior, posterior, lateral

3. Subendocardial infarction (ST-T changes): _____
   circle location(s): anterior, inferior, posterior, lateral

b) Circle complications: CHF   Low BP or Shock   VT - VF - AF -
   PVCs - Heart Block - Pacemaker

c) Last admission occurred: (day, month, year) _____

Pertinent Details: _____

2) The patient has had coronary angiography performed.

☐ Yes   ☐ No

Number of times _____

Dates (month, year): _____

The last study showed: (Prior to coronary surgery if performed)

LV GRAM	H = Hypokinesis A = Akinesis D = Dyskinesis (paradoxical)				Ejection Fraction:
☐ Yes ☐ No ☐ Normal ☐ Abnormal	Inf	Ant	Apical	Post	_____ %

PERCENT DIAMETER REDUCTION				
Circ or Marg	LAD Before Second Perf	Distal LAD or Diagonal	Left Main	RCA

Pertinent Details: _____

3) Patient had Coronary Artery Bypass surgery.

☐ Yes   ☐ No

Date(s) (mo., day, year): _____

	LAD	Diagonal	LCX	Marginal	RCA
Check bypass location					
If angio performed post-op enter P for patent; O for obstructed.					

Complications of surgery: _____

4) History of chest pain that is possibly ischemic:
(Check all applicable)

☐ Yes   ☐ No

☐ Atypical
☐ Typical angina pectoris
☐ Typical partially controlled by medications
☐ Typical controlled by medications
☐ Had angina but it disappeared

Pertinent Details: _____

5) The patient is on medications (Check and enter all applicable):

☐ Yes   ☐ No

FOR ANGINA:
☐ NTG (Number per day) _____ /day
☐ Inderal _____ mg _____ x/day
☐ Long acting NTG _____ mg _____ x/day
☐ (name) _____ mg _____ x/day

FOR DISRHYTHMIAS:
☐ Quinidine/Pronestyl _____ mg _____ x/day
☐ Inderal _____ mg _____ x/day
☐ Other (name) _____ mg _____ x/day
☐ (name) _____ mg _____ x/day

FOR CONGESTIVE HEART FAILURE
☐ Diuretic (name) _____ mg _____ x/day
☐ (name) _____ mg _____ x/day
☐ Digoxin _____ mg _____ x/day
☐ Other (name) _____ mg _____ x/day

FOR HIGH BLOOD PRESSURE
☐ Diuretic (name) _____ mg _____ x/day
☐ Inderal _____ mg _____ x/day
☐ Other (name) _____ mg _____ x/day
☐ (name) _____ mg _____ x/day

Others:

6) MEDICAL HISTORY

?	No	Past	Current	
☐	☐	☐	☐	1) Dysrhythmias (circle: VT, PVCs, Heart Block, SVT, AF)
☐	☐	☐	☐	2) Congestive Heart Failure (circle: signs/symptoms
☐	☐	☐	☐	3) Claudication or other peripheral vascular disease

?	No	Past	Current	
☐	☐	☐	☐	4) Hypertension
☐	☐	☐	☐	5) Hyperlipidemia
☐	☐	☐	☐	6) Moderate or severe lung disease
☐	☐	☐	☐	7) Episode requiring resuscitation
☐	☐	☐	☐	8) Loss of consciousness
☐	☐	☐	☐	9) TIAs or CVA neurological defect
☐	☐	☐	☐	10) Diabetes Mellitus
☐	☐	☐	☐	11) Other:

Explain Responses:

7) Occupational Status
☐ Employed   ☐ Unemployed   ☐ Disabled   ☐ Retired
Most recent occupation:

8) Criteria for program entry include (check all applicable)
☐ Angina   ☐ Myocardial Infarct   ☐ Abnl coronary angiogram
☐ Coronary surgery   ☐ Abnl. exercise test   ☐ Asymptomatic, high risk

9) Referred By

B 093 (3-78) SIC 600   ORIGINAL - Medical Record   WHITE - Physician   CANARY - Exercise Class   GREEN - Rehabilitation

CARDIAC UCSD REHAB

UNIVERSITY HOSPITAL
University of California Medical Center
San Diego

CARDIOVASCULAR HISTORY
AND
EXERCISE TEST SUMMARY

NAME: _____

ID #: _____

AGE: _____ HT: _____ in. WT: _____ lbs.

PHONE #: H / W _____

PHYSICIAN: _____ Phone #: _____

RELATIVE/PHONE #: _____

HISTORY

☐ YES The patient has been hospitalized for ischemic episode(s):
☐ NO   (specify type)
    ☐ Myocardial infarct   ☐ Angina
    ☐ Unstable angina   ☐ "Rule out" infarct or uncertain

Last admission occurred: (day, month, year) _____

Pertinent Details: _____

☐ YES History of chest pain that is possibly ischemic:
☐ NO   (Check all applicable)
    ☐ Atypical   ☐ Typical controlled
    ☐ Typical angina pectoris   by medications
    ☐ Typical partially controlled   ☐ Had angina but it
    by medications   disappeared

Pertinent Details: _____

☐ YES The patient has had coronary angiography performed.
☐ NO   Number of times _____
    Date(s) (month, year): _____
    Check if > 50% obstruction: ☐ RCA ☐ LAD ☐ LCX

Pertinent Details: _____

☐ YES Patient had Coronary Artery Bypass surgery.
☐ NO   Date(s) (mo., day, year): _____
Complications of surgery: _____

Criteria for program entry include (check all applicable)
☐ Angina ☐ Myocardial Infarct ☐ Abnl coronary angiogram
☐ Coronary surgery ☐ Abnl exercise test ☐ Asymptomatic, high risk

LV function: _____

MEDICAL HISTORY

?	No	Past	Current		?	No	Past	Current	
☐	☐	☐	☐	1) Dysrhythmias (circle: VT, PVCs, Heart Block, SVT, AF)	☐	☐	☐	☐	4) Hypertension
☐	☐	☐	☐	2) Congestive Heart Failure (circle: signs/symptoms)	☐	☐	☐	☐	5) Hyperlipidemia
☐	☐	☐	☐	3) Claudication or other peripheral vascular disease	☐	☐	☐	☐	6) Moderate or severe lung disease
					☐	☐	☐	☐	7) Episode requiring resuscitation
					☐	☐	☐	☐	8) Loss of consciousness
					☐	☐	☐	☐	9) TIAs or CVA neurological defect
					☐	☐	☐	☐	10) Diabetes Mellitus
					☐	☐	☐	☐	11) Other:

Explain Responses:

☐ YES
☐ NO

Medication	Dosage		Medication	Dosage	
_____	____ mg	____ x/Day	_____	____ mg	____ x/Day
_____	____ mg	____ x/Day	_____	____ mg	____ x/Day
_____	____ mg	____ x/Day	_____	____ mg	____ x/Day

☐ YES Patient has orthopedic problems:
☐ NO
Describe: _____

EXERCISE TEST RESPONSES	Date ___ / ___ / ___

Test Type: ☐ Treadmill ☐ Bike

   Supine Standing

HR rest _____   HR peak _____

BP rest ___ / ___ | ___ / ___   BP peak ___ / ___

RPP peak _____

Peak Workload: _____ mph _____ % grade _____ kpm
_____ METS

ST Changes: _____

Angina: _____

Medications: _____

Dysrhythmias: _____

Other: _____

Reason(s) for stopping: 1 _____
    2 _____

Exercise Rx:

HR _____ METS _____

Walk/Run _____

Onset of signs or symptoms:

HR _____ RPP _____ METS _____

Describe: _____

D1180(8-79)3

HISTORY/PHYSICAL FORM

NAME [   ]   DATE [   ]

PERFEXT# [   ] BIRTHDATE [   ] AGE [   ] SEX [   ] GROUP [   ]

SOCIAL SECURITY #   1=M; 2=F   1 = CONTROL
                                                               2 = TRAINED.

PATIENT WAS HOSPITALIZED FOR: (1 = No; 2 = Yes; 3 = Suspected)
                                          DATE OF EVENT
[   ] Q-WAVE MI   [   ]
[   ] NON Q-WAVE MI   [   ]
[   ] UNSTABLE ANGINA   [   ]
[   ] CARDIAC CATH   [   ]
[   ] CABG   [   ]

[   ] LOCATION OF Q-WAVE MI:
       0 = None; 1 = Inferior; 2 = Anterior; 3 = Posterior; 4 = Lateral

[   ] COMPLICATION(S) OF MI (Q AND NON Q-WAVE):
       0 = None; 1 = CHF; 2 = Shock; 3 = Ectopy; 4 = Heart Block; 5 = CPR

[   ] CATH SHOWS SIGNIFICANT (<50% OCCLUSION) IN:
0 = None; 1 = RCA; 2 = LAD; 3 = LCX; 4 = LM; 5 = Marginal; 6 = Diagonal

[   ] LV GRAM   [   ] EF
(1 = Not Done; 2 = Normal; 3 = Abnormal)

[   ] CURRENT MEDICATIONS:
0 = None; 1 = Beta Blockers; 2 = NTG; 3 = Long NTG; 4 = Diuretic;
5 = Digoxin; 6 = Anti-Dysrhythmics; 7 = Anti-Hypertensives;
8 = Other_____   _____

[   ] HISTORY OF CHEST PAIN:
1 = None; 2 = Atypical; 3 = Typical; 4 = Typical-partially controlled;
5 = Typical-controlled; 6 = Previously but disappeared

HISTORY OF (1 = No; 2 = Yes; 3 = Suspected):
[   ] Dysrhythmias   [   ] Lung Disease
[   ] CHF   [   ] Resuscitation
[   ] Claudication   [   ] Loss of Consciousness
[   ] Hypertension   [   ] TIA/CVA
[   ] Hyperlipidemia   [   ] Diabetes
                                    [   ] Other
                                             _____

SMOKING HISTORY:
[   ] Ever Smoke   (1 = No; 2 = Yes; 3 = Suspected)
[   ] Smoking Now   (1 = No; 2 = Yes)
[   ] Pack/Years   [   ] Packs/Day
[   ] Number of Years Ago Quit

[   ] Occupational Status:
          1 = Employed; 2 = Unemployed; 3 = Disabled; 4 = Retired
                                    _____
PHYSICAL EXAM: (1 = No; 2 = Yes)
[   ] Bulge
[   ] Murmur
[   ] **Bruits**
[   ] <Pulses
[   ] Gallops

[   ] STATUS   1 = In Program; 2 = Drop-out
                         Date [   ]

UNIVERSITY HOSPITAL
University of California
Medical Center, San Diego

**CARDIOVASCULAR HISTORY
AND EXERCISE TEST RESPONSES**

Name _____

MD _____ Phone_____

Relative_____ Phone_____

HISTORY	**MEDICATIONS**	
	Medication	Dosage

☐ Angina _____ _____ _____mg _____x/day

☐ MI_____ _____ _____mg _____x/day

☐ CABS_____ _____ _____mg _____x/day

☐ CATH_____ _____ _____mg _____x/day

☐ HBP_____ _____ _____mg _____x/day

☐ CHF _____ _____ _____mg _____x/day

☐ Dysrhythmias_____ _____ _____mg _____x/day

☐ Claudication_____ ☐ Orthopedic Problems:

☐ COPD_____ _____

☐ TIAs_____ _____

☐ LV Function_____ _____

Comments: _____

_____

_____

EXERCISE TEST RESPONSES　　Date_____

	REST	PEAK EXER	**ONSET OF SIGNS OR SYMPTOMS**

HR _____ _____　　HR _____METS _____

BP _____ _____　　Describe _____

Functional Capacity_____METS　　_____

Test End Point(s) 1_____　　Test Meds. _____

　　　　　　　　2_____　　_____

☐ ST △_____　　Exercise Rx: HR _____METS _____

☐ Angina_____　　Comments: _____

☐ Dysrhythmias_____　　_____

D697(1-81)6

UNIVERSITY HOSPITAL
University of California
Medical Center, San Diego

CARDIAC REHABILITATION
EXERCISE TRAINING REPORT
WORKSHEET

REFERRING MD

Source   Date   Patient Identification

REPORTING PERIOD   ATTENDANCE

From (m/d/y):   To (m/d/y):   out of   sessions   (% =   )

COMPARE THE RESTING HR AND BP AND THE RESPONSES TO EXERCISE BETWEEN THE TWO DATES

RESULTS FOR (m/d/y)   RESULTS FOR (m/d/y)

BODY WEIGHT   % BODY FAT   BODY WEIGHT   % BODY FAT

RESTING HR   RESTING BP   RESTING HR   RESTING BP

EXERCISE DEVICE	WORKLOAD	METS	HEART RATE	HR/METS	WORKLOAD	METS	HEART RATE	HR/METS

AVERAGE   AVERAGE

TARGET HR   TARGET HR

METS = MULTIPLES OF THE RESTING ENERGY REQUIREMENT (1 MET = 3.5 cc O_2/Kg-min)
HR/METS = CARDIOVASCULAR RESPONSE – ENERGY DEMAND RATIO

SUMMARY AND COMMENTS:

D1138(4-79)6

WORKLOAD RECORD

NAME	
TARGET HEART RATE	

EXERCISE DEVICE	WORKLOAD
TREADMILL	MPH % GRADE
ARM ERG	KPM
STEP	METR S/MIN
ROW ERG	METR R/MIN
BIKE	KPM ( ) KP ( )
AIR DYNE	
WEIGHTS	LBS L/MIN

D738(R10-80)6   **UCSD Medical Center**

CARDIAC
UCSD **REHAB**

UNIVERSITY HOSPITAL
University of California
Medical Center, San Diego

MONTH & YEAR

Weight	Date

10 SEC

PHASE III
DAILY EXERCISE
TRAINING FORM

D1188 (R11 80)6

DATE	EXERCISE			Rest	1	2	3	4	$\bar{X}/\Sigma$	√'	Rec
	Run	Walk	HR								
			D								
A-	BP /										

1 MIN

DATE	EXERCISE			Rest	1	2	3	4	$\bar{X}/\Sigma$	√	Rec
	Run	Walk	HR								
			D								
A-	BP /										

EXERCISE HR:

DATE	EXERCISE			Rest	1	2	3	4	$\bar{X}/\Sigma$	√	Rec
	Run	Walk	HR								
			D								
A-	BP /										

DATE	EXERCISE			Rest	1	2	3	4	$\bar{X}/\Sigma$	√	Rec
	Run	Walk	HR								
			D								
A-	BP /										

DATE	EXERCISE			Rest	1	2	3	4	$\bar{X}/\Sigma$	√	Rec
	Run	Walk	HR								
			D								
A-	BP /										

DATE	EXERCISE			Rest	1	2	3	4	$\bar{X}/\Sigma$	√	Rec
	Run	Walk	HR								
			D								
A-	BP /										

PATIENT NAME

MONTHLY SUMMARY:

PATIENT NO.

UNIVERSITY HOSPITAL
University of California
Medical Center, San Diego

NAME _____

UCSD CARDIAC REHABILITATION PROGRAM
PHYSICAL ACTIVITY DIARY

TARGET HEART RATE:_____ bpm _____ /10 sec.   NOTE: USE REVERSE SIDE FOR COMMENTS.

DATE	PHYSICAL ACTIVITY Type, Distance & Time	HEART RATE					PE	Stretching & Strength Exercises
		Rest	EX 1	EX 2	EX 3	Recovery		

PERCEIVED LEVEL OF EXERTION (PE): Rate the effort for the physical activity by recording the one number that best describes it.

Very,Very Light		Very Light		Light		Somewhat Hard		Hard		Very Hard		Very, Very Hard	
6	7	8	9	10	11	12	13	14	15	16	17	18	19	20

D709(R1-81)6

NAME _____

UCSD CARDIAC REHABILITATION   ID# _____

STRENGTH AND FLEXIBILITY ASSESSMENT

DATE ⬜/⬜/⬜

GRIP STRENGTH:

Dominant: ⬜ R   ⬜ L

⬜ Kg.   ⬜ Kg.

SIT AND REACH
FLEXIBILITY SCORE:

⬜ IN.

KRAUS-WEBER TESTS:

	PASS	FAIL
1-SIT-UP		
2-SIT-UP (HOOK LYING)		
3-LEG LIFT		
4-TRUNK LIFT		
5-LEG EXTENSION		
6-TRUNK FLEXION		

DATE ⬜/⬜/⬜

GRIP STRENGTH:

Dominant: ⬜ R   ⬜ L

⬜ Kg.   ⬜ Kg.

Δ⬜ Kg.   Δ⬜ Kg.

SIT AND REACH
FLEXIBILITY SCORE:

⬜ IN.

Δ⬜ IN.

KRAUS-WEBER TESTS:

	PASS	FAIL
1-SIT-UP		
2-SIT-UP (HOOK LYING)		
3-LEG LIFT		
4-TRUNK LIFT		
5-LEG EXTENSION		
6-TRUNK FLEXION		

DATE ⬜/⬜/⬜

GRIP STRENGTH:

Dominant: ⬜ R   ⬜ L

⬜ Kg.   ⬜ Kg.

Δ⬜ Kg.   Δ⬜ Kg.

SIT AND REACH
FLEXIBILITY SCORE:

⬜ IN.

Δ⬜ IN.

KRAUS-WEBER TESTS:

	PASS	FAIL
1-SIT-UP		
2-SIT-UP (HOOK LYING)		
3-LEG LIFT		
4-TRUNK LIFT		
5-LEG EXTENSION		
6-TRUNK FLEXION		

PERFEXT

SYMPTOM CHECKLIST

Has the patient experienced any of the following symptoms in the past month? (✓ for
a yes response)*

	Month	1	2	3	4	5	6	7	8	9	10	11	12
	Date												
1.	Lightheadedness or dizziness												
2.	Lightheadedness or dizziness with standing												
3.	Short term memory loss												
4.	Clouded sensorium												
5.	Hallucinations												
6.	Visual disturbances												
7.	Disorientation to time and/or place												
8.	Insomnia												
9.	Depression												
10.	Anxiety												
11.	Emotional lability												
12.	Lassitude or fatigue												
13.	Weakness												
14.	Nausea												
15.	Vomiting												
16.	Epigastric distress												
17.	Abdominal cramps												
18.	Diarrhea												
19.	Constipation												
20.	Pharyngitis (sore throat)												
21.	Wheezing												
22.	Orthopnea												
23.	Shortness of breath at rest												
24.	Excessive dyspnea on exertion												
25.	Angina: New onset Frequency (↑, ↓ or 0) Episodes/week Severity (↑, ↓ or 0) Lasting > 30 min. NTG/week												

* Comments on symptoms should be made on reverse side

UNIVERSITY HOSPITAL
University of California
Medical Center, San Diego

UCSD CARDIAC REHABILITATION
EXERCISE TRAINING FORM #1

NAME

BIRTHDATE

HEIGHT _____ (in.) WEIGHT _____ (lbs.)

ID =

TARGET HR

CODES*

ST ↓ or ↑   ST DISPLACEMENT
PVCs VT PACs SVT LBBB RBB HB   ECG Δs
ANG   ANGINA - SEE REVERSE SIDE
DYS   DYSPNEA - ANGINA EQUIVALENT
LH   LIGHTHEADEDNESS
MED   CHANGED OR ADMINISTERED
Δ   ABSENT - SEE REVERSE SIDE
QP   OTHER PROBLEMS

*Use Comments to explain coding

TXT SUMMARY

PEAK METS _____   DATE ___/___/___
HR: REST _____   HR: PEAK EX _____
BP: REST ___/___   BP: PEAK EX ___/___
ST CHANGES _____
ANGINA _____
ARRHYTHMIAS _____
OTHER COMMENTS _____
MED _____

SESSION #

EXERCISE DEVICE	WORK LOAD	EXER HR	CODE	EXER HR	CODE	EXER HR	CODE	WORK LOAD	EXER HR	CODE	EXER HR	CODE	EXER HR	CODE	WORK LOAD	EXER HR	CODE	EXER HR	CODE	EXER HR	CODE
DATE	CODE																				
REST HR	CODE																				
REST BP																					
TREADMILL	MPH %							MPH %							MPH %						
ARM ERG	KPM							KPM							KPM						
STEP	M							M							M						
ROW ERG	M R/M							M R/M							M R/M						
BIKE	KPM							KPM							KPM						
AIR DYNE	KP							KP							KP						
AVE EX HR								WEIGHT							WEIGHT						
COOL DOWN HR																					
COOL DOWN BP								DATE							DATE						

COMMENTS:
(Use back of page for additional comments)

D714(R10-90)5

CODES:

ANGINA: ANY UNUSUAL PAIN SHOULD BE REPORTED IN WRITING. ANGINA WILL BE GRADED AS MILD (1), MODERATE (2), OR SEVERE (3). IF IT LASTS OVER 2-3 MINUTES AFTER CESSATION OF EXERCISE OR DOES NOT RESPOND TO NITRO, A PHYSICIAN SHOULD BE CALLED.

ABSENT:
A - B = BUSINESS CONFLICT
A - E = EXERCISED ON THEIR OWN
A - I = INJURY RELATED TO EXERCISE
A - M = POOR MOTIVATION
A - P = PERSONAL OR FAMILY CONFLICT
A - R = RECREATION CONFLICT
A - S = SICKNESS NOT RELATED TO EXERCISE
A - U = UNDETERMINED REASON

ADDITIONAL COMMENTS:

SESSION	DATE	COMMENTS

D714(R10-80)/6

Name_____

ACTIVITY PREFERENCE FORM

1. Do you enjoy exercising?   [ ] yes   [ ] no   [ ] sometimes

2. What type(s) of exercises or sports do you presently participate in? How often?

3. What type(s) of exercises or sports would you like to participate in? How often?

calisthenics	[ ]	____days/week
walking	[ ]	____
jogging	[ ]	____
swimming	[ ]	____
tennis	[ ]	____
sailing	[ ]	____
golf	[ ]	____
other _____	____	
other _____	____	

calisthenics	[ ]	____days/week
walking	[ ]	____
jogging	[ ]	____
swimming	[ ]	____
tennis	[ ]	____
sailing	[ ]	____
golf	[ ]	____
other _____	____	
other _____	____	

Comments:_____

4. Do you prefer to exercise

   [ ] alone   [ ] with a partner   [ ] with a group

5. Considering your daily schedule of activities, when is the most convenient time for you to exercise?

   [ ] morning   [ ] mid-day   [ ] late afternoon or evening

   time_____   time_____   time_____

Name_____

Date____/____/____

UCSD CARDIAC REHABILITATION

PHYSICAL ACTIVITY GUIDELINES

Exercise Prescription: Target Heart Rate_____bpm

(10 second pulse rate_____)

Activity:_____

Frequency_____non-consecutive days per week.

Warm-Up: 5-10 minutes, progressively increase the level of exertion.

Sustained:_____minutes, Maintain heart rate within 10 beats per minute
of targer by pulse checks every 5-10 minutes. Do not exceed a heart rate of
_____bpm_____10".

Cool-Down: 10-15 minutes, Gradually decrease the level of exertion. Stretching
for the legs, back, and shoulders are recommended. Rhythmic exercises for the
abdomen, back, arms and shoulders using light resistance should also be included.
Avoid activity requiring heavy lifting or straining.

Special Considerations:

Medications: Should be taken at the same time in relation to the exercise
training session.

Exercise Intensity: 1) Pace yourself to maintain the target heart rate. 2) If
you are unable to talk while exercising you are working too hard. 3) Sore muscles
and joints suggest you are working too hard- use moderation- particularly in the
initial weeks.

Contraindications: Avoid food, caffeine containing beverages, alcohol, and
cigarettes for 2 or more hours before exercise (moderate fluid intake is okay
and is advisable during hot and humid weather).

Avoid activity during temerature extremes- use moderation.

Avoid activity when air quality is poor.

Avoid hot showers or saunas before and after exercise.

Avoid activity when ill or excessively tired.

Avoid activity when unusual symptoms appear, i.e., excessive shortness of breath,
chest pain- CONSULT YOUR PHYSICIAN.

Avoid competitive activity with others. Your activity has been individually
determined and excessive effort may be harmful.

Clothing: Comfortable, loose fitting. Wear as little as possible in warmer
weather. Warm-up suit for colder temperatures. Shoes with good support and
cushioned heels and soles.

Travelers or commuters: Take your exercise clothing with you. Opportunities
to exercise are frequent if you are prepared.

UCSD CARDIAC REHABILITATION PROGRAM WARNING SYMPTOMS

1. These symptoms suggest that your activity level is too fast. Slow down to an activity level that avoids these symptoms:

    - chest pain or discomfort during or following activity.

    - palpitations or awareness of pounding or irregular heart beat during or following activity.

    - shortness of breath; if more than you would expect for a particular activity.

2. Seek IMMEDIATE medical attention if you notice:

    - severe chest pain not relieved by rest or nitroglycerine (pain may radiate to neck, arms, jaw).

    - fainting or blackout spell.

3. Call your physician within 24 hours if you notice:

    - recent onset of shortness of breath or an increase in shortness of breath.

    - awakening at night because of shortness of breath.

    - a need to sleep on more pillows than before.

    - an unexplained episode of dizziness or lightheadedness.

    - the onset of chest pain (angina pectoris) or a change in chest pain pattern (more frequent, more severe, or new occurrence at night or at rest).

    - palpitations, or awareness of a pounding or irregular heart - not related to exercise.

    - an unexplained episode of weakness and sweating.

4. Dr. Froelicher should be informed of any warning symptoms or your need for medical care. He can be reached at:

    294-6274 office
        ·6737 nights and weekends
        ·6782 rehab center

    I _____ on ____/____/____ have read and understand the above list of warning symptoms. Any questions about these symptoms have been answered to my satisfaction by a member of the UCSD Cardiac Rehabilitation Staff.

UNIVERSITY HOSPITAL

INFORMED CONSENT FOR EXERCISE TREATMENT

I desire to engage voluntarily in the _____
exercise program in order to attempt to improve my cardiovascular
function. This program has been recommended to me by my physician.

Before I enter this exercise program I will have a clinical
evaluation. This evaluation will include a medical history and
physical examination consisting of, but not limited to, measurements
of heart rate and blood pressure, electrocardiogram at rest and
with effort. The purpose of this evaluation is to attempt to detect
any condition that would indicate that I should not engage in this
exercise program.

The program will follow an exercise prescription approved by

_____.

I understand that activities are designed to place a gradually
increasing work load on the circulation and thereby to attempt to
improve its function. The reaction of the cardiovascular system
to such activities cannot be predicted with complete accuracy.
There is a risk of certain changes occurring during or following
the exercise. These changes include abnormalities of blood pressure
or heart rate, or ineffective "heart function," and possibly in
some instances, "heart attacks" or "cardiac arrest."

I realize that it is necessary for me to report promptly to
the supervisor of exercises any signs or symptoms indicating any
abnormality or distress. I consent to the administration of any
immediate resuscitation measures deemed advisable by the supervisor
of exercise.

I have read the foregoing and I understand it. Any questions
that have arisen or occurred to me have been answered to my
satisfaction.

DATE_____

PATIENT SIGNATURE_____

PHYSICIAN SIGNATURE_____

WITNESS_____

<u>YOU ARE PERFEXT!</u>

Thank you for volunteering for this important scientific investigation. Now that you have completed the preliminary exercise tests we would like to further clarify your involvement in the year ahead. The diagram below summarizes your participation.

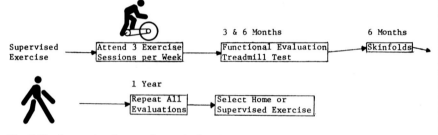

The following topics frequently need clarification:

<u>Medications</u> are important in your management as well as determining your response to exercise. Please try to be consistent in taking medications in relation to exercise sessions and exercise tests. We will advise you on special adjustments necessary for testing. If your medications change, please advise us of this as soon as possible. Medication cards are available for you to help us keep track of your medicines and dosages.

<u>Appointments</u> for sessions or testing are sometimes just impossible to make due to unforseen problems like business or car problems, among others. Please advise us of these conflicts as soon as possible.

<u>Vacations</u> are healthy for everyone and we anticipate that many participants will spend time away from San Diego. It is extremely important that you continue to stay active during these periods. Please let us know when you plan to be away so we can advise you on an exercise program.

<u>Attendance</u> at exercise sessions or regularity of home exercise are extremely important. Exercise is only of functional benefit if done regularly. You will not benefit and your participation in the project will be meaningless if you do not exercise regularly.

We are committed to providing you with close medical supervision over the next year. The PERFEXT project can only be as good as your participation. We look forward to working with you in the year ahead.

Sincerely,

Rehab Staff
294-6782

YOU ARE PERFEXT!

Thank you for volunteering for this important scientific investigation. Now that you have completed the preliminary exercise tests we would like to further clarify your involvement in the year ahead. The diagram below summarizes your participation.

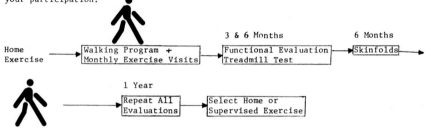

Please be assured that if you are selected as a home exerciser you will be offered a free supervised exercise program at the end of the year.

The following topics frequently need clarification:

Medications are important in your management as well as determining your response to exercise. Please try to be consistent in taking medications in relation to exercise sessions and exercise tests. We will advise you on special adjustments necessary for testing. If your medications change, please advise us of this as soon as possible. Medication cards are available for you to help us keep track of your medicines and dosages.

Appointments for sessions or testing are sometimes just impossible to keep due to unforseen problems like business or car problems, among others. Please advise us of these conflicts as soon as possible.

Vacations are healthy for everyone and we anticipate that many participants will spend time away from San Diego. It is extremely important that you continue to stay active during these periods. Please let us know when you plan to be away so we can advise you on an exercise program.

We are committed to providing you with close medical supervision over the next year. The PERFEXT project can only be as good as your participation. We look forward to working with you in the year ahead.

Sincerely,

Rehab Staff
294-6782

UNIVERSITY OF CALIFORNIA SAN DIEGO

School Of Medicine

EXERCISE LABORATORIES AND CARDIAC REHABILITATION

Certificate Of Appreciation

Given To

FOR CONTRIBUTIONS TO SCIENTIFIC KNOWLEDGE
MADE BY SERVING AS A SUBJECT IN MEDICAL
STUDIES PERFORMED BETWEEN

_____ AND _____

Index

Absolute spatial vector velocity (ASVV), 224–225
Activity status, oxygen consumption and, 115
Adenosine triphosphatase (ATPase) activity, chronic exercise and, 190
Aerobic capacity, 22
Aerobic exercise, 39, 179–180, 198–199; *see also* Chronic exercise
Age
    chronic exercise and, 182–183
    oxygen consumption and, 39, 115
    screening apparently healthy individuals and, 99, 101
Air Force School of Aerospace Medicine (USAFSAM) protocol, 12
Alpha decay/rays, 139, 140
Anaerobic capacity, 198
Analog input window, 30, 32–34
Analog *vs* digital data processing, 23
Aneurysms, left ventricular, 276
Angina pectoris, 82, 204–205
Angiographic coronary disease, angina pectoris and, 82
Angiography
    cold-spot imaging correlation with, 145–151
        table of, 146
    computerized, 308
    in diagnosis
        limitation of, 75
        sensitivity for coronary artery disease, 78–79
    observer agreement, 71–72
    prognosis and, 84–87
    radionuclide

        dynamic, 169–170
        gated, 72
        left ventricular, 105–107
        ventricular, during bicycle exercise, 151–162; *see also* Radionuclide exercise testing, ventricular angiography during bicycle exercise
    with thallium, 169–170
    screening apparently healthy individuals with, 102–103
Arterial baroreflex, 3–4
Arteriography, coronary artery calcification and, 108
Asymptomatic individuals
    coronary disease in, prognosis of, 110–111
    motivational effects of treadmill test on, 112
    screening of, *see* Screening of apparently healthy individuals
Atherosclerosis, 193–196, 253
Athletes
    cyclists, 248
    echocardiographic studies of, 210–212
    former, 251
    runners, *see* Runners
Attenuation, left ventricular volume and, 164–167

Baroreflex, arterial, 3–4
Baseline discontinuity, averaging signals containing, 313
Baseline wander, cubic spline technique to smooth, 311
Bayes's theorem, 81
Beat averaging for noise removal, 36–37

Beta blockers, 284, 285
Beta rays, 139, 140
Bicycle ergometer, 10
Bicycle exercise
    radionuclide ventricular angiography
        during, 151–162; *see also*
        Radionuclide exercise testing,
        ventricular angiography during bicycle
        exercise
    supine, radionuclide report form for, 300,
        301
    supine *vs* erect, 154, 156
    training effect, 222
    treadmill testing *vs*, 11
Blood flow, exercise program and peripheral,
    196
Blood pressure, 20, 42–43
Blood pressure–heart rate product, 65–66
Bradycardia, training, 208
Bypass surgery, patient selection for, 84–87

Cables for electrocardiograph, 14–15
CADENZA, 109
Cardiac mechanical performance, exercise
    program and, 187–191
Cardiac metabolic performance, exercise
    program and, 187–191
Cardiac output
    chronic exercise effects on, 209
    diagnostic value of maximal, 39–41
    total body oxygen consumption and, 1
Cardiac rehabilitation studies, 254–262,
    269–289; *see also* Radionuclide evaluation
        of cardiac rehabilitation
    complications of, 260–261
    conclusions, 262–263
    early ambulation after acute myocardial
        infarction, 254–258
    follow-up studies, 259–260
    hemodynamic changes, 262
    intervention studies, 259–260
    National Exercise and Heart Disease
        Project (NEHPD), 259–260
    prognostic indicators, 258
    radionuclide evaluation of, 269–289; *see
        also* Radionuclide evaluation of
        cardiac rehabilitation
    summary, 261–262
    training forms, *see* Training forms
    work capacity changes, 262
Cardiokymography, 107–108
Cardiomegaly, 207
Cardiovascular function, type of exercise and,
    198

Cardiovascular rehabilitation training forms, *see*
    Training forms
Cardiovascular response to exercise, 2–4
Care during test, 7–8
Central nervous system, excitation hypothesis, 4
Chair treatment, 254
Chemoreflex hypothesis, 4
Chest pain, 68, 82, 98; *see also* Angina pectoris
Chest x-rays, 109
Cholesterol levels, exercise and, 193–196, 249
Chronic exercise (exercise program/physical
        conditioning/training), 179–227
    adenosine triphosphatase (ATPase)
        activity, 190
    age and, 182–183
    animal studies of, 181–186
    atherosclerosis and, 193–196
    bicycle testing and, 222
    cardiac mechanical and metabolic
        performance and, 187–191
    cardiovascular function and type of
        exercise, 198
    cholesterol and, 193–196
    complications of, 260–261
    conclusions, 227
    coronary artery size and, 184
    coronary collateral circulation and,
        184–187
    coronary heart disease and, 216–217
    definition of, 179
    echocardiographic studies of, 210–220;
        see also Echocardiographic effects of
        exercise program
    electrocardiographic studies of, 220–227;
        see also Electrocardiographic effects
        of exercise program
    end results, factors influencing, 197
    evaluation for individualized program of, 89
    heart size and, 215
    heart volume and, 215
    hemodynamic studies, 197–210; *see also*
        Hemodynamic effects of exercise
        program
    introduction, 179–181
    ischemia and, response to, 189
    left ventricular dimensions and, 212,
        214–215
    maximal oxygen consumption and, 220,
        221
    metabolic alterations, 180
    morphologic changes, 180
    myocardial fiber hyperplasia and, 182
    myocardial hypertrophy and, 181–182
    myocardial infarction and, 183

myocardial microcirculatory changes, 182–183
myocardial perfusion, 187
oxygen consumption and, 216, 220, 221
PERFEXT program of, 283–288; *see also* PERFEXT
peripheral blood flow response to exercise and, 196
QRS complex, 224–227
radionuclide evaluation of rehabilitative, 280–283, 287–288
results, 180
risk factors, 193–196
skeletal muscle mitochondria and respiratory enzyme changes, 191
ST-segment changes, 216–217, 220–222, 225–227
structure of program, 197–198
summary, 196, 220
training forms, *see* Training forms
triglycerides and, 195
type of exercise, 198, 199
Chronotopic incompetence, 42, 116
Circulation during exercise, 3
Cold-spot exercise imaging (myocardial imaging with potassium-like radionuclides), 141–151
angiographic correlation with, 145–151 table of, 146
of coronary occlusions, 142–143
methods, 141–142
normal subjects, 143–144
results of studies, 142–145
uses of, 141
Computer analysis of thallium images, 105, 281–283
Computer probability estimates, 109
Computer storage unit, 29–30
Computerized electrocardiographic analysis, 23–38, 222–227
amount of data and, 24
analog input window, 30, 32–34
analog-to-digital conversion, 29, 32
CASE, 27–29
criteria for, 315
digital *vs* analog data processing, 23
forms and illustrations, 304, 308
ischemia, criteria for, 31
LSI–11 computer (CASE), 27–29
mathematical constructs, 34
microprocessor-based commercial system, 27–28
next decade, 38
noise in electrocardiogram and, 24, 34, 36–37
offset and onset points, identification of, 37–38
PDP-8E computer, 26
principles and approaches, 29
review of literature, 24–29
sampling rate, 29–30, 32–34
signal resolution, 30, 32–34
ST segment, 24–29
standard techniques *vs*, 29
Status 1000, 27–28
storage unit, 29–30
USAFSAM and University of Indiana system, 25
Viagraph system, 28
Consent form, 7, 333
Contact noise, 36
Contraindications to exercise testing, 5
Coronary angiography, *see* Angiography
Coronary arteriography, coronary artery calcification and, 108
Coronary artery bypass surgery, patient selection for, 84–87
Coronary artery calcification, fluoroscopic examination of, 108
Coronary artery disease, diagnostic value of test for, *see* Diagnostic value of tests
Coronary artery size, exercise program and, 184
Coronary collateral circulation, exercise program and, 184–187
Coronary heart disease (CHD), 237–263
asymptomatic, screening for, *see* Screening apparently healthy individuals
cardiac rehabilitation, *see* Cardiac rehabilitation studies
diagnostic tools for, 45; *see also* Diagnostic value of tests
echocardiogram effects of chronic exercise, 216–217
electrocardiographic criteria for, 103–104, 115
evaluation of severity of, 114
hemodynamic effects of chronic exercise on, 202–207
physical inactivity as risk factor, *see* Physical inactivity as risk factor
Coronary occlusions, cold-spot imaging of, 142–143
Cubic spline technique, 311
Cyclists, physical risk and, 248

Diagnostic value of tests, 75–82

angiography
    limitations of, 75
      sensitivity of, 78–79
    chest pain, 82
    choice of discriminant value, 76–77
    definitions and calculation of terms for, 76, 79
    electrocardiography
      criteria for CHD, 103–104
        sensitivity and specificity of, 46
    false positives, 63–66, 79, 113
    population tested, 77
    probability of patient having disease given test result, 80–81
    risk, relative, 76, 79
    sensitivity of tests, 76–80
    specificity of tests, 46, 76–80
    ST-segment changes, 84
    use of clinical events and pathologic end points, 75
Diastolic blood pressure, 42
Diet, physical risk and, 248
Digital *vs* analog data processing, 23
Digital electrographic data, mathematical constructs applied to, 34
Digoxin, 284, 285
Dynamic exercise (isotonic), 2–3, 10, 179
    cardiovascular adjustments to, 2–3
    definition of, 10
Dynamic radionuclide angiography, 169–170
Dysrhythmias, evaluation of, 88–89

Echocardiographic effects of exercise program, 210–220
    before and after, 212–217
      table of, 213–214
    coronary heart disease and, 216–217
    cross-sectional studies, comparing normals and athletes, 210–212
    discussion, 217–220
    left ventricular mass, estimation of, 217–218
    observer agreement, 69–70
    subjective nature of interpretation of, 219–220
Ejection fraction response to exercise, 116, 271
    chronic exercise, 281, 283
    ischemia and, 288–289
    observer agreement, 72
    prognosis and, 116
    radionuclide ventricular angiography and, 156–158, 161–162
    reproducibility, 278
    right ventricular, 161–162

    in valvular heart disease, 162
Electrocardiographic effects of exercise program, 220–227, 270–277
    ASVV, 224–225
    data acquisition and processing for, 222–226
    dynamic categorization of patients, 274–275
    ejection response, reproducibility of, 278
    ischemia and, 276–277
    J junction, 225
    myocardial infarction patients, 271–275
    P wave, 225
    patient subgroups, 273, 275
    physiologic results, 270, 271
    Q waves, 271–273, 276–277
    QRS complex, 224–225
    scar, 276–277
    ST changes, 273–277
    static categorization of patients, 271–273
    symptomatic results, 271
    T wave, 225
    thallium ischemia, 275
    thallium redistribution defects, 277
Electrocardiographic recorders, 8–10
Electrocardiography; *see also* entries beginning Electrocardiographic
    amount of data, 24
    cables, 14–15
    computerized, *see* Computerized electrocardiographic analysis
    criteria for CHD, 103–104, 315
    electrodes, 14–15
    factors contributing to change in, 49
    fasting and, 64
    interpretation of, 45–57; *see also* Interpretation of standard exercise tests
    lead systems, 15–20, 87
      bipolar, 15
      Dalhousie square, 19
      Frank system, 19, 309, 310
      Mason-Likar torso-mounted, 16–18
      multiple, 18–19
      for multivessel disease detection, 87
      recording, 19–20
      results using 12-lead system, 18
      sensitivity and specificity of, 18
      three-dimensional or vectorcardiographic, 19
      treadmill test interpretation and multiple, 18–19
      Wilson's central terminal for precordial, 17–18

noise in, 24, 34, 36–37, 312
normal changes, interpretation of, *see*
    Interpretation of standard exercise
    testing, normal electrocardiogram
    changes
observer agreement, 70–71
PERFEXT and, 287
postinfarct monitoring with, 255
predictive value of, 111–112
Q waves, 46–47, 271–273, 276–277
QRS complex, 45–46, 224–225
R wave, 47
S wave, 47
sensitivity and specificity for CHD, 46
skin preparation, 14
ST segment, 227
T wave, 225
thallium imaging *vs*, 271
Electrodes, 14–15
Electrolytes, electrocardiographic interpretation
    and, 48–49
Endurance, 22
Erect *vs* supine exercise testing, 10–11, 154,
    156
Exercise, types of, 10, 179
Exercise physiology, basic, 1–4
Exercise program (training), *see* Chronic
    exercise
Exercise test modalities, 10
Exercise test predictors, 101
Exercise testing forms and illustrations,
    291–315
    angiographic studies, computerized, 308
    averaging signals containing baseline
        discontinuity, 313
    computerized analysis, 308, 315
    cubic spline technique to smooth baseline
        wander, 311
    ECG criteria, computerized, 315
    Eigen plane, 310
    fiducial placement and average waveform,
        311
    Frank plane
        frontal, 309
        horizontal, 310
    Frank X lead, 309
    heart function, 302, 303
    left main disease, 307
    noise averaging, 312
    radionuclide, 298
    ST-segment vectors, effect of changing
        discriminant value of sensitivity and
        specificity, 314
    supine bike radionuclide test, 300, 301

thallium, 297, 299
treadmill, 292–296
women, 306

FAI (functional aerobic impairment), 21, 115
False-positive exercise test, 63–66, 79, 113
Fasting ECG, 64
Fluoroscopic examination of coronary artery
    calcification, 108
Functional aerobic impairment (FAI), 21, 115
Functional capacity, 38–41, 87–88

Gated chest x-rays, 109
Gated radionuclide studies, 72, 154, 287
Glucose ingestion, 64

HDL (high-density lipoprotein) cholesterol, 249
Heart, mechanical reserve of (functional), 114
Heart function, 302, 303
Heart rate
    impairment, 42, 116
    interpretation of, 41–45
    maximal, 41–42
Heart size
    echocardiogram, exercise program and,
        215
Heart volume, 215; *see also* Left ventricular
    volume, radionuclide determination of
Hemodynamic effects of exercise program,
    197–210, 262
    aerobic performance, training patterns,
        198–199
    anaerobic capacity, 198
    angina patient, 204–205
    AV O_2 difference, 208–209
    cardiac output, 209
    discussion of, 207–210
    impaired ventricular function patients,
        205–206
    long-term exercise program, 204
    myocardial infarction patients, 203, 204,
        206, 207
    normal subjects, 200–202, 209
    peripheral response, 208
    submaximal testing results, 208
    techniques for evaluation of, 199–200
    training bradycardia, 208
High-density lipoprotein (HDL) cholesterol, 249
High-risk patients, identification of, 87
Home exercise, 335
Hypercapnea, cold-spot imaging of, 143
Hyperemia, cold-spot imaging of, 143
Hyperkalemia, cold-spot imaging of, 48

Hypertension, 65–66
Hypoxia, cold-spot imaging of, 143

Informed consent of patients, 7, 333
Interpretation of standard exercise testing,
    38–74
    blood pressure response, 41–45
    chest pain, 68
    echocardiography, 219–220
    electrolytes and electrocardiogram, 48–49
    false positives, 63–66, 79, 113
    functional capacity, 38–41
    heart rate, 41–45
    myocardial oxygen consumption, 44–45
    normal electrocardiogram changes, 49–57
        J-junction depression, 52–56
        Q wave, 50–52
        R wave, 50–52, 56–57
        S wave, 50–52
        ST segment, 52–56
        T wave, 52–56
    observer agreement (reliability), 68–73,
        278–280; see also Observer
        agreement in interpretation
    physical examination, 68, 69
    review of literature, 45–49
    ST-segment changes, 52–63, 68
        normal, 52–56
        not due to coronary artery disease,
            63–66
    subjective response, 67–68
    summary, 74
    various test responses, 43
    ventricular dysrhythmias, 66–67
Ischemia
    chronic exercise and, 189
    cold-spot imaging of, 143
    ejection fraction response and, 288–289
    radionuclide evaluation of rehabilitation,
        276–277
    ST-segment elevation vs, 288
Ischemic heart disease, criteria for, 26, 31
Ischemic myocardium, amount of, 114
Isometric exercise, 10, 179
Isotonic exercise, see Dynamic exercise

J junction
    chronic exercise and, 225
    normal changes in, 52–56

Lactic acid production, 116
Lead systems, see Electrocardiography, lead
    systems

Left main coronary disease, 84–85, 307
Left ventricular aneurysms, 276
Left ventricular angiography, radionuclide,
    105–107
Left ventricular dimension, 212, 214–215; see
    also Left ventricular mass; Left ventricular
    volume, radionuclide determination of
Left ventricular function, radionuclide analysis
    of, see Radionuclide exercise testing,
    ventricular angiography during bicycle
    exercise
Left ventricular hypertrophy, 64–65
Left ventricular imaging, gated radionuclide, 287
Left ventricular mass, echocardiographic
    methods of estimating, 217–218
Left ventricular volume, radionuclide
    determination of, 162–168
    attenuation and, 164–167
    equilibrium gated technique, 163–168
    exercise response, 167–168
    first-pass method, 162–163
    important factors, 164
Legal implications of exercise testing, 7–8
Line-frequency noise, 34, 36
Lipid screening, 109

Marathon hypothesis, 253–254
Maximal exercise tests
    definition of, 13–14
    submaximal vs, 12–14, 95–102
Maximal oxygen uptake ($\dot{V}O_2$ max), see Oxygen
    consumption, maximal
Measurement, variability in, 70; see also
    Observer agreement in interpretation
Mechanical reserve of heart, 114
Metabolic alterations, exercise program and,
    180
Methodology of standard exercise testing, 4–38
    blood pressure, 20
    care during test, 7–8
    consent of patients, 7
    lead systems, 15–20; see also
        Electrocardiography, lead systems
    legal implications, 7–8
    maximal oxygen uptake, measurement or
        estimation of, 20–22
    postexercise period, 22–23
    protocols, 12
    recording instruments, 8–10
    safety precautions, 4–7
    skin preparation, 14
    submaximal vs maximal exercise testing,
        12–14
    supine vs erect exercise testing, 10–11

termination of treadmill test, indications for, 23
treadmill testing, 6, 23
Microcirculatory changes, exercise program and myocardial, 182–183
Mitochondrial changes, exercise program and, 191
Morphologic changes, exercise program and, 180
Multivessel disease detection, 87
Muscle chemoreceptor hypothesis, 4
Muscle noise, 36
Muscle strength, 198
Muscular exercise, dynamic, *see* Dynamic exercise
Myocardial fiber hyperplasia, exercise program and, 182
Myocardial hypertrophy, exercise program and, 181–182
Myocardial imaging with radionuclides, *see* Cold-spot exercise imaging
Myocardial infarction and postinfarction patient
  ambulation after, early, 254–258
  cardiac rehabilitation/chronic exercise program, 103, 203, 204, 206, 207, 254–258, 271–275
    hemodynamic effects, 203, 204, 206, 207
    radionuclide evaluation of, 271–275
  chair treatment, 254
  chronic exercise, *see* cardiac rehabilitation/chronic exercise program *above*
  clinical variables *vs* exercise test, 93
  criteria for complicated acute, 256
  electrocardiographic monitoring, 255
  exercise testing as therapy, 93
  exercise testing soon after, 89–93
  intervention studies, 259
  long-term risk of subendocardial *vs* transmural, 256
  physical inactivity as risk factor, 242–243
  preventing deconditioning after, 257–258
  prognostic indicators, 258
  progressive activity program, 254–255
  radionuclide evaluation of rehabilitation, 271–275
  treadmill testing after, 90–92, 255
  uncomplicated, 256–257
Myocardial mass, 47
Myocardial microcirculatory changes, exercise program and, 182–183
Myocardial oxygen consumption
  as diagnostic tool, 45
  estimation of, 209–210, 220

interpretation of, 44–45
measurement of, 2
Myocardial perfusion, exercise program and, 198

National Exercise and Heart Disease Project (NEHPD), 259–260
Nitrates, 285
Noise in electrocardiogram, 34, 36–37, 312
Nuclear cardiology methods, *see* Radionuclide evaluation of cardiac rehabilitation

Observer agreement in interpretation (reliability), 68–73, 278–280
  coronary angiograms, 71–72
  echocardiogram, 69–70
  ejection fraction response, 72
  electrocardiogram, 70–71
  gated radionuclide angiography, 72
  location of abnormality, 73
  modes for improvement, 73
  physical examination, 69
  thallium scans, 72–73
  variance component model, 70
  vectorcardiogram, 70–71
  ventricular volume, 72
  wall motion abnormalities, 71–72
Occupational activity and CHD, *see* Physical inactivity as risk factor
Ohm's law, definition of, 3
Orthostatic abnormalities, 65
Oxygen consumption ($\dot{V}O_2$)
  cardiovascular and respiratory response relationship to, 3–4
  definition of, 1
  echocardiographic effects of chronic exercise, 216
  estimation of, 115–117
  maximal ($\dot{V}O_2$ max), 1
    aerobic training and, 39
    age and, 39
    cardiac output and, 1
    chronic exercise and, 220, 221
    diagnostic value of, 39–41
    estimation of, 20–22
    habitual physical activity and, 39
    interpretation of, 39–41
    maximal heart rate and, 41
    measurement of, 20–22, 114–115
    reasons for obtaining, 114
    treadmill work load and, 21, 22
  measurement of, 1
  myocardial, *see* Myocardial oxygen

consumption

P wave, chronic exercise and, 225
PERFEXT (Perfusion and Performance Exercise
    Trial), 283–288, 327, 334
    criteria for patient selection, 284–285
    electrocardiographic techniques and, 287
    exercise testing, 287
    exercise training, 287–288
    protocol, 284
    radionuclide left ventricular imaging, gated,
        287
    randomization of patients, 285
    specific purposes of, 285
    symptom checklist, 327
    vectorcardiographic techniques and, 287
Peripheral blood flow, exercise program and,
    196
Physical activity
    maximal oxygen uptake and, 39
    risk and, see Physical inactivity as risk
        factor
Physical conditions, see Chronic exercise
Physical examination, 6–8, 68, 69
Physical inactivity as risk factor, 237
    bias in relationship, 237
    cyclists, 248
    diet and, 248
    elimination of specific risk factors, 249–250
    epidemiologic studies, 239–241
    exercise during leisure time, 247–249
    former athletes, 251
    high-risk characteristics, 251
    job classification and, 239–241
    marathon hypothesis, 253–254
    postmortem studies, 252–253
    prevalence or cross-sectional studies,
        243–245
    prospective studies, 245–252
    retrospective studies, 238–243
    runners, 249
    Seven Countries Coronary Artery Disease
        Study, 246–247
    social class and, 238–239
    for specific occupational groups, 241–242
    for specific populations, 242–243
    treadmill performance and, 248–249
    urban and rural, 248
Physiology of exercise, basic, 1–4
Postexercise period, 22–23, 68
Postinfarction patient, see Myocardial infarction
    and postinfarction patient
Potassium, 48–49
Potassium-like radionuclides, 141–151; see also

Cold-spot exercise imaging
    comparison of, 142–143
    hypercapnea and, 143
    hyperemia and, 143
    hypoxia and, 143
    ischemia and, 143
    respiratory acidosis and, 143
Predictive value of test, 76, 79; see also
    Prognosis, determination of
    of maximal exercise electrocardiograph,
        111–112
    of ST-segment depression, 103–104
    of treadmill testing, 101
Preparation for exercise testing, 5–6
Prognosis, determination of, 82–87; see also
    Predictive value of test
    in asymptomatic coronary disease,
        110–111
    coronary angiography in, 84–87
    ejection fraction response, 116
    electrocardiographic lead system for
        multivessel disease detection, 87
    high-risk patients, identification of, 87
    myocardial infarction patients, 91–92
    ST-segment response, 84, 90
    patient selection for bypass surgery, 84–87
    total body functional capacity, 116
    treadmill testing, 84–85, 91–92
    work load, 82–83
Public safety, screening asymptomatic
    individuals for, see Screening of apparently
    healthy individuals

Q wave
    chronic exercise rehabilitation program
        and, 271–273, 276–277
    computer analysis of, 46–47
    normal, 50–52
QRS complex
    chronic exercise and, 224–227
    computer analysis of, 45–46

R wave
    computer analysis of, 47
    normal, 50–52, 56–57
Radiation dose, 170
Radiation-measuring devices, 140–141
Radiation physics, 137–141
Radioactivity, 138–141
Radionuclide evaluation of cardiac
    rehabilitation, 269–289
    conclusions, 288–289
    correlative and validation studies, 270–280
    dynamic categorization of patients,

274–275
ejection response, reproducibility of, 278
electrocardiographic responses, 270–277;
    see also Electrocardiographic effects
    of exercise program
exercise training, 280–283, 287–288
ischemia, 276–277
myocardial infarction patients, 271–275
patient subgroups, 273, 275
PERFEXT, *see* PERFEXT
physiologic results, 270, 271
Q waves, 271–273, 276–277
reliability, 278–280
reproducibility of results, 278
scar, 276–277
ST changes, 273–277
static categorization of patients, 271–273
symptomatic results, 271
thallium ischemia, 275
thallium redistribution defects, 277
Radionuclide exercise testing, 137–171, 298;
    see also Radionuclide evaluation of cardiac
    rehabilitation
angiography, *see* Angiography,
    radionuclide
conclusions, 168–171
dynamic angiography, with thallium,
    169–170
introduction, 141
left ventricular imaging, 105–107, 287
left ventricular volume, 162–168; *see also*
    Left ventricular volume, radionuclide
    determination of
methodologic problems, 170
methods, 163–169
    equilibrium, 169
    equilibrium gated technique, 163–168
    first-pass, 162–163, 169
    gated, 154, 163–168
myocardial imaging with potassium-like
    radionuclides, 141–151; *see also*
    Cold-spot exercise imaging
present uses, 170–171
radiation dose, 170
radiation physics, 137–141
thallium in conjunction with, 169–170; *see*
    also Thallium exercise test
ventricular angiography during bicycle
    exercise, 151–162
    ejection fraction response, 156–158,
        161–162
    equilibrium techniques for, 153
    first-transit studies, 152–153
    gated radionuclide studies, 154

methods, 151–152
right ventricular ejection fraction
    response, 161–162
99mTc-labeled radiopharmaceuticals
    for, 152
wall motion abnormalities, 158–161
Radionuclides, potassium-like, 141–151; *see*
    also Cold-spot exercise imaging;
    Potassium-like radionuclides
Recording instrument, 8–10
Recovery period, postexercise, 68
Reliability, 278–280; *see also* Observer
    agreement in interpretation
Reproducibility, ejection fraction response and,
    278
Respiratory enzyme changes, exercise program
    and, 191
Respiratory response to exercise, oxygen
    consumption and cardiovascular
    relationship to, 3–4
Risk
    of exercise, 4–5
    of exercise program, 293–296
    informed consent of patient and, 7
    physical inactivity as, *see* Physical inactivity
        as risk factor
    relative, 76, 79
    runners and, 249, 253–254
Runners
    atherosclerosis, 253
    marathon hypothesis, 253–254
    risk and, 249, 253–254

S wave
    computer analysis of, 47
    normal, 50–52
Safety precautions, 4–7
    contraindications to exercise testing, 5
    physical examination, 6–7
    preparations for exercise testing, 5–6
    risk levels for exercise, 4–5
    treadmill test, 5–6
Sample size (heart), noise reduction and, 37
Sampling rate, 29–30, 32–34
Scar, identification of, 276–277
Screening apparently healthy individuals,
    93–114
    age, and, 99, 101
    ancillary techniques, 103
    atypical chest pain, 98
    cardiokymography, 107–108
    chest x-rays, gated, 109
    computer probability estimates, 109
    coronary angiography, 102–103

criteria for selection of patients, 94
false positives, 113
fluoroscopic examination, coronary artery
   calcification and, 108
lipid, 109
maximal exercise test as, 102–103, 112
maximal vs submaximal tests, 95–102
new electrocardiographic criteria, 103–104
predictive value, 111–112
progressive continuous exercise, 95
radionuclide left ventricular angiography,
   105–107
Seattle Heart Watch, 101–102
selection of procedures, 112–113
sensitivity of various factors, 111
ST-segment abnormalities, 99–101
summary, 111–114
systolic time intervals, 110
thallium scans, 104–105
treadmill test, 97–98, 101
women, 99, 101
Seattle Heart Watch, 101–102
Sedentary life-style, see Physical inactivity as
   risk factor
Sensitivity of test, 76–80
   for angiographic coronary artery disease,
     78–79
   definition and calculation of, 76, 77
   specificity and, 79–80
   of ST-segment depression, 78, 314
   of various screening factors, 111
Seven Countries Coronary Artery Disease
   Study, 246–247
Sexual gender, oxygen consumption and, 115
Signal resolution, 30, 32–34
Skeletal muscle mechanoreceptor hypothesis, 4
Skeletal muscle mitochondria changes,
   exercise program and, 191
Skin preparation, 14
Specificity, 46, 76–80
   definition and calculation of, 76, 77
   sensitivity and, 79–80
   of ST response, 78, 80, 314
ST index, 25
ST-segment analysis, 16, 48, 57–63; see also
   ST-segment depression; ST-segment
   elevation
   cancellation effect, 60–61
   chronic exercise program and, 216–217,
     220–222, 225–227, 273–277
     electrocardiogram, 227
      radionuclide evaluation of, 273–277
   computerized electrocardiographic, 24–29
   diagnostic value of, 84

interpretation of, 57–63, 68
   normal, 52–56
not due to coronary artery disease,
   63–66
maximal exercise and, 24–25
normal, 52–56
normalization of, 60–61
prognosis and, 84, 90
screening, 99–101
sensitivity of, 78, 314
specificity of, 78, 80, 314
ST-segment depression, 61–63, 74, 288
   associated ST-segment elevation, 59
   cold-spot imaging of, 144–145
   criteria for, 30
   echocardiographic effects of chronic
     exercise program, 216–217
   not due to coronary artery disease,
     63–66
   predictive value of, 103–104
   sensitivity and specificity of, 78
ST-segment elevation, 57–59, 74, 276, 288
   associated ST-segment depression, 59
   ischemia and, 288
   left ventricular aneurysms, 276
Standard exercise testing, 1–117
   applications, 74–75
   computer approaches vs, 29
   conclusions, 114–117
   diagnostic value of, 75–82; see also
     Diagnostic value of tests
   dysrhythmias, evaluation of, 88–89
   exercise program evaluation, 89
   functional capacity, 87–88
   interpretation, 38–74; see also
     Interpretation of standard exercise
     tests
   introduction, 1–4
   methodology, 4–38; see also Methodology
     of standard exercise testing
   myocardial infarction, soon after, 89–93
   prognosis, determination of, 82–87; see
     also Prognosis, determination of
   screening apparently healthy individuals,
     93–114; see also Screening
     apparently healthy individuals
   treatment, evaluation of, 88
Storage unit, computer, 29–30
Subjective response, 67–68
Submaximal vs maximal exercise testing,
   12–14, 95–102
Supine bicycle radionuclide test, 300, 301
Supine vs erect exercise testing, 10–11, 154,
   156